GYNAECOLOGY | 20th EDITION

by Ten Teachers

GYNAECOLOGY | 20th EDITION

by Ten Teachers

Edited by

Helen Bickerstaff MD, MRCOG

Senior Lecturer in Medical Education

King's College London

London, UK

and

Honorary Consultant Obstetrician and Gynaecologist

Guy's and St Thomas' NHS Foundation Trust

London, UK

Louise C Kenny MBChB (Hons), MRCOG, PhD

Professor of Obstetrics and Gynaecology

University College Cork

Cork, Ireland

and

Director

The Irish Centre for Fetal and Neonatal Translational Research (INFANT)

Cork, Ireland

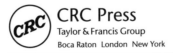

CRC Press

Taylor & Francis Group

Boca Raton   London   New York

CRC Press is an imprint of the
Taylor & Francis Group, an **informa** business

CRC Press
Taylor & Francis Group
6000 Broken Sound Parkway NW, Suite 300
Boca Raton, FL 33487-2742

© 2017 by Taylor & Francis Group, LLC
CRC Press is an imprint of Taylor & Francis Group, an Informa business

No claim to original U.S. Government works

Printed in Great Britain by Ashford Colour Press Ltd

International Standard Book Number-13: 978-1-4987-4428-7 (Pack – Book and Ebook)
International Standard Book Number-13: 978-1-4987-4461-4 (Paperback; restricted territorial availability)

Visit the Taylor & Francis Web site at
http://www.taylorandfrancis.com

and the CRC Press Web site at
http://www.crcpress.com

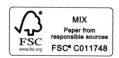

Dedication

This book is dedicated to the first and best teachers we ever had:

My Dad, Frank (HB)
My Mum, Elizabeth (LCK)

Contents

Preface

Gynaecology by Ten Teachers was first published in 1919 as 'Diseases of Women' and is one of the oldest, most respected and accessible texts on the subject. *Gynaecology by Ten Teachers* has informed generations of gynaecologists, and now has a wide international audience. There is great responsibility in revising this landmark 20th edition, to ensure its accessibility and relevance are maintained into the next century.

The 20th edition has been almost entirely rewritten to reflect both changing undergraduate medical curricula and changing diagnostic and management protocols in gynaecology. The 'Ten Teachers' are all internationally renowned experts in their fields and all actively involved in the delivery of undergraduate and postgraduate teaching in the UK. This volume has been edited carefully to ensure consistency of structure, style and level of detail, in common with those of its sister text *Obstetrics by Ten Teachers*. The books can therefore be used together or independently as required. New self assessment sections are presented consistently throughout, with detailed clinical scenarios for each subject in a structure similar to those used in most medical schools.

The global status of women's and girls' sexual and reproductive health and rights is disturbing. Millions of women have no access to contraception, undergo female genital mutilation and receive no gynaecological care. It is fitting, therefore, that the 20th edition, published almost 100 years after the first, maintains a global aspect throughout.

The aim of the text now, as it was a century ago, is to prepare students for their undergraduate examinations, and to continue to be useful afterwards in postgraduate studies and clinical practice. It is a text that the editors used as students, which inspired us to practice and teach in the specialty, and which we still enjoy reading because it is concise yet comprehensive. We hope that in addition to supporting medical students throughout their studies, general practitioners, trainees and allied health care professionals will find it useful in their work.

It has been a privilege and an honour to be the editors of this textbook as it approaches this important milestone; we echo a century of previous editors in hoping that this book will enthuse a new generation of doctors to become gynaecologists and work to improve the health and the safety of women through all reproductive ages.

Helen Bickerstaff
Louise C Kenny

Contributors

Helen Bickerstaff MD, MRCOG
Senior Lecturer in Medical Education
King's College London
and
Honorary Consultant Obstetrician and Gynaecologist
Guy's and St Thomas' NHS Foundation Trust
London, UK

Sharon Cameron MD, MFSRH, FRCOG
Consultant Gynaecologist and Clinical Lead for
    Sexual Health Services
NHS Lothian Chalmers Centre
Edinburgh, UK

T Justin Clark MB ChB, MD(Hons), FRCOG
Consultant Gynaecologist
Birmingham Women's Hospital
and
Honorary Professor in Gynaecology
University of Birmingham
Birmingham, UK

Emma J Crosbie BSc, MB ChB, PhD, MRCOG
Senior Lecturer and Honorary Consultant
    Gynaecological Oncologist
University of Manchester
St Mary's Hospital
Manchester, UK

Leila CG Frodsham, MB ChB, MRCOG
Consultant Gynaecologist
Chair of the Institute of Psychosexual Medicine
    (2012–15)

Andrew Horne PhD, FRCOG
Personal Chair in Gynaecology and Reproductive
    Sciences
Honorary Consultant Gynaecologist
MRC Centre for Reproductive Health
University of Edinburgh
Edinburgh, UK

Margaret Kingston BMBS, BMed Sci, FRCP,
    DipGUM, DFSRH MSc
Consultant Physician
Genitourinary Medicine and Associate
    Medical Director
Central Manchester Foundation Trust
Manchester, UK

Stuart Lavery MBBCh, MSc, FRCOG
Consultant Gynaecologist
Director IVF Hammersmith
and
Queen Charlotte's and Chelsea Hospital
and
Honorary Senior Lecturer Imperial College
    London
London, UK

Edward Morris MD, FRCOG
Consultant Gynaecologist
Norfolk and Norwich University Hospital NHS
    Foundation Trust
Norwich, UK
and
Vice President, Clinical Quality
Royal College of Obstetricians and Gynaecologists
London, UK

Douglas G Tincello BSc, MBChB, MD, FRCOG, FHEA
Professor of Urogynaecology
Department of Health Sciences
College of Medicine, Biological Sciences and
    Psychology
University of Leicester
Leicester, UK

Abbreviations

AFC	antral follicle count	D&C	dilatation and curettage
AFP	α-fetoprotein	DHEA	dehydroepiandrosterone
AIDS	acquired immune deficiency syndrome	DHT	dihydrotestosterone
ALO	actimomyces-like organism	DNA	deoxyribonucleic acid
AMH	anti-Müllerian hormone	DO	detrusor overactivity
APS	antiphospholipid syndrome	DSD	disorders of sexual development
ART	assisted reproductive treatment	DUB	dysfunctional uterine bleeding
AUB	abnormal uterine bleeding		
AUC	area under the curve	EB	endometrial biopsy
AZF	azoospermic factor	EC	emergency contraception
		ECG	electrocardiography
BBV	blood-borne virus	EGF	epidermal growth factor
BEO	bleeding of endometrial origin	EIA	enzyme immunoassay
BEP	bleomycin, etoposide and cisplatin	EP	ectopic pregnancy
BMD	bone mineral density	EVA	electrical vacuum aspiration
BMI	body mass index		
BNF	British National Formulary	FAB	fertility awareness-based method
BOT	borderline ovarian tumour	FBC	full blood count
BRCA	breast ovarian cancer syndrome	FGF	fibroblast growth factor
BSO	bilateral salpingo-oophorectomy	FGM	female genital mutilation
BV	bacterial vaginosis	FH	fetal heartbeat
		FIGO	International Federation of Gynecology and Obstetrics
CAH	congenital adrenal hyperplasia		
CAIS	complete androgen insensitivity syndrome	FSH	follicle-stimulating hormone
CBT	cognitive-behavioural therapy	GFR	glomerular filtration rate
CGIN	cervical glandular intraepithelial neoplasia	GnRH	gonadotrophin-releasing hormone
		GP	general practitioner
CHC	combined hormonal contraception	GTA	gynaecology teaching associate
CIN	cervical intraepithelial neoplasia	GTD	gestational trophoblastic disease
CL	corpus luteum		
CLIA	chemiluminescence immunoassay	HAART	highly active retroviral therapy
CNS	central nervous system	(β) hCG	(beta-) human chorionic gonadotrophin
COCP	combined oral contraceptive pill	HDL	high-density lipoprotein
COX	cyclooxygenase	HFEA	Human Fertilisation and Embryo Authority
CPP	chronic pelvic pain		
CRP	C-reactive protein	HIV	human immunodeficiency virus
CT	computed tomography	HMB	heavy menstrual bleeding
Cu-IUD	copper intrauterine device	HNPCC	hereditary non-polyposis colorectal cancer
CVD	cardiovascular disease	HPO	hypothalamo–pituitary–ovarian (axis)

HPV	human papilloma virus		OAB	overactive bladder
HRT	hormone replacement therapy		OCP	oral contraceptive pill
HSG	hysterosalpingography		17-OHP	17-hydroxyprogesterone
HSIL	high-grade squamous intraepithelial (lesion)		OHSS	ovarian hyperstimulation syndrome
HSV	herpes simplex virus		OI	ovulation induction
HVS	high vaginal swab		OPH	outpatient hysteroscopy
HyCoSy	hysterocontrast synography			
			PAC	preassessment clinic
ICSI	intracytoplasmic sperm injection		PAF	platelet activating factor
Ig	immunoglobulin		PCB	postcoital bleeding
IGF	insulin-like growth factor		PCOS	polycystic ovary syndrome
IMB	intermenstrual bleeding		PCR	polymerase chain reaction
ISD	intrinsic sphincter deficiency		PG	prostaglandin
IUD	intrauterine device		PGD	preimplantation genetic diagnosis
IUI	intrauterine insemination		PGI	prostacyclin
IUS	intrauterine releasing system		PID	pelvic inflammatory disease
IVF	in-vitro fertilization		PMB	postmenopausal bleeding
			PMS	premenstrual syndrome
LARC	long-acting reversible methods of contraception		POCT	point of care test
LAVH	laparoscopic-aided vaginal hysterectomy		POF	premature ovarian failure
			POI	premature ovarian insufficiency
LBC	liquid-based cytology		POP	progestogen-only pill
LDL	low-density lipoprotein		PPC	primary peritoneal carcinoma
LH	luteinizing hormone		PPH	postpartum haemorrhage
LLETZ	large loop excision of transformation zone		PUL	pregnancy of unknown location
LMP	last menstrual period		REM	rapid eye movement
LMWH	low-molecular weight heparin		RCOG	Royal College of Obstetricians and Gynaecologists
LNG-IUS	levonorgestrel intrauterine system		RMI	Risk of Malignancy Index
LOD	laparoscopic ovarian drilling		RNA	ribonucleic acid
			RPOC	retained products of conception
MAS	minimal access surgery		RPR	rapid plasma reagin
MBL	mean blood loss		RR	relative risk
MDT	multidisciplinary team			
MEC	medical eligibility criteria		SCJ	squamocolumnar junction
MRI	magnetic resonance imaging		SERM	selective oestrogen receptor modulator
MRKH	Mayer–Rokitansky–Kuster–Hauser syndrome		SFA	semen fluid analysis
MSU	midstream urine sample		SHBG	sex hormone-binding globulin
MTCT	mother-to-child transmission		SIS	saline instillation sonography
MVA	manual vacuum aspiration		SPRM	selective progesterone receptor modulator
			SSR	surgical sperm retrieval
NAAT	nucleic acid amplification test		SSRI	selective serotonin-reuptake inhibitor
NICE	National Institute for Health and Care Excellence		STI	sexually-transmitted infection
			STIC	serous tubal intraepithelial carcinoma
NSAID	non-steroidal anti-inflammatory drug		STOP	surgical termination of pregnancy

TAUSS	transabdominal ultrasound scan		UPT	urinary pregnancy test
TCRF	transcervical resection of fibroid		USS	ultrasound scan
TED	thromboembolic stocking			
TGF	transforming growth factor		VaIN	vaginal intraepithelial neoplasia
TLH	total laparoscopic hysterectomy		VDRL	Venereal Disease Reference Laboratory
TOT	transobturator tape		VEGF	vascular endothelial growth factor
TPHA	*T. pallidum* haemagglutination assay		VIN	vulval intraepithelial neoplasia
TPPA	*T. pallidum* particle assay		VTE	venous thromboembolism
TV	*Trichomonas vaginalis*			
TVT	tension-free vaginal tape		WCC	white cell count
TVUSS	transvaginal ultrasound scan		WHI	Women's Health Initiative
TZ	transformation zone		WHO	World Health Organization
UAE	umbilical/uterine artery embolization			
UPA	ulipristal acetate			

eResources

You can access the resources (video clips and still images) that are referenced above and in the text directly via the ebook that accompanies this print edition: follow the instructions printed on the inside the front cover. From the ebook click on the list above or use the links from the chapters, indicated in the text by the icon: ▶

In addition, the videos and images from this book can be accessed via the companion website that accompanies this textbook www.routledge.com/cw/kenny where you will also find resources for the sister volume, *Obstetrics by Ten Teachers, 20th Edition*. Additional video clips and still images will be added to this library over time.

The development and anatomy of the female sexual organs and pelvis

HELEN BICKERSTAFF

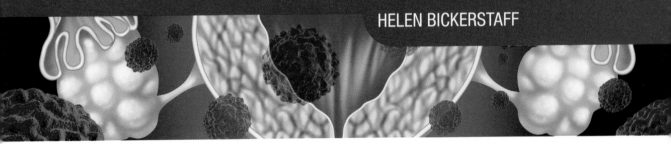

LEARNING OBJECTIVES

- Understand that sexual differentiation and development begin in early embryonic life.
- Understand the embryonic development and the anatomy of the perineum, the vagina, cervix and uterus, the adnexa and ovary and the bladder and ureters.
- Describe the blood supply and lymphatics of the perineum and pelvis.

- Understand the innervation of the perineum and pelvis.
- Understand the vulnerability of certain structures in gynaecological surgery.
- Describe the structural anomalies resulting from Müllerian tract disorders.

Sexual differentiation of the fetus and development of sexual organs

The gonadal rudiments appear as the 'genital ridge' overlying the embryonic kidney in the intermediate mesoderm during the fourth week of embryonic life, and they remain sexually indifferent until the seventh (**Figure 1.1**). The undifferentiated gonad has the potential to become either a testis or an ovary, and hence is termed bipotential, and the chromosomal complement of the zygote determines whether the gonad becomes a testis or an ovary. The development of either the testis or ovary is an active gene-directed process. In the male the activity of the SRY gene (sex-determining region of the Y chromosome)

causes the gonad to begin development into a testis. In the past, ovarian development was considered a 'default' development due solely to the absence of SRY, but in the last 10 years ovarian-determining genes have also been found that actively lead to the development of a female gonad.

The fetus has two sets of structures called the Müllerian (or paramesonephric) ducts and Wolffian (or mesonephric) ducts, which have the potential to develop into male or female internal and external genitalia respectively.

Development of the male sexual organs

As the gonad develops into a testis, it differentiates into two cell types. The Sertoli cells produce

1

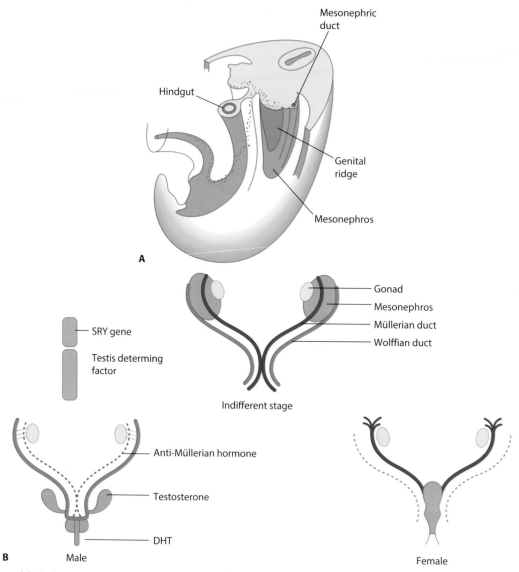

Figure 1.1 A: Cross-section diagram of the posterior abdominal wall showing the genital ridge; **B**: diagrammatic representation of the embryological pathways of male and female development. (DHT: dihydrotestosterone.)

anti-Müllerian hormone (AMH) and the Leydig cells produce testosterone. AMH suppresses further development of the Müllerian ducts whereas testosterone stimulates the Wolffian ducts to develop into the vas deferens, epididymis and seminal vesicles. In addition, in the external genital skin, testosterone is converted by the enzyme 5-alpha-reductase into dihydrotestosterone (DHT). This acts to virilize the external genitalia. The genital tubercle becomes the penis and the labioscrotal folds fuse to form the scrotum.

The urogenital folds fuse along the ventral surface of the penis and enclose the urethra so that it opens at the tip of the penis.

Development of the female sexual organs

In the primitive ovary granulosa cells, derived from the proliferating coelomic epithelium, surround the germ cells and form primordial follicles.

Each primordial follicle consists of an oocyte within a single layer of granulosa cells. Theca cells develop from the proliferating coelomic epithelium and are separated from the granulosa cells by a basal lamina. The maximum number of primordial follicles is reached at 20 weeks' gestation when there are six to seven million primordial follicles present. The numbers of these reduce by atresia and at birth only 1–2 million remain. Atresia continues throughout life and by menarche only 300,000–400,000 are present, and by menopause none.

The development of an oocyte within a primordial follicle is arrested at the prophase of its first meiotic division. It remains in that state until it undergoes atresia or enters the meiotic process preceding ovulation.

In the female, the absence of testicular AMH allows the Müllerian structures to develop and the female reproductive tract develops from these paired ducts. The proximal two-thirds of the vagina develop from the paired Müllerian ducts, which grow in a caudal and medial direction and fuse in the midline. The midline fusion of these structures produces the uterus, cervix and upper vagina, and the unfused caudal segments form the Fallopian tubes, as shown in **Figure 1.2**.

Cells proliferate from the upper portion of the urogenital sinus to form structures called the 'sinovaginal bulbs'. The caudal extension of the Müllerian ducts projects into the posterior wall of the urogenital sinus as the Müllerian tubercle. The Müllerian tubercles and the urogenital sinus fuse to form the vaginal plate, which extends from the Müllerian ducts to the urogenital sinus. This plate begins to canalize, starting at the hymen and proceeding upwards to the cervix in the sixth embryonic month.

External female genitalia

The external genitalia do not virilize in the absence of testosterone. Between the fifth and seventh weeks of life, the cloacal folds, which are a pair of swellings adjacent to the cloacal membrane, fuse anteriorly to become the genital tubercle. This will become the clitoris. The perineum develops and divides the cloacal membrane into an anterior urogenital membrane and a posterior anal membrane. The cloacal folds anteriorly are called the urethral folds, which form the labia minora. Another pair of folds within the cloacal membrane form the labioscrotal folds that eventually become the labia majora. The urogenital sinus becomes the vestibule of the vagina. The external genitalia are recognizably female by the end of the twelfth embryonic week.

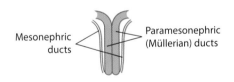

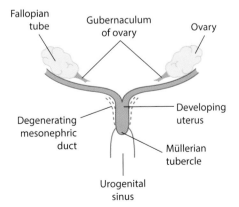

Figure 1.2 Caudal parts of the paramesonephric ducts (top) fuse to form the uterus and Fallopian tubes.

> ## 🔑 KEY LEARNING POINTS
>
> - The primitive gonad is first evident at 5 weeks of embryonic life and forms on the medial aspect of the mesonephric ridge.
> - The undifferentiated gonad has the potential to become either a testis or an ovary.
> - The paramesonephric duct, which later forms the Müllerian system, is the precursor of female genital development.
> - The lower end of the Müllerian ducts fuse in the midline to form the uterus and upper vagina.
> - Most of the upper vagina is of Müllerian origin, while the lower vagina forms from the sinovaginal bulbs.
> - Primordial follicles contain an oocyte arrested in prophase surrounded by granulosa cells separated by a basement membrane from Leydig cells.
> - The maximum number of primordial follicles is reached at 20 weeks' gestation. These reduce by atresia throughout childhood and adult life.

Female anatomy

External genitalia

The external genitalia are commonly called the vulva and include the mons pubis, labia majora and minora, the vaginal vestibule, the clitoris and the greater vestibular glands. The mons pubis is a fibro-fatty pad covered by hair-bearing skin that covers the bony pubic ramus.

The labia majora are two folds of skin with underlying adipose tissue lying either side of the vaginal opening. They contain sebaceous and sweat glands and a few specialized apocrine glands. In the deepest part of each labium is a core of fatty tissue continuous with that of the inguinal canal and the fibres of the round ligament, which terminate here.

The labia minora are two thin folds of skin that lie between the labia majora. These vary in size and may protrude beyond the labia major where they are visible, but may also be concealed by the labia majora. Anteriorly, they divide in two to form the prepuce and frenulum of the clitoris (clitoral hood). Posteriorly, they divide to form a fold of skin called the fourchette at the back of the vagina introitus. They contain sebaceous glands, but have no adipose tissue. They are not well developed before puberty and atrophy after the menopause. Both the labia minora and labia majora become engorged during sexual arousal.

The clitoris is an erectile structure measuring approximately 0.5–3.5 cm in length. The body of the clitoris is the main part of the visible clitoris and is made up of paired columns of erectile tissue and vascular tissue called the 'corpora cavernosa'. These become the crura at the bottom of the clitoris and run deeper and laterally. The vestibule is the cleft between the labia minora. It contains openings of the urethra, the Bartholin's glands and the vagina. The vagina is surrounded by two bulbs of erectile and vascular tissue that are extensive and almost completely cover the distal vaginal wall. These have traditionally been named the bulb of the vaginal vestibule, although recent work on both dissection and magnetic resonance imaging (MRI) suggests that they may be part of the clitoris and should be renamed 'clitoral bulbs'. Their function is unknown but they probably add support to the distal vaginal wall to enhance its rigidity during penetration.

The Bartholin's glands are bilateral and about the size of a pea. They open via a 2 cm duct into the vestibule below the hymen and contribute to lubrication during intercourse.

The hymen is a thin covering of mucous membrane across the entrance to the vagina. It is usually perforated, which allows menstruation. The hymen is ruptured during intercourse and any remaining tags are called 'carunculae myrtiformes'.

Internal reproductive organs (Figure 1.3)

The vagina

The vagina is a fibromuscular canal lined with stratified squamous epithelium that leads from the uterus to the vulva. It is longer in the posterior wall (approximately 9 cm) than in the anterior wall (approximately 7 cm). The vaginal walls are normally in apposition, except at the vault where they are separated by the cervix. The vault of the vagina is divided into four fornices: posterior, anterior and two lateral.

The midvagina is a transverse slit while the lower vagina is an H-shape in transverse section. The vaginal walls are lined with transverse folds. The vagina has no glands and is kept moist by secretions from the uterine and cervical glands and by transudation from its epithelial lining. The epithelium is thick and rich in glycogen, which increases in the postovulatory phase of the cycle. However, before puberty and after the menopause, the vagina is devoid of glycogen due to the lack of oestrogen. Doderlein's bacillus is a normal commensal of the vaginal flora and breaks down glycogen to form lactic acid, producing a pH of around 4.5. This has a protective role for the vagina in decreasing the growth of pathogenic bacteria.

The upper posterior wall forms the anterior peritoneal reflection of the pouch of Douglas. The middle third is separated from the rectum by pelvic fascia and the lower third abuts the perineal body. Anteriorly, the vagina is in direct contact with the base of the bladder, while the urethra runs down the lower half in the midline to open into the vestibule. Its muscles fuse with the anterior

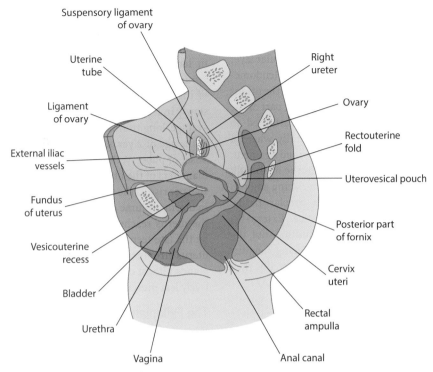

Figure 1.3 Sagittal section of the female pelvis.

vagina wall. Laterally, at the fornices, the vagina is related to the cardinal ligaments. Below this are the levator ani muscles and the ischiorectal fossae. The cardinal ligaments and the uterosacral ligaments, which form posteriorly from the parametrium, support the upper part of the vagina.

At birth, the vagina is under the influence of maternal oestrogens so the epithelium is well developed. After a couple of weeks, the effects of the oestrogen disappear and the pH rises to 7 and the epithelium atrophies. At puberty, the reverse occurs and finally at the menopause the vagina tends to shrink and the epithelium atrophies once again.

The uterus

The uterus is shaped like an inverted pear tapering inferiorly to the cervix and in its non-pregnant state is situated entirely within the pelvis. It is hollow and has thick, muscular walls. Its maximum external dimensions are approximately 7.5 cm long, 5 cm wide and 3 cm thick. An adult uterus weighs approximately 70 g. In the upper part, the uterus is termed the body or 'corpus'. The area of insertion of

each Fallopian tube is termed the 'cornu' and that part of the body above the cornu is called the 'fundus'. The uterus tapers to a small constricted area, the isthmus, and below this is the cervix, which projects obliquely into the vagina. The longitudinal axis of the uterus is approximately at right angles to the vagina and normally tilts forward. This is called 'anteversion'. In addition, the long axis of the cervix is rarely the same as the long axis of the uterus. The uterus is also usually flexed forward on itself at the isthmus – antiflexion. However, in around 20% of women, the uterus is tilted backwards – retroversion and retroflexion. This has no pathological significance in most women, although retroversion that is fixed and immobile may be associated with endometriosis. This has relevance in gynaecological surgery and is referred to again in Chapter 2, Gynaecological history, examination and investigations.

The cavity of the uterus is the shape of an inverted triangle and when sectioned coronally the Fallopian tubes open at lateral angles The constriction at the isthmus where the corpus joins the cervix is the anatomical os. Seen microscopically, the site of the histological internal os is where the mucous membrane of the isthmus becomes that of the cervix.

The uterus consists of three layers: the outer serous layer (peritoneum), the middle muscular layer (myometrium) and the inner mucous layer (endometrium). The peritoneum covers the body of the uterus and posteriorly it covers the supravaginal part of the cervix. The peritoneum is intimately attached to a subserous fibrous layer, except laterally where it spreads out to form the leaves of the broad ligament.

The muscular myometrium forms the main bulk of the uterus and is made up of interlacing smooth muscle fibres intermingling with areolar tissue, blood vessels, nerves and lymphatics. Externally, the muscle fibres are mostly longitudinal, but the thicker intermediate layer has interlacing longitudinal, oblique and transverse fibres. Internally, they are mainly longitudinal and circular.

The inner endometrial layer has tubular glands that dip into the myometrium. The endometrial layer is covered by a single layer of columnar epithelium. Ciliated prior to puberty, this epithelium is mostly lost due to the effects of pregnancy and menstruation. The endometrium undergoes cyclical changes during menstruation, as described in Chapter 3, Hormonal control of the menstrual cycle and hormonal disorders, and varies in thickness.

The cervix

The cervix is narrower than the body of the uterus and is approximately 2.5 cm in length. Lateral to the cervix lies cellular connective tissue called the parametrium. The ureter runs about 1 cm laterally to the supravaginal cervix within the parametrium. The posterior aspect of the cervix is covered by the peritoneum of the pouch of Douglas.

The upper part of the cervix mostly consists of involuntary muscle, whereas the lower part is mainly fibrous connective tissue. The mucous membrane of the cervical canal (endocervix) has anterior and posterior columns from which folds radiate out, the 'arbour vitae'. It has numerous deep glandular follicles that secrete clear alkaline mucus, the main component of physiological vaginal discharge. The epithelium of the endocervix is columnar and is also ciliated in its upper two-thirds. This changes to stratified squamous epithelium around the region of the external os and the junction of these two types of epithelium is called the 'squamocolumnar junction'.

Age changes to anatomy

The disappearance of maternal oestrogens from the circulation after birth causes the uterus to decrease in length by around one-third and in weight by around one-half. The cervix is then twice the length of the uterus. During childhood, the uterus grows slowly in length, in parallel with height and age. The average longitudinal diameter ranges from 2.5 cm at the age of 2 years, to 3.5 cm at 10 years. After the onset of puberty, the anteroposterior and transverse diameters of the uterus start to increase, leading to a sharper rise in the volume of the uterus. The increase in uterine volume continues well after menarche and the uterus reaches its adult size and configuration by the late teenage years. After the menopause, the uterus atrophies, the mucosa becomes very thin, the glands almost disappear and the wall becomes relatively less muscular.

The Fallopian tubes

The Fallopian tube extends outwards from the uterine cornu to end near the ovary. At the abdominal ostium, the tube opens into the peritoneal cavity, which is therefore in communication with the exterior of the body via the uterus and the vagina. This is essential to allow the sperm and egg to meet. The Fallopian tubes convey the ovum from the ovary towards the uterus and promote oxygenation and nutrition for sperm, ovum and zygote should fertilization occur.

The Fallopian tube runs in the upper margin of the broad ligament, known as the mesosalpinx, which encloses the tube so that it is completely covered with peritoneum, except for a narrow strip along this inferior aspect. Each tube is about 10 cm long and is described in four parts:

- The interstitial portion.
- The isthmus.
- The ampulla.
- The infundibulum or fimbrial portion.

The interstitial portion lies within the wall of the uterus, while the isthmus is the narrow portion adjoining the uterus. This passes into the widest and longest portion, the ampulla. This, in turn, terminates in the extremity known as the 'infundibulum'. The opening of the tube into the peritoneal cavity is surrounded by finger-like processes, known as fimbria, into which the muscle coat does not extend. The inner surfaces of the fimbriae are covered by ciliated epithelium that is similar to the lining of the Fallopian tube itself. One of these fimbriae is longer than the others and extends to, and partially embraces, the ovary. The muscular fibres of the wall of the tube are arranged in an inner circular and an outer longitudinal layer.

The tubal epithelium forms a number of branched folds or plicae that run longitudinally; the lumen of the ampulla is almost filled with these folds. The folds have a cellular stroma, but at their bases the epithelium is only separated from the muscle by a very scanty amount of stroma. There is no submucosa and there are no glands. The epithelium of the Fallopian tubes contains two functioning cell types: the ciliated cells, which act to produce constant current of fluid in the direction of the uterus, and the secretory cells, which contribute to the volume of tubal fluid. Changes occur under the influence of the menstrual cycle, but there is no cell shedding during menstruation.

The ovaries

The size and appearance of the ovaries depends on both age and stage of the menstrual cycle. In a child, the ovaries are small structures approximately 1.5 cm long; however, they increase to adult size in puberty due to proliferation of stromal cells and commencing maturation of the ovarian follicles. In the young adult, they are almond-shaped and measure approximately 3 cm long, 1.5 cm wide and 1 cm thick. After the menopause, no active follicles are present and the ovary becomes smaller with a wrinkled surface. The ovary is the only intra-abdominal structure not to be covered by peritoneum. Each ovary is attached to the cornu of the uterus by the ovarian ligament and at the hilum to the broad ligament by the mesovarium, which contains its supply of nerves and blood vessels. Laterally, each ovary is attached to the suspensory ligament of the ovary with folds of peritoneum that becomes continuous with that of the overlying psoas major.

Anterior to the ovaries lie the Fallopian tubes, the superior portion of the bladder and the uterovesical pouch. Posterior to the ovary lies the ureter where it runs downwards and forwards in front of the internal iliac artery.

Structure of the ovary

The ovary has a central vascular medulla consisting of loose connective tissue containing many elastin fibres and non-striated muscle cells. It has an outer thicker cortex, denser than the medulla, consisting of networks of reticular fibres and fusiform cells, although there is no clear-cut demarcation between the two. The surface of the ovaries is covered by a single layer of cuboidal cells, the germinal epithelium. Beneath this is an ill-defined layer of condensed connective tissue called the 'tunica albuginea', which increases in density with age. At birth, numerous primordial follicles are found, mostly in the cortex, but some are found in the medulla. With puberty, some form each month into the graafian follicles under gonadotrophic control, to ovulate and subsequently form corpus lutea and ultimately the atretic follicles, the corpora albicans.

The bladder, urethra and ureter

The bladder

The bladder wall is made of involuntary muscle arranged in an inner longitudinal layer, a middle circular layer and an outer longitudinal layer. It is lined with transitional epithelium and has an average capacity of 400 ml.

The ureters open into the base of the bladder after running medially for about 1 cm through the bladder wall. The urethra leaves the bladder below the ureteric orifices. The triangular area lying between the ureteric orifices and the internal meatus of the urethra is known as the 'trigone'. At the internal meatus, the middle layer of muscle forms anterior and posterior loops round the neck of the bladder, some fibres of the loops being continuous with the circular muscle of the urethra.

The base of the bladder is adjacent to the cervix, with only a thin layer of tissue intervening. It is separated from the anterior vaginal wall below by the pubocervical fascia that stretches from the pubis to the cervix.

The urethra

The female urethra is about 3.5 cm long and is lined with transitional epithelium. It has a slight posterior angulation at the junction of its lower and middle thirds. The smooth muscle of its wall is arranged in outer longitudinal and inner circular layers. As the urethra passes through the two layers of the urogenital diaphragm, it is embraced by the striated fibres of the deep transverse perineal muscle (also known as the compressor urethrae) and some of the striated fibres of this muscle form a loop on the urethra. Between the muscular coat and the epithelium is a plexus of veins. There are a number of tubular mucous glands and in the lower part a number of crypts that occasionally become infected. In its upper two-thirds, the urethra is separated from the symphysis by loose connective tissue, but in its lower third it is attached to the pubic ramus on each side by strong bands of fibrous tissue called the 'pubourethral tissue'. Posteriorly, it is firmly attached in its lower two-thirds to the anterior vaginal wall. This means that the upper part of the urethra is mobile, but the lower part is relatively fixed.

Medial fibres of the pubococcygeus of the levator ani muscles are inserted into the urethra and vaginal wall. When they contract, they pull the anterior vaginal wall and the upper part of the urethra forwards forming an angle of about 100° between the posterior wall of the urethra and the bladder base. On voluntary voiding of urine, the base of the bladder and the upper part of the urethra descend and the posterior angle disappears so that the base of the bladder and the posterior wall of the urethra come to lie in a straight line.

The ureter

As the ureter crosses the pelvic brim, it lies in front of the bifurcation of the common iliac artery. It runs downwards and forwards on the lateral wall of the pelvis to reach the pelvic floor and then passes inwards and forwards attached to the peritoneum of the back of the broad ligament to pass beneath the uterine artery. It next passes forward through a fibrous tunnel, the ureteric canal, in the upper part of the cardinal ligament. Finally, it runs close to the lateral vaginal fornix to enter the trigone of the bladder.

Its blood supply is derived from small branches of the ovarian artery, from a small vessel arising near the iliac bifurcation, from a branch of the uterine artery where it crosses beneath it and from small branches of the vesical artery.

Box 1.1 Ureteric damage during hysterectomy

Because of its close relationship to the cervix, the vault of the vagina and the uterine artery, the ureter may be damaged during hysterectomy. Apart from being cut or tied, in radical procedures, the ureter may undergo necrosis because of interference with its blood supply. It may be displaced by scar tissue or by fibromyomata or cysts that are growing between the layers of the broad ligament and may suffer injury if its position is not noticed at surgery.

The rectum

The rectum extends from the level of the third sacral vertebra to a point about 2.5 cm in front of the coccyx where it passes through the pelvic floor to become continuous with the anal canal. Its direction follows the curve of the sacrum and is about 11 cm in length. The front and sides are covered by the peritoneum of the rectovaginal pouch. In the middle third only the front is covered by peritoneum. In the lower third there is no peritoneal covering and the rectum is separated from the posterior wall of the vagina by the rectovaginal fascial septum. Lateral to the rectum are the uterosacral ligaments, beside which run some of the lymphatics draining the cervix and vagina.

The pelvic muscles, ligaments and fascia
The pelvic diaphragm (Figure 1.4)

The pelvic diaphragm is formed by the levator ani muscles, which are broad, flat muscles the fibres of which pass downwards and inwards. The two muscles, one on either side, constitute the pelvic diaphragm. The muscles arise by linear origin from the following points:

- The lower part of the body of the os pubis.

- The internal surface of the parietal pelvic fascia along the white line.

- The pelvic surface of the ischial spine.

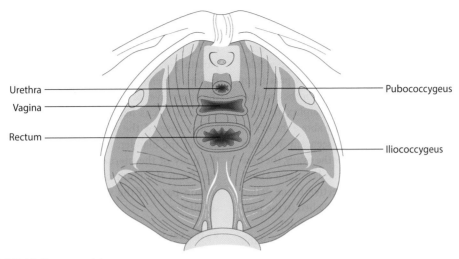

Figure 1.4 Pelvic floor musculature.

The levator ani muscles are inserted into the following points:

- The preanal raphe and the central point of the perineum, where one muscle meets the other on the opposite side.
- The wall of the anal canal, where the fibres blend with the deep external sphincter muscle.
- The postanal or anococcygeal raphe, where again one muscle meets the other on the opposite side.
- The lower part of the coccyx.

The muscle is described in two parts:

- The pubococcygeus, which arises from the pubic bone and the anterior part of the tendinous arch of the pelvic fascia (the 'white line').
- The iliococcygeus, which arises from the posterior part of the tendinous arch and the ischial spine.

The medial borders of the pubococcygeus muscle pass on either side from the pubic bone to the preanal raphe. They thus embrace the vagina and on contraction have some sphincteric action. The nerve supply is from the third and fourth sacral nerves. The pubococcygeus muscles support the pelvic and abdominal viscera, including the bladder. The medial edge passes beneath the bladder and runs laterally to the urethra, into which some of its fibres are inserted. Together with the fibres from the opposite muscle, they form a loop that maintains the angle between the posterior aspect of the urethra and the bladder base. During micturition, this loop relaxes to allow the bladder neck and upper urethra to open and descend.

Urogenital diaphragm

The urogenital diaphragm (also known as the triangular ligament) is made up of two layers of pelvic fascia that fill the gap between the descending pubic rami and lies beneath the levator ani muscles. The deep transverse perineal muscles (compressor urethrae) lie between the two layers and the diaphragm is pierced by the urethra and vagina.

The perineal body

This is a mass of muscular tissue that lies between the anal canal and the lower third of the vagina. Its apex is at the lower end of the rectovaginal septum at the point where the rectum and posterior vaginal walls come into contact. Its base is covered with skin and extends from the fourchette to the anus. It is the point of insertion of the superficial perineal muscles and is bounded above by the levator ani muscles where they come into contact in the midline between the posterior vaginal wall and the rectum.

The pelvic peritoneum

The peritoneum is reflected from the lateral borders of the uterus to form, on either side, a double fold of peritoneum – the broad ligament. Despite the name, this is not a ligament but a peritoneal fold and it does not support the uterus. The Fallopian tube runs in the upper free edge of the broad ligament as far as the point at which the tube opens into the peritoneal cavity. The part of the broad ligament that is lateral to the opening is called the 'infundibulopelvic fold' and in it the ovarian vessels and nerves pass from the side wall of the pelvis to lie between the two layers of the broad ligament. The mesosalpinx, the portion of the broad ligament that lies above the ovary, is layered; between its layers are seen any Wolffian remnants that may remain. Below the ovary, the base of the broad ligament widens out and contains a considerable amount of loose connective tissue called the 'parametrium'. The ureter is attached to the posterior leaf of the broad ligament at this point.

The ovary is attached to the posterior layer of the broad ligament by a short mesentry (the mesovarium) through which the ovarian vessels and nerves enter the hilum.

The ovarian ligament and round ligament (Figure 1.5A)

The ovarian ligament lies beneath the posterior layer of the broad ligament and passes from the medial pole of the ovary to the uterus just below the point of entry of the Fallopian tube.

The round ligament is the continuation of the same structure and runs forwards under the anterior leaf of peritoneum to enter the inguinal canal, ending in the subcutaneous tissue of the labium major.

The pelvic fascia and pelvic cellular tissue (Figure 1.5B)

Connective tissue fills the irregular spaces between the various pelvic organs. Much of it is loose cellular tissue, but in some places it is condensed to form strong ligaments that contain some smooth muscle fibres and which form the fascial sheaths that enclose the various viscera. The pelvic arteries, veins, lymphatics, nerves and ureters run through it. The cellular tissue is continuous above with the extraperitoneal tissue of the abdominal wall, but below it is cut off from the ischiorectal fossa by the pelvic fascia and the levator ani muscles. The pelvic fascia may be regarded as a specialized part of this connective tissue and has parietal and visceral components.

The parietal pelvic fascia lines the wall of the pelvic cavity covering the obturator and pyramidalis muscles. The thickened tendinous arch (known as

the white line) lies on the side wall of the pelvis. It is here that the levator ani muscle arises and the cardinal ligament gains its lateral attachment. Where the parietal pelvic fascia encounters bone, as in the pubic region, it blends with the periosteum. It also forms the upper layer of the urogenital diaphragm.

Each viscus has a fascial sheath that is dense in the case of the vagina and cervix and at the base of the bladder, but is tenuous or absent over the body of the uterus and the dome of the bladder. From the point of view of the gynaecologist, certain parts of the visceral fascia are important, as follows:

- The cardinal ligaments (transverse cervical ligaments) provide the essential support of the uterus and vaginal vault. These are two strong fan-shaped fibromuscular bands that pass from the cervix and vaginal vault to the side wall of the pelvis on either side.

- The uterosacral ligaments run from the cervix and vaginal vault to the sacrum. In the erect position, they are almost vertical in direction and support the cervix.

- The bladder is supported laterally by condensations of the vesical pelvic fascia, one each side, and by a sheet of pubocervical fascia, which lies beneath it anteriorly.

The blood supply (Figure 1.6)
Arteries supplying the pelvic organs

Because the ovary develops on the posterior abdominal wall and later migrates down into the pelvis, it carries its blood supply with it directly from the abdominal aorta. The ovarian artery arises from the aorta just below the renal artery and runs downwards on the surface of the psoas muscle to the pelvic brim, where it crosses in front of the ureter and then passes into the infundibulopelvic fold of the broad ligament. The artery divides into branches that supply the ovary and tube and then run on to reach the uterus, where they anastamose with the terminal branches of the uterine artery.

The internal iliac (hypogastric) artery
This vessel is about 4 cm in length and begins at the bifurcation of the common iliac artery in front of the sacroiliac joint. It soon divides into anterior

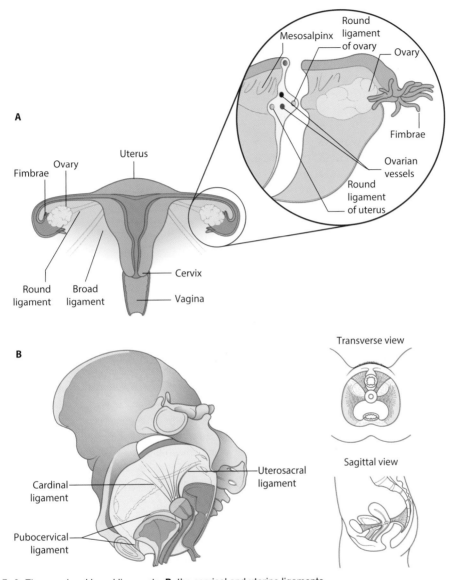

Figure 1.5 A: The round and broad ligaments; **B**: the cervical and uterine ligaments.

and posterior branches; the branches that supply the pelvic organs are all from the anterior division and are as follows:

- The uterine artery provides the main blood supply to the uterus. The artery first runs downwards on the lateral wall of the pelvis, in the same direction as the ureter. It then turns inward and forwards lying in the base of the broad ligament. On reaching the wall of the uterus, the artery turns upwards to run tortuously to the upper part of the uterus, where it anastamoses

with the ovarian artery. In this part of its course, it sends many branches into the substance of the uterus. The uterine artery supplies a branch to the ureter as it crosses it and shortly afterwards another branch is given off to supply the cervix and upper vagina.

- The vaginal artery runs at a lower level to supply the vagina.
- The vesical arteries are variable in number and supply the bladder and terminal ureter. One usually runs in the roof of the ureteric canal.

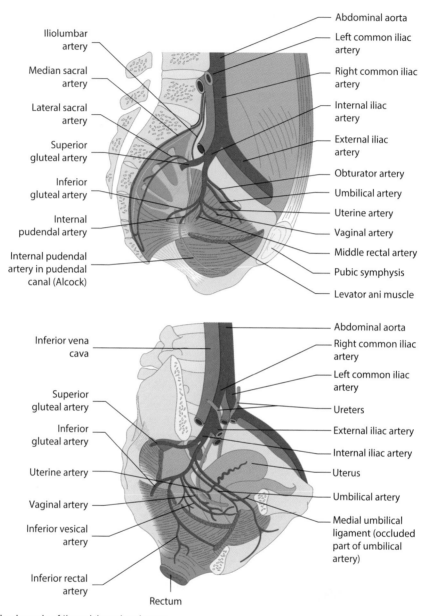

Figure 1.6 Blood supply of the pelvis and perineum.

- The middle rectal artery often arises in common with the lowest vesical artery.
- The pudendal artery leaves the pelvic cavity through the sciatic foramen and, after winding round the ischial spine, enters the ischiorectal fossa where it gives off the inferior rectal artery. It terminates in the perineal and vulval arteries, supplying the erectile tissue of the vestibular bulbs and clitoris.

The superior rectal artery

This artery is the continuation of the inferior mesenteric artery and descends in the base of the mesocolon. It divides into two branches that run on either side of the rectum and supply numerous branches to it.

The pelvic veins

The veins around the bladder, uterus, vagina and rectum form plexuses that intercommunicate freely.

Venous drainage from the uterine, vaginal and vesical plexus is chiefly into the internal iliac veins. Venous drainage from the rectal plexus is via the superior rectal veins to the inferior mesenteric veins, and the middle and inferior rectal veins to the internal pudendal veins and so to the iliac veins.

The ovarian veins on each side begin in the pampiniform plexus, which lies between the layers of the broad ligament. At first, there are two veins on each side accompanying the corresponding ovarian artery. Higher up the vein becomes single, with that on the right ending in the inferior vena cava and that on the left in the left renal vein.

Lymphatics

The pelvic lymphatics (Figure 1.7)

Lymph draining from all the lower extremities and the vulva and perineal regions is all filtered through the inguinal and superficial femoral nodes before continuing along the deep pathways on the side wall of the pelvis. One deep chain passes upwards lateral to the major blood vessels, forming in turn the external iliac, common iliac and para-aortic groups of nodes.

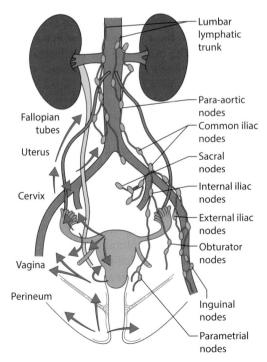

Figure 1.7 Lymphatic drainage of the pelvis and perineum.

Medially, another chain of vessels passes from the deep femoral nodes through the femoral canal to the obturator and internal iliac groups of nodes. These last nodes are interspersed among the origins of the branches of the internal iliac artery receiving lymph directly from the organs supplied by this artery, including the upper vagina, cervix and body of the uterus.

From the internal iliac and common iliac nodes, afferent vessels pass up the para-aortic chains, and finally all lymphatic drainage from the legs and pelvis flows into the lumbar lymphatic trunks and cisterna chyli at the level of the second lumbar vertebra. From here, all the lymph is carried by the thoracic duct through the thorax with no intervening nodes to empty into the junction of the left subclavian and internal jugular veins.

Tumour cells that penetrate or bypass the pelvic and para-aortic nodes are rapidly disseminated via the great veins at the root of the neck.

Lymphatic drainage from the genital tract

The lymph vessel from individual parts of the genital tract drain into this system of pelvic lymph nodes in the following manner:

- The vulva and perineum medial to the labiocrural skin folds contain superficial lymphatics that pass upwards towards the mons pubis, then curve laterally to the superficial and inguinal nodes. Drainage from these is through the fossa ovalis into the deep femoral nodes. The largest of these, lying in the upper part of the femoral canal, is known as the node of Cloquet.

- The lymphatics of the lower third of the vagina follow the vulval drainage to the superficial lymph nodes, whereas those from the upper two-thirds pass upwards to join the lymphatic vessels of the cervix.

- The lymphatics of the cervix pass either laterally in the base of the broad ligament or posteriorly along the uterosacral ligaments to reach the side wall of the pelvis. Most of the vessels drain to the internal iliac obturator and external iliac nodes, but vessels also pass directly to the common iliac and lower para-aortic nodes. Radical surgery for carcinoma of the cervix should include removal of all these node groups on both sides of the pelvis.

- Most of the lymphatic vessels of the body of the uterus join those of the cervix and therefore reach similar groups of nodes. A few vessels at the fundus follow the ovarian channels and there is an inconsistent pathway along the round ligament to the inguinal nodes.

- The ovary and Fallopian tube have a plexus of vessels that drain along the infundibulopelvic fold to the para-aortic nodes on both sides of the midline. On the left, these are found around the left renal pedicle, while on the right there may only be one node intervening before the lymph flows into the thoracic duct, thus accounting for the rapid early spread of metastatic carcinoma to distant sites such as the lungs.
- The lymphatic drainage of the bladder and upper urethra is to the iliac nodes, while those of the lower part of the urethra follow those of the vulva.
- Lymphatics from the lower anal canal drain to the superficial inguinal nodes and the remainder of the rectal drainage follows pararectal channels accompanying the blood vessels to both the internal iliac nodes (middle rectal artery) and the para-aortic nodes and the origin of the inferior mesenteric artery.

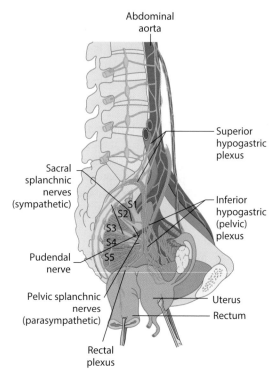

Figure 1.8 Nerve supply of the pelvis and perineum.

The nerves (Figure 1.8)

Nerve supply of the vulva and perineum

The pudendal nerve arises from the second, third and fourth sacral nerves. As it passes along the outer wall of the ischiorectal fossa, it gives off an inferior rectal branch and divides into the perineal nerve and dorsal nerve of the clitoris. The perineal nerve gives the sensory supply to the vulva and also innervates the anterior part of the external anal canal and the levator ani and the superficial perineal muscles. The dorsal nerve of the clitoris is sensory. Sensory fibres from the mons and labia also pass in the ilioinguinal and genitofemoral nerves to the first lumbar root. The posterior femoral cutaneous nerve carries sensation from the perineum to the small sciatic nerve and thus to the first, second and third sacral nerves. The main nerve supply of the levator ani muscles comes from the third and fourth sacral nerves.

Nerve supply of the pelvic viscera

The innervation of the pelvic viscera is complex and not well understood. All pelvic viscera receive dual innervation (i.e both sympathetic and parasympathetic). Nerve fibres of the preaortic plexus of the sympathetic nervous system are continuous with those of the superior hypogastric plexus, which lies in front of the last lumber vertebra and is wrongly called the 'presacral nerve'. Below this, the superior hypogastric plexus divides and on each side its fibres are continuous with fibres passing beside the rectum to join the uterovaginal plexus (inferior hypogastric plexus or plexus of Frankenhauser). This plexus lies in the loose cellular tissue posterolateral to the cervix, below the uterosacral folds of peritoneum. Parasympathetic fibres from the second, third and fourth sacral nerves join the uterovaginal plexus. Fibres from (or to) the bladder, uterus, vagina and rectum join the plexus. The uterovaginal plexus contains a few ganglion cells, so it is likely that a few motor cells also have their relay stations there and then pass onward with the blood vessels onto the viscera.

The ovary is not innervated by the nerves already described, but from the ovarian plexus that surrounds the ovarian vessels and joins the preaortic plexus high up.

KEY LEARNING POINTS

- An adult uterus consists of three layers: the perito-neum, myometrium and endometrium.
- The cervix is narrower than the body of the uterus and is approximately 2.5 cm in length. The ureter runs about 1 cm lateral to the cervix.
- The ovary is the only intraperitoneal structure not covered by peritoneum.
- The main supports to the pelvic floor are the connective tissue and levator ani muscles. The main supports of the uterus are the uterosacral and cardi-nal ligaments, which are condensations of connective tissue.
- The ovarian arteries arise directly from the aorta, while the right ovarian vein drains into the vena cava and the left into the left renal vein.
- The major nerve supply of the pelvis comes from the pudendal nerves, which arise from the second, third and fourth sacral nerves.

Structural problems of pelvic organs

Müllerian anomalies

These are common, occurring in up to 6% of the female population, and may be asymptomatic. The aetiology is unknown, although associated renal anomalies are present in up to 30%. Several classi-fications are used that have relevance to the clinical management. **Figure 1.9** represents the classification used in Europe.

Müllerian obstruction

Failure of complete canalization of the Müllerian structures can lead to menstrual obstruction. The obstruction most commonly occurs at the junc-tion of the lower third of the vagina at the level of the hymen, although more proximal obstruction can occur. Presentation with an imperforate hymen

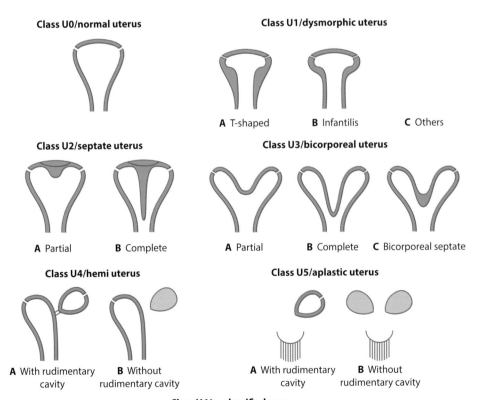

Figure 1.9 Müllerian structural abnormalities.

is usually with increasing abdominal pain in a girl in early adolescence. The retained menstrual blood stretches the vagina, causing a haematocolpus. This can cause a large pelvic mass and in addition can usually be seen as a bulging membrane at the vaginal entrance. Treatment is simple with a surgical incision of the hymen and drainage of the retained blood.

Müllerian duplication

Duplication of the Müllerian system can occur, resulting in a wide range of anomalies. It may be a complete duplication of the uterus, cervix and vagina, but may be simply a midline uterine septum in otherwise normal internal genitalia. Second uterine horns may also occur and can be rudimentary or functional.

Müllerian agenesis

In approximately 1 in 5,000 to 1 in 40,000 girls, the Müllerian system does not develop, resulting in an absent or rudimentary uterus and upper vagina. This condition is known as Rokitansky syndrome or Mayer–Rokitansky–Kuster–Hauser syndrome (MRKH). The ovaries function normally and so the most common presentation is with primary amenorrhoea in the presence of otherwise normal pubertal development. The aetiology of this condition is not known, although possible factors include environmental, genetic, hormonal or receptor factors. On examination, the vagina will be blind ending and is likely to be shortened in length. An ultrasound scan will confirm the presence of ovaries, but no functioning uterus will be present.

Treatment options focus on psychological support and on the creation of a vagina comfortable for penetrative intercourse, as discussed in Chapter 3, Hormonal control of the menstrual cycle and hormonal disorders. There is currently no treatment available to transplant a uterus in humans, although there is extensive ongoing research being undertaken in this area. Women with MRKH syndrome may have their own genetic children, using ovum retrieval and assisted conception techniques, and a surrogate mother.

Vestigial structures

Vestigial remains of the mesonephric duct and tubules are always present in young children, but are variable structures in adults. The epoophoron, a series of parallel blind tubules, lies in the broad ligament between the mesovarium and the Fallopian tube. The tubules run to the rudimentary duct of the epoophoron, which runs parallel to the lateral Fallopian tube. Situated in the broad ligament between the epoophoron and the uterus, a few rudimentary tubules are occasionally seen, the paroophoron. In a few individuals, the caudal part of the mesonephric duct is well developed, running alongside the uterus to the internal os. This is the duct of Gartner.

Further reading

Netter FH (2011) *Atlas Of Human Anatomy*. Philadelphia, PA: Saunders/Elsevier.
Setchell M, Hudson CN (2013) *Shaw's Textbook Of Operative Gynaecology*. New Delhi: Elsevier.

Self assessment

CASE HISTORY

A 15-year-old girl was seen in gynaecology clinic with her mother. She had not yet started her periods. She described breast development at age 12 and pubic hair development. All her friends had started their periods and she wondered what was wrong.

She also described abdominal pain that had started a couple of years ago. Initially she had ignored it but now it was interfering with sport. It was intermittent and on questioning she wondered if it was coming about monthly. It was a cramping lower abdominal pain.

She had a boyfriend but was not sexually active. Medically there were no problems, no previous operations and no allergies. Socially she was doing well at school.

On examination there was normal breast development and distribution of pubic hair. There was a hard swelling in the lower abdomen that was quite tender. On observation of the genitalia, a blue swelling at the level of the hymen was seen.

A What is the most likely diagnosis?

B Which investigations(s) should be performed and what is the differential diagnosis?

ANSWERS

A The most likely diagnosis is a haematocolpos from an imperforate hymen. Menstrual fluid had been collecting above the hymen as it could not escape. Over time this had distended the vagina and filled the uterine cavity. This was causing the swelling and the cyclical pain.

B An ultrasound should be performed to confirm the diagnosis and exclude any Müllerian structural alterations. The important differential is obstruction due to a horizontal vaginal plate at a higher level. In this case the ultrasound would not show blood filling the vagina down to the introitus because the site of an imperforate plate is higher in the vagina and is due to imperforate urogenital sinus. The additional finding of the blue vaginal swelling also points to the hymen being the level of obstruction.

The girl was admitted for day case surgery. An incision was made in the hymen under general anaesthetic. 700 ml of old blood was evacuated. She made a good recovery and her periods commenced shortly afterwards.

SBA QUESTIONS

1 Which of the following statements is true about the round ligament? Choose the single best answer.

A The round ligament lies posterior to the uterus.

B The round ligament supports the fundus of the uterus.

C The round ligament is a vestigial structure.

D The round ligament ends distally in the inguinal canal.

E The round ligament contains the neuromuscular bundle supplying the ovary.

ANSWER

D The round ligament lies anterior to the uterus. It does not physically support the uterus and is not a vestigial structure. It runs from the cornu of the uterus from the anterior leaf of the broad ligament, to the inguinal canal. The round ligament does not contain the vascular bundle of the ovary; this runs in the mesovarian.

2 Which of the following statements is true about the Fallopian tube? Choose the single best answer.

A The Fallopian tube is 20 cm long.

B The Fallopian tube has a glandular submucosa.

C The Fallopian tube is independent of hormonal influence.

D The Fallopian tube is lined by ciliated epithelium.

E The Fallopian tube lies in the round ligament.

ANSWER

D The Fallopian tube is about 10 cm long. It runs in the upper margin of the broad ligament. The epithelium is responsive to hormones and has two types of cell: ciliated and secretory cells. There is no submucosa nor glands.

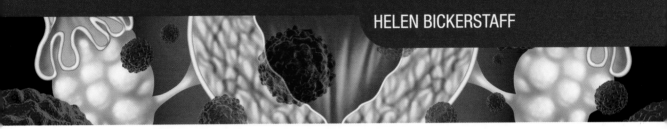

Gynaecological history, examination and investigations

HELEN BICKERSTAFF

LEARNING OBJECTIVES

- To understand that a detailed and structured gynaecological history is vital for making a diagnosis, and will place the patient's symptoms in her social context.
- To understand that the gynaecological examination will be customized by the history to elicit the appropriate signs.
- Imaging in gynaecology may include ultrasound, magnetic resonance imaging (MRI) and computed tomography (CT) scanning.
- Biochemical, haematological and microbiological investigations will be guided by the history and examination findings.

History

The gynaecological consultation should ideally be held in a closed room with adequate facilities and privacy. Some women will feel anxious or apprehensive about the forthcoming consultation, so it is important that the student or doctor establishes initial rapport with the patient and puts them at ease. The practitioner should introduce themselves by name and status, and should check the patient's details. Ideally, there should be no more than one other person in the room, but any student or attending nurse should be introduced by name and their role briefly explained.

A number of women attend with their partner, close family member or friend. Provided the patient herself consents to this, there is no reason to exclude them from the initial consultation, but this should be limited to one person. In some instances, the additional person may be required to be a key

 eResource 2.1

The gynaecological consultation
http://www.routledgetextbooks.com/textbooks/tenteachers/gynaecologyv2.1.php

part of the consultation (i.e. if there is a language or comprehension difficulty). However, an independent interpreter should always be used to ensure the patient's best interests are being presented. At least some part of the consultation or examination should be with the woman alone, to allow her to answer any specific queries more openly.

It is important to be aware of the different attitudes to women's health issues in a religious and culturally diverse population. Appropriate respect and sensitivity should always be shown.

Enough time should be allowed for the patient to express herself and the doctor's manner should be one of interest and understanding, while guiding her with appropriate questioning. A history that is taken with sensitivity will often encourage the patient to reveal more details that may be relevant to future management. While there are number of terms used in gynaecology (**Box 2.1**), care should be taken to avoid medicalized language, using lay terms where possible.

A set template should be used for history taking, as this prevents the omission of important points and will help direct the consultation (**Box 2.2**). Some clinics employ a template routinely to ensure all questions are covered.

Social history

Sensitive enquiry should be made about the woman's social situation including details of her occupation, who she lives with, her housing and whether or not she is in a stable relationship. A history regarding smoking and alcohol intake should also be obtained. Any pertinent family or other relevant social problems should be briefly discussed. If admission and surgery are being contemplated it is necessary to establish what support the woman has at home, particularly if she is elderly or frail.

Box 2.1 Glossary

Menarche	Start of menstruation
Last menstrual period (LMP)	Date of last menstrual bleed
Amenorrhoea	Absence of bleeds for more than 6 months in women of reproductive age, see Chapter 3, Hormonal control of the menstrual cycle and hormonal disorders
Oligomenorrhoea	Infrequent menstrual bleeds more than 35 days apart, see Chapter 3, Hormonal control of the menstrual cycle and hormonal disorders
Dysmenorrhoea	Painful menstrual bleeding (primary or secondary) see Chapter 4, Disorders of menstrual bleeding
Menorrhagia	Now called heavy menstrual bleeding (HMB), see Chapter 4, Disorders of menstrual bleeding
Abnormal uterine bleeding (AUB)	Includes postcoital bleeding (PCB)/intermenstrual bleeding (IMB), see Chapter 4, Disorders of menstrual bleeding
Dyspareunia	Painful intercourse, superficial or deep, see Chapter 13, Benign conditions of the vulva and vagina, psychosexual disorders and female genital mutilation
Incontinence	Involuntary loss of urine, stress, urge or mixed, see Chapter 10 Urogynaecology and pelvic floor problems
Prolapse	Feeling of something coming down in the vagina, see Chapter 10, Urogynaecology and pelvic floor problems

---

Box 2.2 Template for gynaecological history taking in suggested order

1 General

Name, age and occupation.

A brief statement of the general nature and duration of the main complaints (try to use the patient's own words rather than medical terms at this stage).

2 History of presenting complaint

This section should focus on the presenting complaint (e.g. menstrual problems, pain, subfertility, urinary incontinence, etc).

3 Menstrual history

This will be explored in all patients except menopausal women:

- usual duration of each period and length of full cycle (how many days from day 1 of bleed to day 1 of next bleed);

- first day of the LMP;

- pattern of bleeding: regular or irregular and length of cycle;

- amount of blood loss: patients will have different ideas as to what constitutes a 'heavy period'.

4 Cervical screening

This will be explored in all patients:

- date of last smear, its outcome and any previous abnormalities, colposcopy or treatments.

5 Sexual and contraceptive history

- present partner(s), sexual orientation;
- contraceptive method or needs.

6 Other gynaecological symptoms

A brief exploration of the following complaints should follow. The detailed questions relating to each complaint are explained in more detail later:

- any irregular bleeding?
- any HMB, IMB, PCB?
- any pelvic pain?
- any problems with fertility?
- any problems with continence?
- any dyspareunia or sexual difficulty?
- any vaginal discharge?
- menopausal history and use of HRT.

7 Previous gynaecological history

This section should include any previous gynaecological treatments or surgery.
Previous obstetric history:

- number of children with ages and birthweights, mode of delivery and any complications;
- number of miscarriages and gestation at which they occurred;
- any terminations of pregnancy with record of gestational age and any complications.

8 Previous medical history

- any serious illnesses or operations with dates.

9 Medication and allergies

- allergies: including to what and the reaction;
- current/previous medications tried.

10 Family history

Significant autoimmune disease, BRAC related cancers and thrombophilias.

11 Systems enquiry

- appetite, weight loss, weight gain;
- bowel function (if urogynaecological complaint, more detail may be required);
- bladder function (if urogynaecological complaint, more detail may be required).

Box 2.3 How to determine if there is HMB

- Is the bleeding more or less than usual?
- Do you use tampons, towels or both?
- How often does soaked sanitary wear need to be changed?
- Is there presence of clots?
- Is the bleeding so heavy (flooding) that it spills over your towel/tampon and onto your pants, clothes or bedding?
- Have you had to take any time off work due to this bleeding?
- Do you ever find you are confined to your house when the bleeding is at its worst?
- Do you feel dizzy or short of breath, particularly after a period, or find it hard to climb stairs?
- Does it constrain your lifestyle?

Specific gynaecological problems require more focussed history taking, and the questions to be asked are detailed below.

Abnormal uterine bleeding (AUB) (see Chapter 4, Disorders of menstrual bleeding)

- Length of time of problem.

- Amount of blood loss.

- Relationships of bleeding to sex and to menstrual cycle, or to the last menstrual bleed in the case of postmenopausal bleeding (PMB).

- For HMB the objective measurement is difficult, see **Box 2.3**.

Early pregnancy problems (see Chapter 5, Implantation and early pregnancy)

- Date of LMP, whether it was normal and the regularity of cycle are used to establish likely gestation.
- Whether contraception used and whether the patient plans to proceed with pregnancy if unintended.
- Pregnancy symptoms.
- Episodes of bleeding or pain in this pregnancy.
- Whether a scan has already been performed to establish viability and site of the pregnancy.
- Whether there are risk factors for an ectopic pregnancy (sexually-transmitted infection [STI], delayed conception, previous ectopics).
- Previous history of miscarriages, the gestation and their management (surgical, medical, conservative).

Contraception and emergency contraception (EC) (see Chapter 6, Contraception and abortion)

- LMP.
- Exact timing of unprotected intercourse(s) if requires EC.
- Contraindications to oestrogen-based contraception (thromboembolism, obesity, smoking, age, migraines with aura).
- Regular or multiple partners.
- Previous sexual health screening.
- Other menstrual problems (which may be improved with certain forms of contraception).

Fertility (see Chapter 7, Subfertility)

- Length of time in present relationship using no contraception.
- Length of time 'trying for pregnancy'.
- Previous tests performed, both male and female.
- Previous STIs.
- Previous fertility treatments attempted.
- Particular attention to length and regularity of menstrual cycle.
- Evidence of uterine problems (HMB, scanty periods, previous surgery, abdominal fullness).

- Evidence of polycystic ovary syndrome (oligomenorrhoea, hirsutism, excess weight, acne).
- Evidence of endocrine problems such as thyroid symptoms (heat sensitivity, weight change, tremor), prolactinomas (galactorrhea, visual field disturbance, headaches).

Menopause (see Chapter 8, The menopause and postreproductive health)

- Date of last period.
- PMB.
- Evidence of any menopausal symptoms (such as hot flushes, sleep disturbance, emotional or psychological difficulty, sexual difficulty, vaginal dryness, bladder symptoms).
- Any hormone replacement therapy (HRT) taken now or previously and any specific cautions such as breast cancer, thromboembolic events, hypertension.

Urogynaecology (see Chapter 10, Urogynaecology and pelvic floor problems)

- Number of times passing urine during the day and at night.
- Difficulty in passing urine.
- Uncontrolled passage of urine on coughing or straining.
- Urgent need to pass urine and loss of urine with urge.
- Exacerbating factors such as alcohol, caffeine.
- Extent to which affects general life such as fluid restricting or planning routes around toilet facilities.
- Incontinence of flatus or faeces.
- Incontinence during sexual intercourse.
- Feeling of something coming down in vagina.
- Risk factors such as number of pregnancies and vaginal and instrumental births.
- Evidence of abdominal masses such as fibroids.
- Menopausal status and HRT.

Sexual health (see Chapter 9, Genitourinary medicine)

- Present sexual partner, regular or not and other partners.
- Vaginal/anal/oral sex.
- Contraception.
- Previous contraception and sexual partners.
- Previous sexual health screening.
- Previous STIs.
- Symptoms of vaginal discharge, its colour and odour.
- Vaginal and perineal discomfort or itching or lesions.

Pelvic pain (see Chapter 11, Benign conditions of the ovary and pelvis)

- Site of pain, its nature and severity.
- Anything that aggravates or relieves the pain – specifically enquire about temporal relationship to menstrual cycle and intercourse.
- Does the pain radiate anywhere or is it associated with bowel or bladder function?
- Is there pain having intercourse and is this deep or superficial and is there associated sexual dysfunction (see Chapter 13, Benign conditions of the vulva and vagina, psychosexual disorders and female genital mutilation)?

Summary

The history should be summarized in one to two sentences before proceeding to the examination to focus the problem and alert the examiner to the salient features.

- Privacy and confidentiality are essential in gynaecological history taking.
- It is important to avoid medical language.
- The symptoms experienced by the patient and the relevance in their lives are both important.
- A systematic and thorough gynaecological history should be asked at each consultation.
- Specific areas of the history should then be explored.

Box 2.4 Sample history

This 32-year-old Afro-Caribbean lady has presented to gynaecology with heavy regular periods. She uses eight towels a day and floods at night. She has symptoms of anaemia. Her periods became heavier 3 years ago. There is no abnormal pain. She has also noted abdominal fullness and frequency of urine during the day.

Her last smear test was 2 years ago and was normal. She has had two full term normal deliveries, her children are aged 6 and 10. She uses condoms with her regular partner for contraception. She would like more children in a few years time. She has had no STIs. She has had no previous surgery and is fit and well, takes no medication, and has no allergies.

Examination

Important information about the patient can be obtained by watching them walk into the examination room. Poor mobility may affect decisions regarding surgery or future management. Any examination should always be carried out with the patient's consent and with appropriate privacy and sensitivity. Check and explain that the door is closed, check the patient's comfort (e.g. is an elderly patient comfortable without the head being raised, is she warm enough) before proceeding. A female chaperone must be present throughout the examination.

It is good practice to perform a general examination, which should include examining the hands and mucous membranes for evidence of anaemia. The supraclavicular area should be palpated for the presence of nodes, particularly on the left side where in cases of abdominal malignancy one might palpate the enlarged Virchow's node (this is also known as Troissier's sign). The thyroid gland should be palpated. The breasts should be examined as part of the examination if indicated by the history or pelvic examination; this is particularly relevant if there is a suspected ovarian mass, as there may be a breast tumour with secondaries in the ovaries known as Krukenburg tumours. In addition, a pleural effusion may be elicited as a consequence of abdominal ascites.

Blood pressure and body mass index (BMI) should be recorded as this will be relevant to medical and surgical management.

Abdominal examination

The patient should empty her bladder before the abdominal examination for comfort. If a urine infection or pregnancy is suspected, a sample should be tested. The patient should be comfortable and lying semi-recumbent with a sheet covering her from the waist down, but the area from the xiphisternum to the symphysis pubis should be left exposed (**Figure 2.1**). Palpation is traditionally performed while standing on the right-hand side of the patient using the right hand. Abdominal examination comprises inspection, palpation, percussion and, if appropriate, auscultation.

Inspection

The contour of the abdomen should be inspected and noted. There may be an obvious distension or mass. The presence of surgical scars, dilated veins or striae gravidarum (stretch marks) should be noted. It is important specifically to examine the umbilicus for laparoscopy scars and just above the symphysis pubis for Pfannenstiel scars (used for caesarean section, hysterectomy, etc). The patient should be asked to raise her head or cough and any hernias or divarication of the rectus muscles will be evident.

Palpation

First, if the patient has any abdominal pain she should be asked to point to the site – the area should not be examined until the end of palpation. Palpation is performed examining the left lower quadrant and proceeding in a total of four steps to the right lower quadrant of the abdomen. Palpation should include examination for masses, the liver, spleen and kidneys. If a mass is present but one can palpate below it, then it is more likely to be an abdominal mass rather than a pelvic mass. It is important to remember that one of the characteristics of a pelvic mass is that it arises from the pelvis, hence one cannot palpate below it. If the patient has pain, her abdomen should be palpated gently and the examiner should look for signs of peritonism (i.e. guarding and rebound tenderness). The patient should also be examined for inguinal hernias and lymph nodes.

Percussion

Percussion is particularly useful if free fluid is suspected. In the recumbent position, ascitic fluid will settle down into a horseshoe shape and dullness in the flanks can be demonstrated. As the patient moves over to her side, the dullness will move to her lowermost side. This is known as 'shifting dullness'. A fluid thrill can also be elicited. An enlarged bladder due to urinary retention will also be dull to percussion.

Auscultation

This method is not specifically useful for the routine gynaecological examination. However, a patient will sometimes present with an acute abdomen, with bowel obstruction or a postoperative patient with ileus, and in this situation listening for bowel sounds will be appropriate.

Pelvic examination

Before proceeding to a vaginal examination, the patient's verbal consent should be obtained and a female chaperone should be present for any intimate examination. It is good practice (and common in most UK medical schools) for a student to have written consent. This is mandatory if the patient will be under anaesthetic for the examination. Non-sterile gloves can be used for the examination unless the patient is pregnant, in which case sterile gloves should be worn. There are three components to the pelvic examination.

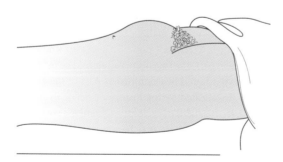

Figure 2.1 A patient in the correct position for abdominal examination, showing obvious abdominal distension.

Inspection

The external genitalia and surrounding skin, including the perianal area, are first inspected under a good light with the patient in the dorsal position, the hips flexed and abducted and knees flexed (**Figure 2.2**). The patient is asked to cough or bear down to enable signs of a prolapse or stress incontinence. Abnormal signs such as skin discolouration, lumps, scars from previous episiotomy, deficient perineum or prolapse (see Chapter 10, Urogynaecology and pelvic floor problems) are noted. Female genital mutilation (FGM) (see Chapter 13, Benign conditions of the vulva and vagina, psychosexual disorders and female genital mutilation) should be described.

Speculum

A sterile speculum is an instrument that is inserted into the vagina to obtain a clearer view of part of the vagina or pelvic organs. There are two principal types in widespread use. The first is a bivalve or Cusco's speculum (**Figure 2.3A**), which holds back the anterior and posterior walls of the vagina and allows visualization of the cervix when opened out (**Figure 2.3B**). It has a retaining screw that can be tightened to allow the speculum to stay in place while a procedure or sample is taken from the cervix (e.g. smear or swab). A Sim's speculum (**Figure 2.4A**) may also be used for examination of prolapse as it allows inspection of the vaginal walls. It is used in the left lateral position (**Figure 2.4B**). The choice of speculum will depend on the patient's presenting problem.

Excessive lubrication should be avoided and if a smear is being taken, lubrication with anything other than water should be avoided as it may interfere with the analysis. Microbiology swabs are taken from the vaginal fornices. Endocervical swabs for chlamydia are taken from the endocervical canal (see Chapter 9, Genitourinary problems).

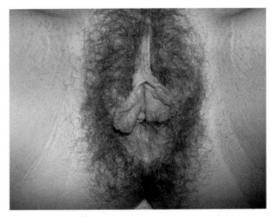

Figure 2.2 The normal vulva.

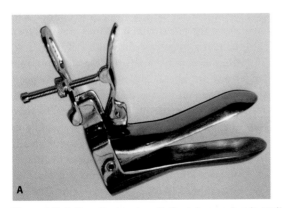

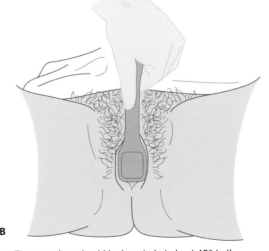

Figure 2.3 A: Cusco's speculum; **B**: Cusco's speculum in position. The speculum should be inserted at about 45° to the vertical and rotated to the vertical as it is introduced. Once it is fully inserted, the blades should be opened up to visualize the cervix.

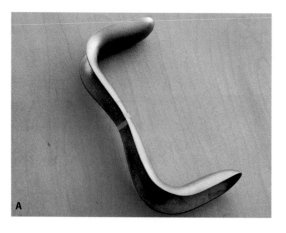

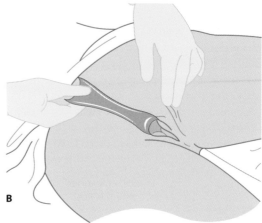

Figure 2.4 A: Sim's speculum; **B**: Sim's speculum inserted with the patient in the left lateral position. The speculum is being used to hold back the posterior vaginal walls to allow inspection of the anterior wall and vault. The speculum can be rotated 180° or withdrawn slowly to visualize the posterior wall.

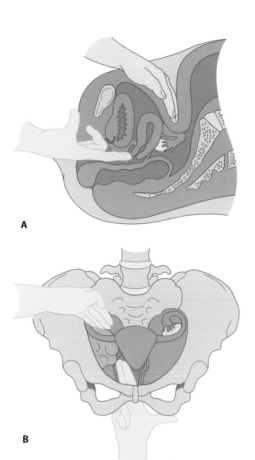

Figure 2.5 A: Bimanual examination of the pelvis assessing the uterine position and size; **B**: bimanual examination of the lateral fornix.

Bimanual examination

This is usually performed after the speculum examination and is performed to assess the pelvic organs. It is a technique that requires practice. There are a variety of 'model pelvises' that can be used to train the student in the basics of the examination. Most UK medical schools employ gynaecology teaching associates (GTAs), who are trained in teaching communication about pelvic examination and use their own bodies to teach the examination process and give feedback. It is customary to use the left hand to part the labia and expose the vestibule and then insert one or two fingers of the right hand into the vagina. The fingers are passed upwards and backwards to reach the cervix (**Figure 2.5A**). The cervix is palpated and any irregularity, hardness or tenderness noted. The left hand is now placed on the abdomen above the pubic symphysis and pressed down into the pelvis to palpate the fundus of the uterus. The size, shape, position, mobility, consistency and tenderness are noted. The normal uterus is pearshaped and about 9 cm in length. It is usually anteverted with the angle of the axis falling forward (see Chapter 1, The development and anatomy of the female sexual organs and pelvis), and normally freely mobile and non-tender. The tips of the fingers are then placed into each lateral fornix to palpate the adenexae (tubes and ovaries) on each side. The fingers are pushed backwards and upwards, while at the same time pushing down in the corresponding area with the fingers of the abdominal hand. It is unusual

Box 2.5 Version and flexion of the uterus

The position as well as the size of the uterus is very important in any patient requiring any type of intrauterine instrumentation (contraceptive coil insertion, hysteroscopy, laparoscopy). The reason for this is the instrument will be guided into the uterus along its axis. It takes some experience to get this correct. If an acutely retroflexed uterus is missed, perforation through the anterior wall with surgical instruments is more likely. If an acutely anteverted uterus is missed, posterior perforation is likely.

The size of an enlarged uterus is described in terms of the size of the uterus in weeks of gestation, for example a '6 weeks size uterus' is a non-pregnant uterus of the size associated with 6 weeks' pregnancy, about the size of a small orange. For very large uteri it can be useful to describe by abdominal landmarks, for example to umbilicus or xiphisternum.

Box 2.7 Professionalism

- Pelvic examination is classed by the Royal College of Obstetricians and Gynaecologists (RCOG) as an 'intimate examination' and as such should be taught initially by simulation, and thereafter with consent.
- Written consent by a student should be taken prior to examination under anaesthetic for teaching practice.
- An explanation of the necessity and procedure of vaginal examination should be given.
- A female chaperone must be present.

a vaginal examination to differentiate between an enterocele and a rectocele or to palpate the uterosacral ligaments more thoroughly. Occasionally, a rectovaginal examination (index finger in the vagina and middle finger in the rectum) may be useful to identify a lesion in the rectovaginal septum.

to be able to feel normal ovaries. Any swelling or tenderness is noted (**Figure 2.5B**). The posterior fornix should also be palpated to identify the uterosacral ligaments, which may be tender or scarred in women with endometriosis.

Rectal examination

In some situations, a rectal examination with specific additional consent can be useful in addition to

Box 2.6 Global context

A rectal examination can be used as an alternative to a vaginal examination in children and in adults who have never had sex, if ultrasound is not available as an investigation. It is less sensitive than a vaginal examination and can be quite uncomfortable, but it will help pick up a pelvic mass.

FGM may be encountered in women of sub-Saharan origin. The presence and type must be recorded. In some cases this will make vaginal examination impossible. The presence of FGM must be recorded in the case notes as a legal requirement.

Some cultures would prohibit examination by a male practitioner except in cases of emergency.

Summary

- The size and consistency of the pelvic organs may indicate the diagnosis and need for further investigations.
- Accurate determination of anteversion or retroversion of the uterus is crucial immediately prior to operations that require dilation of the uterine cervix to reduce the chance of perforation. This takes experience.
- Extreme reluctance to a vaginal examination, even with a qualified female doctor, should alert the practitioner to psychological issues that should be explored.
- Some women will be reluctant to be examined while bleeding. They should be reassured and encouraged if this is part of the presenting complaint. Some women will prefer to return when not bleeding.

Investigations

Once the examination is complete, the patient should be given the opportunity to dress in privacy and come back into the consultation room to sit down and discuss the findings. You should now be able to give a summary of the whole case and formulate a differential diagnosis. This will then determine the appropriate further investigations (if any) that should be needed. Swabs and smears and urine sample will have been taken earlier in the examination. The urine should be kept and checked for beta-HCG if intrauterine examination is required. Further tests are outlined later in this chapter.

Imaging

Ultrasound imaging in gynaecology has become uniformly available in the UK. Basic competence in gynaecological ultrasound is part of the RCOG Curriculum for Training Doctors. Ultrasound imaging of the uterus and adnexa is part of the investigations of nearly all gynaecological problems, perhaps with the exception of contraception and sexual health screening in asymptomatic women.

Pelvic ultrasound using a transvaginal ultrasound scan (TVUSS) is performed for adult women and is the investigation of choice for most problems. The probe is cleaned in the presence of the patient and covered with a probe cover (or commonly a latex-free condom), containing ultrasound gel on the inside and outside. The probe is inserted into the

Box 2.8 Clinical context

- Ultrasound imaging of the pelvic organs has become part of routine assessment in gynaecology in the UK, but should not replace pelvic examination.
- TVUSS has excellent resolution and is inexpensive, and can enable accurate and instant diagnosis of most gynaecological problems, including acute and early pregnancy problems.
- The availability of ultrasound before or during a gynaecological consultation can often avoid the need for a patient to return to see the practitioner.
- Uterine and ovarian pathologies have specific appearances and can be diagnosed with accuracy.
- More expensive tests such as MRI are usually not needed in gynaecology. Increasingly, 3D ultrasound is used to diagnose uterine and adnexal abnormalities.
- Increased BMI can cause difficulty in visualization

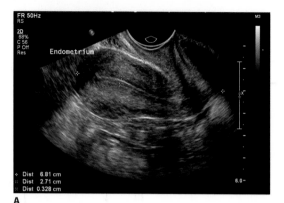

Figure 2.6

▶ eResource 2.2

Ultrasound imaging in gynaecology
http://www.routledgetextbooks.com/textbooks/tenteachers/gynaecologyv2.2.php

vagina while the images are viewed on a screen. The images can be shared with the patient once the correct image has been determined. The presence of pain and the correlation with images can be useful diagnostically. The resolution of TVUSS is high, particularly if the organ lies close to the probe, and the depth of images visible is around 12 cm. Excellent images of the uterus and adnexa, including the internal architecture of the myometrium, endometrium, Fallopian tubes *when abnormal* and ovaries are achievable (**Figure 2.6A–D**), as well as images of early intrauterine pregnancies. For women who have not been sexually active, children and teenagers and some elderly women, an abdominal ultrasound is more appropriate. In some women with a large pelvic mass both types of ultrasound may be utilized.

Instillation of saline through the cervix (saline instillation sonography, SIS) allows distension of the cavity of the uterus to enable the detection of abnormalities such as endometrial polyps and submucosal fibroids. 3D TVUSS improves the ability to diagnose structural abnormalities in the uterus.

T2-weighted MRI, although expensive, may be requested to distinguish fibroid change from adenomyosis and to delineate ovarian cysts and assess malignancy. It can also be used to identify structural abnormalities in the genital tract (**Figure 2.7A–C**). Increasingly, expert 3D TVUSS is used as a cheaper

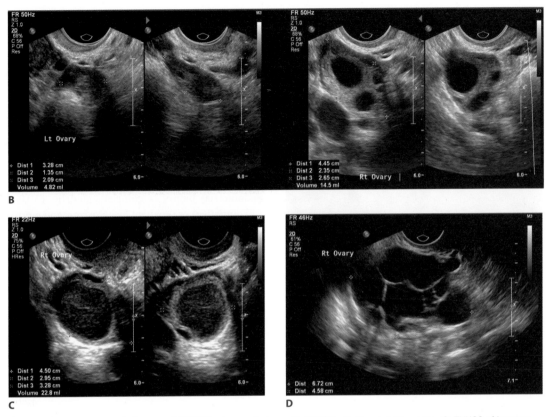

Figure 2.6 **A**: Transvaginal ultrasound (TVUSS) of normal uterus. **B**: TVUSS of left and right ovaries; **C**: TVUSS of haemorrhagic cyst; **D**: TVUSS of multiseptated cyst.

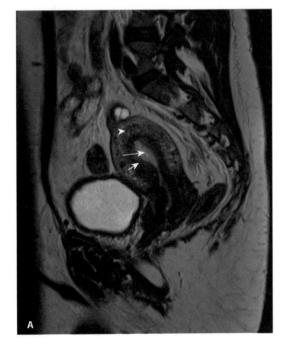

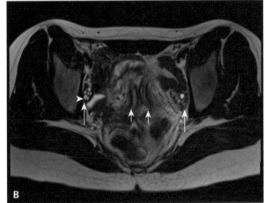

Figure 2.7 **A**: Magnetic resonance imaging (MRI) of normal pelvis (long arrow, endometrium; short arrow, inner myometrium and cervix; arrowhead, outer myometrium); **B**: axial MRI of pelvis in a patient with uterus didelphys and double cervices (long arrows, ovaries; short arrows, cervices; arrowhead, follicle).   *(Continued)*

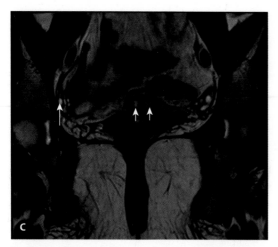

Figure 2.7 *(Continued)* **C**: coronal MRI in a patient with uterus didelphys (long arrow, right ovary; short arrows, cervices). (Images courtesy of Dr Sarah Natas, Consultant Radiologist.)

alternative. When malignancy has been identified CT may be indicated to determine the stage of the disease.

Endometrial biopsy

Biopsy of the endometrium can be performed without anaesthetic in most women, and is indicated for some women over 45 with menstrual symptoms, including HMB and PCB, after ensuring that the woman is not pregnant (see Chapter 4, Disorders of menstrual bleeding) (**Figure 2.8** and **Box 2.9**). Endometrial biopsy is complemented by TVUSS, and outpatient or inpatient hysteroscopy and guided biopsy, where indicated.

In addition to imaging and histology there are a number of investigations that are common in gynaecology (*Table 2.1*).

Table 2.1 Common investigations in gynaecology

Investigation	Relevant condition	Result
FBC and haematinics in anaemic patients	Suspected anaemia from heavy bleeding Preoperative assessment	Low haemoglobin, low MCV and low iron stores
FSH/LH/E2 should be taken during early follicular phase, further described in Chapter 3, Reproductive endocrinology	Irregular menstrual cycle, menopausal symptoms	Raised gonadotrophs in ovarian failure Low oestrogen in ovarian failure High LH in PCOS Low FSH/LH/E2 in hypogonadotrophic hypogonadism
Progesterone, further described in Chapter 7, Subfertility	Mid-luteal phase progesterone, day 21 in a 28 day cycle, 7 days before menstruation in a longer cycle	Confirmation of ovulation
HVS for microbiology, endocervical swab for chlamydia, further described in Chapter 9, Genitourinary medicine and HIV	Vaginal discharge or risk of STI	Culture positive
Endocrine tests, further described in Chapter 3, Reproductive endocrinology	Irregular bleeds with systemic symptoms	Abnormal thyroid function, raised prolactin, raised androgens may indicate endocrine disturbance
AMH further described in Chapter 7, Subfertility	Ovarian reserve	Indicates high, medium or low fertility potential
Beta-HCG, further described in Chapter 5, Implantation and early pregnancy	Pregnancy	May be used in cases of pregnancy of unknown location

AMH, anti-Müllerian hormone; E2, oestrogen; FBC, full blood count; FSH, follicle-stimulating hormone; HIV, human immunodeficiency virus; HVS, high vaginal swab; LH, luteinizing hormone; MCV, mean corpuscular volume; PCOS, polycystic ovary syndrome; STI sexually transmitted infection.

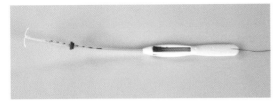

Figure 2.8 Endometrial sampler.

Box 2.9 Perfoming an endometrial biopsy

An endometrial biopsy can be performed in the outpatient setting. It is performed as follows:

- Speculum examination is carried out and the cervix is completely visualized.
- A vulsellum instrument may be required to grasp the cervix and provide gentle traction, thereby straightening the endocervical canal.
- The endometrial sampler is carefully inserted through the cervical os until it reaches the fundus of the uterus. The length of the uterus is noted.
- The inner part of the sampler is withdrawn to create a vacuum and the device is gently moved in and out to obtain a sample of endometrial tissue.
- The sampler is removed and the tissue is expelled into a histopathology container of formalin.

Further reading

RCOG Training in Ultrasound. https://www.rcog.org.uk/en/careers-training.

Self assessment

🔑 KEY LEARNING POINTS

- The consultation should be performed in a private environment and in a sensitive fashion.
- The practitioner should introduce him/herself, be courteous and explain what is about to happen and why.
- The practitioner should be familiar with the history template and use it regularly to avoid omissions.
- Remember to summarize the history to the patient before proceeding to the examination.
- A female chaperone should always be present for an intimate examination.
- The practitioner should be sensitive to the patient's needs and anxiety and respect her privacy and dignity.
- The examination should always begin with a general assessment of the patient.
- The patient should be asked to inform the practitioner if the examination is uncomfortable.
- The practitioner should reassure the patient during the examination and give feedback about what is being done.
- After the examination, the practitioner should make sure that the patient is comfortable and allow her to get dressed in privacy.
- The practitioner should explain the findings to the patient in suitable language and give her the opportunity to ask questions.
- Prepare a differential diagnosis and order any appropriate investigations.
- TVUSS scanning is inexpensive and accurate to aid diagnosis of most gynaecological conditions.
- Further imaging modalities may be used to aid more complex diagnoses.
- Biochemistry and haematology may complete these findings plus smear/swabs/urine.
- Histological specimens from endometrial or superficial biopsy may be required.

CASE HISTORY

A 32-year-old Afro-Caribbean teacher has come to clinic to see you. She has had increasingly heavy periods over the last 18 months. Her periods are regular and there is no IMB or PCB, bleeding is for 5 days every 28 days. On the second and third day of bleeding she uses tampons and towels together, which get soaked in blood within 1 hour. In classes she has had to run out when she had flooding, and passed clots about 4 cm in size. This is really embarrassing with the school children and she has taken to wearing nappies just in case. She is avoiding classroom teaching while she has a period but can not explain why to her male head teacher. When her period finishes she feels 'washed out' and gets short of breath exercising easily. She has not tried any treatment so far.

She has never been pregnant and hoped to get pregnant soon after her marriage last year, but nothing has happened in the last 8 months. She has never had an STI, is in her only and stable sexual relationship and has no abnormal vaginal discharge, and her smears have always been normal, the last was 2 years ago.

On questioning she admits to feeling full in the abdomen when she lies on her stomach. There is no pain as such and sex is not painful. She has never had surgery, has a healthy life style, does not smoke or drink much alcohol and has no medical conditions. There is no family history of illnesses. She is not allergic to any prescribed medicines.

On examination the abdomen is distended by a hard mass rising from the pelvis and coming half way between the pubic symphysis and umbilicus. It is not tender. Cuscoe speculum shows that the cervix is normal. Bimanual examination reveals the anteverted uterus to be enlarged to the size of a grapefruit (about 12 weeks' size for a pregnant uterus).

A *What are the important parts of the history?*

B *Which investigations should be commenced?*

C *What treatment would you suggest?*

ANSWERS

A   Important parts of the history here are a clear history of menstrual disturbance and the time scale over which it occurred. There are three issues: the heavy embarrassing periods, the likely symptoms of anaemia and the desire to get pregnant so far without success. The healthy life style and lack of previous surgery are important in case surgery is required. Lack of drug allergies is very important to know for medications.

B   Investigations should include:

Full blood count to exclude anaemia. Without a personal or family history of thyroid disease, biochemical thyroid function is not indicated. As the cycle is regular no other hormonal tests are indicated at this stage.

Transvaginal ultrasound scan. The scan shows that the uterus is enlarged with fibroids. There are three fibroids of which the largest is 6 cm × 8 cm at the fundus. There is a 2 cm × 2.5 cm submucosal fibroid in the uterine cavity.

Smear or swabs are not required as there are no symptoms of discharge or IMB and last smear is normal.

C   Treatments should be discussed with the patient as described in later chapters. This patient will benefit from a transcervical resection of her submucosal fibroid, which is probably causing both her heavy menstrual bleeding and also her subfertility.

SBA QUESTION

1 A 32-year-old woman has come to the gynaecology clinic complaining of heavy menstrual bleeding. On examination the uterus is anteverted and bulky. What is the best imaging modality to further investigate her symptoms? Choose the single best answer.

A   Abdominal ultrasound scan.

B   CT.

C   Hysterosalpingogram (HSG).

D   MRI.

E   TVUSS.

ANSWER

E   TVUSS provides excellent resolution, is inexpensive and allows immediate diagnosis of uterine and adnexal pathology.

Hormonal control of the menstrual cycle and hormonal disorders

CHAPTER

3

HELEN BICKERSTAFF

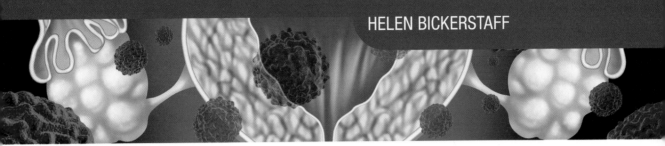

LEARNING OBJECTIVES

- Describe the features of the normal menstrual cycle and the ovarian and endometrial changes that accompany them.
- Describe the normal changes of puberty and the secondary sexual differentiation that accompanies it.
- Understand the classification and causes of abnormal puberty and disorders of sexual development (DSD).

- Describe the causes and investigation of primary and secondary amenorrhoea and oligomenorrhoea.
- Understand the epidemiology and effects of polycystic ovary syndrome (PCOS), its diagnosis and management.
- Describe the common effects and management of premenstrual syndrome (PMS).
- Describe premature cessation of periods.

Introduction

This chapter considers hormonal control of the menstrual cycle and the abnormalities that may affect the physiological initiation, regulation and cessation of the cycle. Abnormalities of uterine bleeding are the subject of the next chapter.

Physiology of the menstrual cycle

The external manifestation of a normal menstrual cycle is the presence of regular vaginal bleeding. This occurs as a result of the shedding of the endometrial lining following failure of fertilization of the oocyte or failure of implantation. The cycle depends on changes occurring after puberty within the ovaries and fluctuation in ovarian hormone levels, which are themselves controlled by the pituitary and hypothalamus within the hypothalamo–pituitary–ovarian axis (HPO). In situations of DSD or hormonal abnormalities, menstruation may not begin.

The hypothalamus

The hypothalamus in the forebrain secretes the peptide hormone gonadotrophin-releasing hormone (GnRH), which in turn controls pituitary hormone secretion. GnRH must be released in a pulsatile fashion to stimulate pituitary secretion of luteinizing hormone (LH) and follicle-stimulating hormone (FSH).

33

The pituitary gland

GnRH stimulation of the basophil cells in the anterior pituitary gland causes synthesis and release of the gonadotrophic hormones FSH and LH. This process is modulated by the ovarian sex steroid hormones oestrogen and progesterone. Low levels of oestrogen have an inhibitory effect on LH production (negative feedback), whereas high levels of oestrogen will increase LH production (positive feedback). The mechanism of action for the positive feedback effect of oestrogen involves an increase in GnRH receptor concentrations, while the mechanism of the negative feedback effect is uncertain. The high levels of circulating oestrogen in the late follicular phase of the ovary act via the positive-feedback mechanism to generate a periovulatory LH surge from the pituitary.

The clinical relevance of these mechanisms is seen in the use of the combined oral contraceptive pill, which artificially creates a constant serum oestrogen level in the negative-feedback range, inducing a correspondingly low level of gonadotrophin hormone release.

Unlike oestrogen, low levels of progesterone have a positive-feedback effect on pituitary LH and FSH secretion (as seen immediately prior to ovulation) and contribute to the LH and FSH surge. High levels of progesterone, as seen in the luteal phase, inhibit pituitary LH and FSH production. Positive-feedback effects of progesterone occur via increasing sensitivity to GnRH in the pituitary. Negative-feedback effects are generated through both decreased GnRH production from the hypothalamus and decreased sensitivity to GnRH in the pituitary. It is known that progesterone can only have these effects on gonadotropic hormone release after priming by oestrogen (**Figure 3.1**).

The ovary

Starting at menarche, the primordial follicles containing oocytes, arrested at the first prophase step in meiotic division, will start to activate and grow in a cyclical fashion, causing ovulation and subsequent menstruation in the event of non-fertilization. In the course of a normal menstrual cycle, the ovary will go through three phases: follicular, ovulatory and luteal.

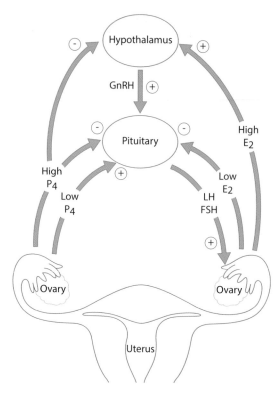

* N.B. the mechanism of action of the negative feedback of oestrogen is uncertain

Figure 3.1 Hypothalamus–pituitary axis. (E2, oestrogen; FSH, follicle-stimulating hormone; GnRH, gonadotrophin-releasing hormone; LH, luteinizing hormone; P4, progesterone.)

Follicular phase

The initial stages of follicular development are independent of hormone stimulation. However, follicular development will fail at the preantral stage, and follicular atresia will ensue if pituitary hormones LH and FSH are absent.

FSH levels rise in the first days of the menstrual cycle, when oestrogen, progesterone and inhibin levels are low. This stimulates a cohort of small antral follicles on the ovaries to grow. Within the follicles, there are two cell types that are involved in the processing of steroids, including oestrogen and progesterone. These are the theca and the granulosa cells, which respond to LH and FSH stimulation, respectively. LH stimulates production of androgens from cholesterol within theca cells. These androgens are converted into oestrogens by the process of aromatization in granulosa cells, under the influence of FSH.

As the follicles grow and oestrogen secretion increases, there is negative feedback on the pituitary to decrease FSH secretion. This assists in the selection of one follicle to continue in its development towards ovulation – the dominant follicle. In the ovary, the follicle that has the most efficient aromatase activity and highest concentration of FSH-induced LH receptors will be the most likely to survive as FSH levels drop, while smaller follicles will undergo atresia.

There are other autocrine and paracrine mediators playing a role in the follicular phase of the menstrual cycle. These include inhibin and activin. Inhibin is secreted by the granulosa cells within the ovaries. It participates in feedback to the pituitary to down-regulate FSH release, and also appears to enhance ongoing androgen synthesis. Activin is structurally similar to inhibin, but has an opposite action. It is produced in granulosa cells and in the pituitary, and acts to increase FSH binding on the follicles.

Insulin-like growth factors (IGF-I, IGF-II) act as paracrine regulators. Circulating levels do not change during the menstrual cycle, but follicular fluid levels increase towards ovulation, with the highest level found in the dominant follicle.

Kisspeptins are proteins that have more recently been found to play a role in regulation of the HPO axis, via the mediation of the metabolic hormone leptin's effect on the hypothalamus. Leptin is thought to be key in the relationship between energy production, weight and reproductive health. Mutations in the kisspeptin receptor, gpr-54, are associated with delayed or absent puberty, probably due to a reduction in leptin-linked triggers for gonadotrophin release.

Ovulation

By the end of the follicular phase, which lasts an average of 14 days, the dominant follicle has grown to approximately 20 mm in diameter. As the follicle matures, FSH induces LH receptors on the granulosa cells to compensate for lower FSH levels and prepare for the signal for ovulation. Production of oestrogen increases until it reaches the necessary threshold to exert a positive feedback effort on the hypothalamus and pituitary to cause the LH surge. This occurs over 24–36 hours, during which time the LH-induced luteinization of granulosa cells in the dominant follicle causes progesterone to be produced, adding further to the positive feedback for LH secretion and causing a small periovulatory rise in FSH. Androgens, synthesized in the theca cells, also rise around the time of ovulation, and this is thought to have an important role in stimulating libido, ensuring that sexual activity is likely to occur at the time of greatest fertility.

The LH surge is one of the best predictors of imminent ovulation, and this is the hormone detected in urine by most over-the-counter 'ovulation predictor' tests. The LH surge has another function in stimulating the resumption of meiosis in the oocyte just prior to its release. The physical ovulation of the oocyte occurs after breakdown of the follicular wall takes place under the influence of LH, FSH and proteolytic enzymes, such as plasminogen activators and prostaglandins (PGs). Studies have shown that inhibition of PG production may result in failure of ovulation. Thus, women wishing to become pregnant should be advised to avoid taking PG synthetase inhibitors, such as aspirin and ibuprofen, which may inhibit oocyte release.

Luteal phase

After the release of the oocyte, the remaining granulosa and theca cells on the ovary form the corpus luteum (CL). The granulosa cells have a vacuolated appearance with accumulated yellow pigment, hence the name CL ('yellow body'). The CL undergoes extensive vascularization in order to supply granulosa cells with a rich blood supply for continued steroidogenesis. This is aided by local production of vascular endothelial growth factor (VEGF).

Ongoing pituitary LH secretion and granulosa cell activity ensure a supply of progesterone, which stabilizes the endometrium in preparation for pregnancy. Progesterone levels are at their highest in the cycle during the luteal phase. This also has the effect of suppressing FSH and LH secretion to a level that will not produce further follicular growth in the ovary during that cycle.

The luteal phase lasts 14 days in most women, without great variation. In the absence of beta-human chorionic gonadotrophin (βhCG) being produced from an implanting embryo, the CL will regress in a process known as luteolysis. The mature

CL is less sensitive to LH, produces less progesterone and will gradually disappear from the ovary. The withdrawal of progesterone has the effect on the uterus of causing shedding of the endometrium and thus menstruation. Reduction in levels of progesterone, oestrogen and inhibin feeding back to the pituitary cause increased secretion of gonadotrophic hormones, particularly FSH. New preantral follicles begin to be stimulated and the cycle begins anew.

The endometrium

The hormone changes effected by the HPO axis during the menstrual cycle will occur whether the uterus is present or not. However, the specific secondary changes in the uterine endometrium give the most obvious external sign of regular cycles (**Figure 3.2**).

The proliferative phase

The endometrium enters the proliferative phase after menstruation, when glandular and stromal growth begin. The epithelium lining the endometrial glands changes from a single layer of columnar cells to a pseudostratified epithelium with frequent mitoses. Endometrial thickness increases rapidly, from 0.5 mm at menstruation to 3.5–5 mm at the end of the proliferative phase.

The secretory phase

After ovulation (generally around day 14), there is a period of endometrial glandular secretory activity. Following the LH surge, the oestrogen-induced cellular proliferation is inhibited and the endometrial thickness does not increase any further. However, the endometrial glands will become more tortuous, spiral arteries will grow and fluid is secreted into glandular cells and into the uterine lumen. Later in the secretory phase, progesterone induces the formation of a temporary layer, known as the decidua, in the endometrial stroma. Histologically, this is seen as occurring around blood vessels. Stromal cells show increased mitotic activity, nuclear enlargement and generation of a basement membrane (**Figure 3.3**).

Apical membrane projections of the endometrial epithelial cells, known as pinopodes, appear after day 21–22 and appear to be a progesterone-dependent stage in making the endometrium receptive for embryo implantation (**Figure 3.4**).

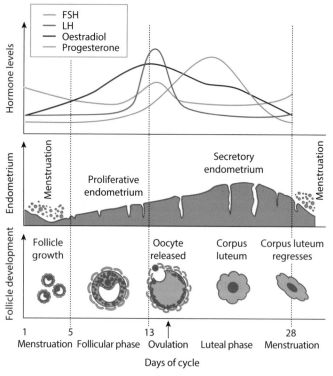

Figure 3.2 Changes in hormone levels, endometrium and follicle development during the menstrual cycle.

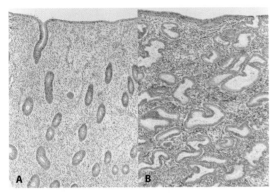

Figure 3.3 Tissue sections of normal endometrium during proliferative (**A**) and secretory (**B**) phases of the menstrual cycle.

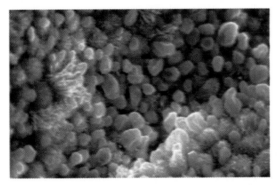

Figure 3.4 Photomicrograph of endometrial pinopods from the implantation window.

Menstruation

Menstruation (day 1) is the shedding of the 'dead' endometrium and ceases as the endometrium regenerates (which normally happens by day 5–6 of the cycle). Immediately prior to menstruation, three distinct layers of endometrium can be seen. The basalis is the lower 25% of the endometrium, which will remain throughout menstruation and shows few changes during the menstrual cycle. The midportion is the stratum spongiosum with oedematous stroma and exhausted glands. The superficial portion (upper 25%) is the stratum compactum with prominent decidualized stromal cells. A fall in circulating levels of oestrogen and progesterone approximately 14 days after ovulation leads to loss of tissue fluid, vasoconstriction of spiral arterioles and distal ischaemia. This results in tissue breakdown and loss of the upper layers, along with bleeding from fragments of the remaining arterioles, seen as menstrual bleeding. Enhanced fibrinolysis reduces clotting.

The effects of oestrogen and progesterone on the endometrium can be reproduced artificially, for example in patients taking the combined oral contraceptive pill or hormone replacement therapy (HRT), who experience a withdrawal bleed during their pill-free week each month.

Vaginal bleeding will cease after 5–10 days as arterioles vasoconstrict and the endometrium begins to regenerate. Haemostasis in the uterine endometrium is different from haemostasis elsewhere in the body as it does not involve the processes of clot formation and fibrosis.

The endocrine influences in menstruation are clear. However, the paracrine mediators are less so. PG F2α, endothelin-1 and platelet activating factor (PAF) are vasoconstrictors that are produced within the endometrium and are thought likely to be involved in vessel constriction, both initiating and controlling menstruation. They may be balanced by the effect of vasodilator agents, such as PG E2, prostacyclin (PGI) and nitric oxide, which are also produced by the endometrium. Recent research has shown that progesterone withdrawal increases endometrial PG synthesis and decreases PG metabolism. The cyclooxygenase (COX)-2 enzyme and chemokines are involved in PG synthesis and this is likely to be the target of non-steroidal anti-inflammatory drugs (NSAIDs) used for the treatment of heavy and painful periods.

Endometrial repair involves both glandular and stromal regeneration and angiogenesis to reconstitute the endometrial vasculature. VEGF and fibroblast growth factor (FGF) are found within the endometrium and both are powerful angiogenic agents. Epidermal growth factor (EGF) appears to be responsible for mediation of oestrogen-induced glandular and stromal regeneration. Other growth factors, such as transforming growth factors (TGFs) and IGFs, and the interleukins may also be important.

Puberty and secondary sexual development

Normal puberty

Puberty is the process of reproductive and sexual development and maturation that changes a child into an adult. During childhood, the HPO axis is suppressed and levels of GnRH, FSH and LH are very low. From the age of 8–9 years GnRH is secreted in pulsations of increasing amplitude and frequency. These are initially sleep-related, but as puberty progresses, these extend throughout the day. This stimulates secretion of FSH and LH by the pituitary glands, which in turn triggers follicular growth and steroidogenesis in the ovary. The oestrogen produced by the ovary then initiates the physical changes of puberty. The exact mechanism determining the onset of puberty is still unknown, but it is influenced by many factors including race, heredity, body weight and exercise. Leptin plays a permissive role in the onset of puberty.

The physical changes occurring in puberty are breast development (thelarche), pubic and axillary hair growth (adrenarche), growth spurt and onset of menstruation (menarche).

The first physical signs of puberty are breast budding and this occurs 2–3 years before menarche. The appearance of pubic hair is dependent on the secretion of adrenal androgens and is usually after thelarche. In addition to increasing levels of adrenal and gonadal hormones, growth hormone secretion also increases, leading to a pubertal growth spurt. The mean age of menarche is 12.8 years and it may take over 3 years before the menstrual cycle establishes a regular pattern. Initial cycles are usually anovulatory and can be unpredictable and irregular. The absence of menstruation is called amenorrhoea and may be primary or secondary (see Box 3.2, page 41). Pubertal development was described by Tanner and the stages of breast and pubic hair development are often referred to as Tanner stages 1–5 (**Figure 3.5**).

Precocious puberty

This is defined as the onset of puberty before the age of 8 in a girl or 9 in a boy. It is classified as either central or peripheral. Central precocious puberty is gonadotrophin dependent. The aetiology is often unknown, although up to 25% are due to central nervous system (CNS) malformations or brain tumours. Peripheral precocious puberty, which is gonadotrophin independent, is always pathological and can be caused by oestrogen secretion, such as exogenous ingestion or a hormone-producing tumour.

Delayed puberty

When there are no signs of secondary sexual characteristics by the age of 14 years this is termed delayed puberty. It is due to either a central defect

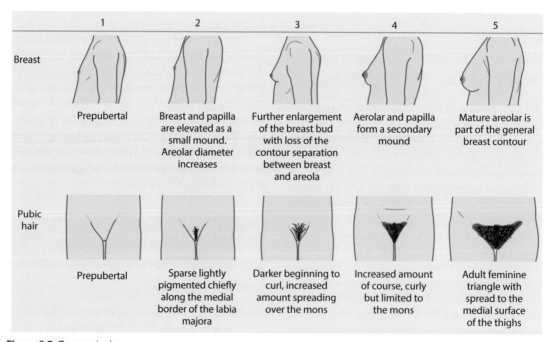

	1	2	3	4	5
Breast	Prepubertal	Breast and papilla are elevated as a small mound. Areolar diameter increases	Further enlargement of the breast bud with loss of the contour separation between breast and areola	Aerolar and papilla form a secondary mound	Mature areolar is part of the general breast contour
Pubic hair	Prepubertal	Sparse lightly pigmented chiefly along the medial border of the labia majora	Darker beginning to curl, increased amount spreading over the mons	Increased amount of course, curly but limited to the mons	Adult feminine triangle with spread to the medial surface of the thighs

Figure 3.5 Tanner staging.

(hypogonadotrophic hypogonadism) or a failure of gonadal function (hypergonadotrophic hypogonadism), which are described below.

> **Box 3.1** Hypo- and hypergonadotrophic hypogonadism
>
> **Hypogonadotrophic hypogonadism**
> - This is central and may be constitutional, but other causes must be excluded: these include anorexia nervosa, excessive exercise and chronic illness, such as diabetes or renal failure. Rarer causes include a pituitary tumour and Kalmans syndrome.
> - Associated with delayed puberty and primary amenorrhoea.
>
> **Hypergonadotrophic hypogonadism**
> - This is caused by gonadal failure.
> - The gonad does not function despite high gonadotrophins.
> - Associated with Turner syndrome and XX gonadal dysgenesis.
> - Premature ovarian failure can occur at any age, including prior to pubertal age, and may be idiopathic, but can also be part of an autoimmune or metabolic disorder or following chemo- or radiotherapy for childhood cancer.
> - Associated with delayed puberty and primary amenorrhoea.
> - Hypergonadotrophic hypogonadism can also occur later in life and will cause secondary amenorrhoea after normal sexual development.

Disorders of sexual development

DSD are conditions where the sequence of events described above does not happen. The clinical consequences of this depend upon where within the sequence the variation occurs. DSD may be diagnosed at birth with ambiguous or abnormal genitalia, but may also be seen at puberty in girls who present with primary amenorrhoea or increasing virilization.

Table 3.1 Summary of terminology for disorders of sex development (DSD)

Previous intersex	Accepted DSD
Male pseudohermaphrodite	46, XY DSD
Undervirilization of XY male	
Undermasculinization of XY male	
Female pseudohermaphrodite	46 XX DSD
Overvirilization of an XX female	
Masculinization of an XX female	
True hermaphrodite	Ovotesticular DSD

There has been change in the terminology used to refer to these conditions over the last 10 years. Older terms, such as 'hermaphrodite' and 'intersex', are confusing to both the clinician and patients, and in addition can be hurtful. The accepted terminology is summarized in *Table 3.1*.

Non-structural causes of DSD

Turner syndrome

The total complement of chromosomes is 45 in Turner syndrome, which results from a complete or partial absence of one X chromosome (45XO). Turner syndrome is the most common chromosomal anomaly in females, occurring in 1 in 2,500 live female births. A mosaic karyotype is not uncommon, leading to a variable presentation. Although there can be variation, the most typical clinical features include short stature, webbing of the neck and a wide carrying angle. Associated medical conditions include coarctation of the aorta, inflammatory bowel disease, sensorineural and conduction deafness, renal anomalies and endocrine dysfunction, such as autoimmune thyroid disease.

In this condition, the ovary does not complete its normal development and only the stroma is present at birth. The gonads are called 'streak gonads' and do not function to produce oestrogen or oocytes. Diagnosis is usually made at birth or in early childhood from the clinical appearance of the baby or due to short stature during childhood. However, in about 10% of women, the diagnosis is not made until adolescence with delayed puberty. The ovaries do not produce oestrogen, so the normal physical changes of puberty cannot happen. In childhood, treatment is focused on growth, but in adolescence it focuses on induction of puberty. Pregnancy is only possible with ovum donation. Psychological input and support is important. In girls with mosaicism the clinical picture can vary and normal puberty and menstruation can occur, with early cessation of periods.

46XY gonadal dysgenesis

In this situation, the gonads do not develop into a testis, despite the presence of an XY karyotype. In about 15% of cases, this is due to a mutation in the SRY gene on the Y chromosome, but in most cases the cause is unknown. In complete gonadal dysgenesis (Swyer syndrome), the gonad remains as a streak gonad and does not produce any hormones. In the absence of anti-Müllerian hormone (AMH), the Müllerian structures do not regress and the uterus, vagina and Fallopian tubes develop normally. The absence of testosterone means the fetus does not virilize. The baby is phenotypically female, although has an XY chromosome. The gonads do not function and presentation is usually at adolescence with delayed puberty. The dysgenetic gonad has a high malignancy risk and should be removed when the diagnosis is made. This is usually performed laparoscopically. Puberty must be induced with oestrogen and pregnancies have been reported with a donor oocyte. Full disclosure of the diagnosis including the XY karytoype is essential, although this can be devastating and specialized psychological input is crucial.

Mixed gonadal dysgenesis is a more complex condition. The karyotype may be 46XX, but XX/XY mosaicism is present in up to 20%. In this situation, both functioning ovarian and testicular tissue can be present and if so, this condition is known as ovotesticular DSD. The anatomical findings vary depending on the function of the gonads. For example, if the testis is functional, then the baby will virilize and have ambiguous or normal male genitalia. The Müllerian structures are usually absent on the side of the functioning testis, but a unicornuate uterus may be present if there is an ovary or streak gonad.

46XY DSD

The most common cause of 46XY DSD, complete androgen insensitivity syndrome (CAIS), occurs in individuals where virilization of the external genitalia does not occur, due to a partial or complete inability of the androgen receptor to respond to androgen stimulation. In the fetus with CAIS, testes form normally due to the action of the SRY gene. At the appropriate time, these testes secrete AMH, leading to the regression of the Müllerian ducts. Hence, CAIS women do not have a uterus. Testosterone is also produced at the appropriate time; however, due to the inability of the androgen receptor to respond, the external genitalia do not virilize and instead undergo female development. The baby is born with normal female external genitalia, an absent uterus and testes that are found somewhere in their line of descent through the abdomen from the pelvis to the inguinal canal. Presentation is usually at puberty with primary amenorrhoea, although if the testes are in the inguinal canal they can cause a hernia in a younger girl. Once the diagnosis is made, initial management is psychological with full disclosure of the XY karyotype and the information that the patient will be infertile.

Gonadectomy is recommended because of the small long-term risk of testicular malignancy, although this can be deferred until after puberty. Once the gonads are removed, long-term HRT will be required. The vagina is usually shortened and treatment will be required to create a vagina suitable for penetrative intercourse. Vaginal dilation is the most effective method of improving vaginal length and entails the insertion of vaginal moulds of gradually increasing length and width for at least 30 minutes a day. Surgical vaginal reconstruction operations are reserved for those women that have not responded to a dilation treatment programme.

In cases of partial androgen insensitivity, the androgen receptor can respond to some extent with limited virilization. The child is usually diagnosed at birth with ambiguous genitalia.

5-Alpha-reductase deficiency

In this condition, the fetus has an XY karyotype and normal functioning testes that produce both testosterone and AMH. However, the fetus is unable to convert testosterone to dihydrotestosterone in the peripheral tissues and so cannot virilize normally. Presentation is usually with ambiguous genitalia at birth, but can also be with increasing virilization at puberty of a female child, due to the large increase in circulating testosterone with the onset of puberty. In the Western world, the child is usually assigned to a female sex of rearing, but there have been descriptions of a few communities where transition from a female to male gender at puberty is accepted.

46XX DSD

The most common cause of 46XX DSD, congenital adrenal hyperplasia (CAH), leads to virilization of a female fetus. It is due to an enzyme deficiency in the corticosteroid production pathway in the adrenal gland, with over 90% being a deficiency in 21-hydroxylase, which converts progesterone to deoxycorticosterone and 17-hydroxyprogesterone (17-OHP) to deoxycortisol. The reduced levels of cortisol being produced drive the negative-feedback loop, resulting in hyperplasia of the adrenal glands. This leads to an excess of androgen precursors and then to elevated testosterone production. Raised androgen levels in a female fetus will lead to virilization of the external genitalia. The clitoris is enlarged and the labia are fused and scrotal in appearance. The upper vagina joins the urethra and opens as one common channel onto the perineum. In addition, two-thirds of children with 21-hydroxylase CAH will have a 'salt-losing' variety, which also affects the ability to produce aldosterone. This represents a life-threatening situation, and those children who are salt-losing often become dangerously unwell within a few days of birth. Affected individuals require life-long steroid replacement, such as hydrocortisone, along with fludrocortisone for salt losers. Once the infant is well and stabilized on their steroid regime, surgical treatment of the genitalia is considered. Traditionally, all female infants with CAH underwent feminizing genital surgery within the first year of life. This management is now controversial as adult patients with CAH are very dissatisfied with the outcome of their surgery and argue that surgery should have been deferred until they were old enough to have a choice. Surgery certainly leaves scarring and may reduce sexual sensitivity, but the alternative of leaving the genitalia virilized throughout childhood can be difficult for parents to consider. At present, cases are managed individually by a multidisciplinary team (MDT) involving surgeons, endocrinologists and psychologists.

Disorders of menstrual regularity

Amenorrhoea and oligomenorrhoea

Amenorrhoea is defined as the absence of menstruation for more than 6 months in the absence of pregnancy in a woman of fertile age, and oligomenorrhoea is defined as irregular periods at intervals of more than 35 days, with only 4–9 periods a year. The causes may be hypothalamic, pituitary, ovarian or endometrial, and both amenorrhoea and oligomenorrhoea may be primary or secondary.

Box 3.2 Amenorrhoea

- Primary amenorrhoea is when girls fail to menstruate by 16 years of age.
- Secondary amenorrhoea is absence of menstruation for more than 6 months in a normal female of reproductive age that is not due to pregnancy, lactation or the menopause.

Hypothalamic disorders

Hypothalamic disorders will give rise to hypogonadotrophic hypogonadism, with the following causes:

- Excessive exercise, weight loss and stress.
- Hypothalamic lesions (craniopharyngioma, glioma), which can compress hypothalamic tissue or block dopamine.
- Head injuries.
- Kallman's syndrome (X-linked recessive condition resulting in deficiency in GnRH causing underdeveloped genitalia).
- Systemic disorders including sarcoidosis, tuberculosis resulting in an infiltrative process in the hypothalamo-hypophyseal region.
- Drugs: progestogens, HRT or dopamine antagonists.

Pituitary disorders

Pituitary disorders will also give rise to hypogonadotrophic hypogonadism, with the following causes:

- Adenomas, of which prolactinoma is most common.
- Pituitary necrosis (e.g. Sheehan's syndrome, due to prolonged hypotension following major obstetric haemorrhage).

- Iatrogenic damage (surgery or radiotherapy).
- Congenital failure of pituitary development.

Ovarian disorders

Anovulation is often due to polycystic ovary syndrome (PCOS), described below. Ovarian failure is the cause of hypergonadotrophic hypogonadism. Premature ovarian failure (POF) is defined as cessation of periods before 40 years of age and is described in Chapter 8, The menopause and postreproductive health.

Endometrial disorders

Primary amenorrhoea may result from Müllerian defects in the genital tract including an absent uterus, or outflow tract abnormalities, leading to a haematocolpos. Secondary amenorrhoea may result from scarring of the endometrium called Asherman syndrome and is described further in Chapter 4, Disorders of menstrual bleeding.

Findings from the history should guide the examination (*Table 3.2*). A general inspection of the patient should be carried out to assess body mass index (BMI), secondary sexual characteristics (hair growth, breast development using Tanner scores) and signs of endocrine abnormalities (hirsutism, acne, abdominal striae, moon face, skin changes). If the history is suggestive of a pituitary lesion, an assessment of visual fields is indicated. External genitalia and a vaginal examination should be performed to detect structural outflow abnormalities or demonstrate atrophic changes consistent with hypo-oestrogenism.

Investigation of amenorrhoea/oligomenorrhoea

Findings from the history and examination should guide the choice and order of investigations. A pregnancy test should be carried out if the patient is sexually active. Blood can be taken for LH, FSH and testosterone; raised LH or raised testosterone could

Table 3.2 History and examination of patient with amenorrhoea/oligomenorrhoea

Information required	Relevant factors	Possible diagnoses
Developmental history including menarche	Delayed/incomplete puberty	Congenital malformation or chromosomal abnormality
Menstrual history	Oligomenorrhoea	PCOS
	Secondary amenorrhoea	POF
Reproductive history	Infertility	PCOS
		Congenital malformation
Cyclical symptoms	Cyclical pain without menstruation	Congenital malformation
		Imperforate hymen
Hair growth	Hirsutism	PCOS
Weight	Dramatic weight loss	Hypothalamic malfunction
	Difficulty losing weight	PCOS
Lifestyle	Exercise, stress	Hypothalamic malfunction
Past medical history	Systemic diseases (e.g. sarcoidosis)	Hypothalamic malfunction
Past surgical history	Evacuation of uterus	Asherman
Drug history	Dopamine agonists, HRT	Hypothalamic malfunction
Headache		Pituitary adenoma
Galactorrhoea		Prolactinoma
Visual disturbance		Pituitary adenoma

HRT, hormone replacement therapy; PCOS, polycystic ovary syndrome; POF, premature ovarian failure.

Table 3.3 Management of amenorrhoea/oligomenorrhoea

Cause	Management
Low BMI	Dietary advice and support
Hypothalamic lesions (e.g. glioma)	Surgery
Hyperprolactinaemia/prolactinoma	Dopamine agonist (e.g. cabergoline or bromocriptine) or surgery if medication fails
POF	HRT or COCP, see Chapter 8
PCOS	COCP, clomiphene, see below
Asherman's	Adhesiolysis and IUD insertion at time of hysteroscopy, see Chapter 17
Cervical stenosis	Hysteroscopy and cervical dilatation, see Chapters 16 and 17

BMI, body mass index; COCP, combined oral contraceptive pill; HRT, hormone replacement therapy; IUD, intrauterine device; PCOS, polycystic ovary syndrome; POF, premature ovarian failure.

be suggestive of PCOS; raised FSH may be suggestive of POF. A raised prolactin level may indicate a prolactinoma. Thyroid function should be checked if clinically indicated. An ultrasound scan can be useful in detecting the classical appearances of polycystic ovaries (**Figure 3.6**) and magnetic resonance imaging (MRI) of the brain should be carried out if symptoms are consistent with a pituitary adenoma. Hysteroscopy is not routine, but is a suitable investigation where Asherman or cervical stenosis is suspected. Karyotyping is diagnostic of Turner's and other sex chromosome abnormalities.

The management of amenorrhoea/oligomenorrhoea is outlined in *Table 3.3*. More specific descriptions of management are detailed in the chapters indicated.

Polycystic ovary syndrome

PCOS is a syndrome of ovarian dysfunction along with the cardinal features of hyperandrogenism and polycystic ovary morphology (**Figure 3.6**). The prevalence of polycystic ovaries seen on ultrasound is around 25% of all women but is not always associated with the full syndrome. Clinical manifestations include menstrual irregularities, signs of androgen excess (e.g. hirsutism and acne) and obesity. Elevated serum LH levels, biochemical evidence of hyperandrogenism and raised insulin resistance are also common features.

PCOS is associated with an increased risk of type 2 diabetes and cardiovascular events. It affects around 5–10% of women of reproductive age. The aetiology of PCOS is not completely clear, although the frequent familial trend points to a genetic cause.

Clinical features

- Oligomenorrhoea/amenorrhoea in up to 75% of patients, predominantly related to chronic anovulation.
- Hirsutism.
- Subfertility in up to 75% of women.

> ▶ **eResource 3.1**
>
> Polycystic ovary syndrome (PCOS)
> http://www.routledgetextbooks.com/textbooks/tenteachers/gynaecologyv3.1.php

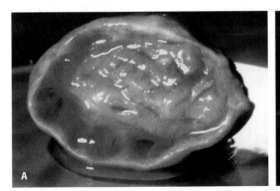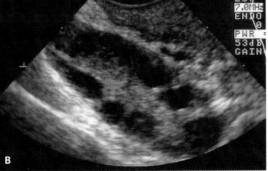

Figure 3.6 Gross appearance of a polycystic ovary (**A**) and transvaginal ultrasound scan image (**B**).

- Obesity in at least 40% of patients.
- Acanthosis nigricans (areas of increased velvety skin pigmentation occur in the axillae and other flexures).
- May be asymptomatic.

Diagnosis

Patients must have two out of the three features below:

- Amenorrhoea/oligomenorrhoea.
- Clinical or biochemical hyperandrogenism.
- Polycystic ovaries on ultrasound. The ultrasound criteria for the diagnosis of a polycystic ovary are eight or more subcapsular follicular cysts <10 mm in diameter and increased ovarian stroma. While these findings support a diagnosis of PCOS, they are not by themselves sufficient to identify the syndrome.

Management

Management of PCOS involves the following:

- Combined oral contraceptive pill (COCP) to regulate menstruation. This also increases sex hormone-binding globulin, which will help reduce androgenic symptoms.
- Cyclical oral progesterone: used to regulate a withdrawal bleed.
- Clomiphene: this can be used to induce ovulation where subfertility is a factor.
- Lifestyle advice: dietary modification and exercise is appropriate in these patients as they are at an increased risk of developing diabetes and cardiovascular disease later in life. Aerobic exercise has been shown to improve insulin resistance.
- Weight reduction.
- Ovarian drilling, a laparoscopic procedure to destroy some of the ovarian stroma that may prompt ovulatory cycles.
- Treatment of hirsutism/androgenic symptoms:
  - eflornithine cream (Vaniqua™) applied topically;
  - cyproterone acetate (an antiandrogen contained in the Dianette™ contraceptive pill, sometimes used alone);

- metformin: this is beneficial in a subset of patients with PCOS, those with hyperinsulinaemia and cardiovascular risk factors. It improves parameters of insulin resistance, hyperandrogenaemia, anovulation and acne in PCOS, and may aid weight loss. It is less effective than clomiphene for ovulation induction and does not improve pregnancy outcome;
- GnRH analogues with low-dose HRT: this regime should be reserved for women intolerant of other therapies;
- surgical treatments (e.g. laser or electrolysis).

Premenstrual syndrome

Premenstrual syndrome (PMS) is the occurrence of cyclical somatic, psychological and emotional symptoms that occur in the luteal (premenstrual) phase of the menstrual cycle and resolve by the time menstruation ceases. Premenstrual symptoms occur in almost all women of reproductive age. In 3–60% symptoms are severe, causing disruption to everyday life, in particular interpersonal relationships.

Aetiology

The precise aetiology of PMS is unknown, but cyclical ovarian activity and the effects of oestradiol and progesterone on certain neurotransmitters, including serotonin, appear to play a role.

History and examination

The patient is likely to complain of some or all of the following: bloating cyclical weight gain, mastalgia, abdominal cramps, fatigue, headache, depression, irritability. The cyclical nature of PMS is the cornerstone of the diagnosis. A symptom chart, to be filled in by the patient prospectively, may help.

Management

The management of PMS is depicted in **Figure 3.7**.

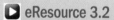 eResource 3.2

PMS patient guidance
http://www.routledgetextbooks.com/textbooks/tenteachers/gynaecologyv3.2.php

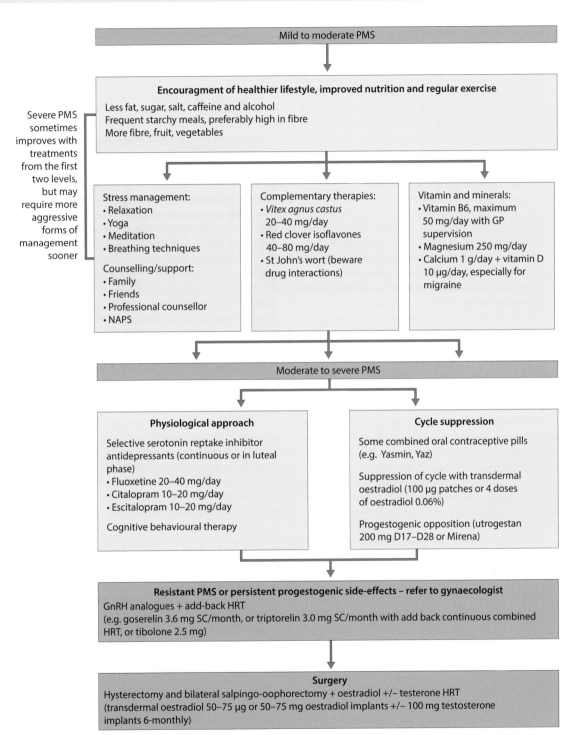

Figure 3.7 Algorithm for the treatment of premenstrual syndrome (PMS). (GP, general practitioner; GnRH, gonadotrophin-releasing hormone; HRT, hormone replacement therapy; NAPS, National Association for Premenstrual Syndrome.) (Adapted with permission from Guidelines for the National Association for Premenstrual Syndrome, www.pms.org.uk.)

- Simple therapies: include stress reduction, alcohol and caffeine limitation and exercise.
- Medical treatments:
  - COCP: the most effective regime appears to be bicycling or tricycling pill packets (i.e. taking two or three packets in a row without a scheduled break);
  - transdermal oestrogen: this has been shown to significantly reduce PMS symptoms, by overcoming the fluctuations of the normal cycle;
  - GnRH analogues are a very effective treatment for PMS as they turn off ovarian activity. To reduce the risk of osteoporosis it is recommended that a continuous combined form of hormone replacement therapy is administered concurrently;
  - selective serotonin-reuptake inhibitors (SSRIs): there is good evidence that this group of drugs significantly improves PMS.
- Hysterectomy with bilateral salpingo-oopherectomy: this procedure obviously completely removes the ovarian cycle. It should only be performed if all other treatments have failed. It is essential for such patients to have a preoperative trial of GnRH analogue as a 'test' to ensure that switching off ovarian function (by removing the ovaries at hysterectomy) will indeed cure the problem.
- Vitamins: initial studies suggest that magnesium, calcium and isoflavones and vitamin B6 may be useful in treating PMS.
- Alternative therapies:
  - initial results of St John's Wort are promising, particularly in improving mood. Although

Evening Primrose oil is commonly used, there is no evidence to support this treatment for PMS;

- cognitive-behavioural therapy (CBT): CBT appears to be particularly effective when combined with SSRIs.

KEY LEARNING POINTS

- The hypothalamus, pituitary, ovary and the end organ endometrium have a subtle interplay.
- Normal puberty and a regular menstrual cycle require function of each organ and healthy hormonal interaction.
- DSD may be diagnosed at birth but some cause delayed puberty or primary amenorrhoea.
- Oligomenorrhoea and amenorrhoea may be primary or secondary and may be caused by hypothalamic, pituitary, ovarian or other hormonal disorders. They can also be caused by endometrial problems.
- PCOS is a common disorder associated with oligomenorrhoea.
- PMS is common and can be treated with simple remedies as well as medical remedies.

Further reading

Balen AH, Conway GS, Homburg R, Legro RS (2005). *Polycystic Ovary Syndrome: A Guide to Clinical Management*. London, New York: Taylor & Francis.

Hughes IA, Houk C, Ahmed SF, Lee PA; LWPES Consensus Group; ESPE Consensus Group (2006). Consensus statement on management of intersex disorders. *Arch Dis Child* 91(7):554–63.

National Association for Premenstrual Syndrome. http://www.pms.org.uk/assets/files/guidelinesfinal60210.pdf.

Self assessment

CASE HISTORY

A 22-year-old woman approached her GP complaining of irregular periods and excess facial hair and spots. She had increased her weight by 5 kg in the last year. Examination was not remarkable, but her BMI was raised at 30.

A What additional features of the history would you seek?

B Outline the investigations and management.

ANSWERS

A In the history it would be important to know the number of periods in the last year, as oligomenorrhoea is a risk factor for endometrial hypertrophy. Although she is only 22, it would be important to know her plans for future children, as many women will have read about polycystic ovaries on the internet and be concerned about the infertility risk. Ask whether she has a partner at the moment and whether she is sexually active. Ask about contraindications to the pill, as even without investigation the possibility of PCOS should have occurred to you because it is the most common cause of anvolution and strongly associated with obesity. You find that she has no contraindications to the pill, has a partner and is sexually active using condoms but does not want children yet.

B You recommend a transvaginal ultrasound scan (TVUSS).

This reveals that the ovaries are enlarged with more than 10 prenatal follicles on each side with a dense stroma. The combination of this and the clinical signs are sufficient to make a diagnosis of PCOS, and you do not need to perform further blood tests at this point.

The first-line medical treatment would be the oral contraceptive pill. This will regulate her bleeds. It will also help reduce facial hair growth by elevating sex hormone-binding globulin (SHBG), hence reducing free testosterone. However, the most important treatment is to reduce her weight and increase her aerobic exercise, as a reduction in weight will promote spontaneous ovulation.

SBA QUESTIONS

1 Menstruation is the shedding of the dead endometrium. Which of the following facts are correct? Choose the single best answer.

A During menstruation the stratum basalis is shed.

B During menstruation the stratum compactum is shed.

C During menstruation fibrinolysis is enhanced.

D Endometrial regeneration begins after ovulation.

E Vasodilation of the spiral arterioles precedes menstruation.

ANSWER

B Prior to menstruation vasoconstriction of the spiral arterioles occurs causing ischaemia.

The stratum basalis remains while the compactum is shed. Fibrinolysis is enhanced to prevent clotting; haemostasis is not the same as elsewhere is the body. Endometrial regeneration begins as the bleed ends.

2 With regards polycystic ovary syndrome (PCOS), which of the following statements is true? Choose the single best answer.

A   PCOS is an unusual cause of anovulation.

B   Ultrasonic evidence of polycystic ovaries is present in 50% of all women.

C   PCOS is associated with obesity in 10% of women.

D   PCOS is associated with acanthosis nigricans.

E   The diagnosis of PCOS can only be made with biochemical evidence of hyperandrogenism.

ANSWER

D   PCOS is the most common cause of anovolution. Based on ultrasound alone, PCOS-type ovaries are seen in 25% of women, some of whom are not symptomatic. More than 40% of women with PCOS are overweight, and PCOS is associated with acanthosis nigricans mediated by high insulin. Women must have two of three diagnostic criteria: ultrasonic evidence of PCOS, clinical or biochemical hyperandrogenism, chronic anovulation.

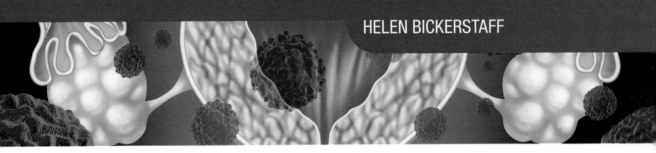

Disorders of menstrual bleeding

HELEN BICKERSTAFF

CHAPTER

4

LEARNING OBJECTIVES

- Understand the symptoms and aetiology of abnormal uterine bleeding (AUB).
- Describe the terminology of AUB.
- Understand the symptoms, investigation and management of heavy menstrual bleeding (HMB).

- Appreciate the impact of HMB on ability to function.
- Understand the causes and investigation of dysmenorrhoea.
- Understand the action of medication used for menorrhagia and dysmenorrhoea.

Introduction

Disorders of menstrual bleeding, now termed AUB, are one of the most common reasons for women to attend their general practitioner (GP) and, subsequently, a gynaecologist. Although rarely life threatening, menstrual disorders can cause major social, psychological and occupational upset. There are several types of abnormal bleeding and their terminology should be known. Heavy menstrual bleeding (HMB), intermenstrual bleeding (IMB), postcoital bleeding (PCB) and postmenopausal bleeding (PMB) should be investigated and treated further as described in the chapters indicated. Initial investigations for each include speculum examination of the cervix, with swabs for microbiology and cervical smear if indicated, and transvaginal ultrasound scan (TVUSS) and endometrial biopsy (EB) as

necessary. Further to this, outpatient hysteroscopy and biopsy may be indicated.

There are several classification systems for AUB, some of which link symptoms to pathology. Such systems help clinicians to adopt a similar categorization of the pathology they are seeing, which helps audit and research. One system that is increasingly recognized is the PALM–COEIN system developed by the International Federation of Gynecology and Obstetrics (FIGO), in which the nemonic **PALM** represents visually objective structural criteria: Polyps, Adenomyosis, Leiomyoma, Malignancy, and **COEIN** for causes unrelated to structural anomalies: Coagulopathy, Ovulatory disorders, Endometrial, Iatrogenic, and Not classified causes (see Further reading). Note that further descriptions in this chapter for causes of AUB do not refer specifically to this system.

Accepted terminology for common types of AUB

- **HMB**: excessive menstrual blood loss (this chapter).
- **IMB**: bleeding between periods, often seen with endometrial and cervical polyps (Chapter 12, Benign conditions of the uterus, cervix and endometrium), also endometriosis (Chapter 11, Benign conditions of the ovary and pelvis).
- **PCB**: bleeding after sex. Often associated with cervical abnormalities (Chapter 16, Premalignant and malignant disease of the lower genital tract).
- **PMB**: bleeding more than 1 year after cessation of periods. Exclude endometrial pathology or vaginal atrophy (Chapter 8, The menopause and postreproductive health and Chapter 15, Malignant disease of the uterus).
- **BEO**: 'bleeding of endometrial origin', a diagnosis of exclusion, has replaced the term 'dysfunctional uterine bleeding' (DUB).

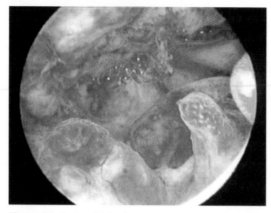

Figure 4.1 Endometrial polyps.

- Coagulation disorders (e.g. von Willebrand disease).
- Pelvic inflammatory disease (PID).
- Thyroid disease.
- Drug therapy (e.g. warfarin).
- Intrauterine devices (IUDs).
- Endometrial/cervical carcinoma.

Other symptoms may be described in the history of women with HMB that may be suggestive of pathology, as shown in *Table 4.1*.

Despite appropriate investigations, often no pathology can be identified. BEO is the diagnosis of exclusion. This replaces the older DUB. Disordered endometrial prostaglandin production has been implicated in the aetiology of BEO, as has abnormalities of endometrial vascular development.

Heavy menstrual bleeding

HMB is the most common type of menstrual bleeding disorder. There has previously been some confusion over the various terminologies used for abnormalities of excessive menstrual blood loss. HMB is now the preferred description as it is simple and easily translatable into other languages. It replaces the older term 'menorrhagia'.

HMB is defined as a blood loss of greater than 80 ml per period. In reality, methods to quantify menstrual blood loss are both inaccurate (poor correlation with haemoglobin level) and impractical, and so a clinical diagnosis based on the patient's own perception of blood loss is preferred.

Of women of reproductive age, 20–30% suffer from HMB. Each year in the UK, 5% of women between the ages of 30 and 49 consult their GP with HMB, with a substantial number being referred on to secondary care.

The aetiology of HBM may be hormonal or structural, with common causes listed below:

- Fibroids: 30% of HMB is associated with fibroids.
- Adenomyosis: 70% of women will have AUB/HMB.
- Endometrial polyps (**Figure 4.1**).

History and examination

The relevant questions to determine heaviness of the period and the extent to which is disrupts the woman's life and causes anaemia have been covered in Chapter 2, Gynaecological history, examination and investigations. In younger women it is important to question whether HMB started at menarche, as this is much less likely to be associated with pathology. The regularity of the menstrual cycle is also important as heavy anovulatory bleeds may be associated with early puberty, polycystic ovary syndrome or the perimenopause.

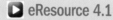 **eResource 4.1**

HMB history and examination
http://www.routledgetextbooks.com/textbooks/tenteachers/gynaecologyv4.php

Table 4.1 Symptoms that may be associated with HMB and related pathologies

Associated symptoms	Suggestive of
Irregular bleeding	Endometrial or cervical polyp or other cervical abnormality
IMB	
PCB	
Excessive bruising/bleeding from other sites	Coagulation disorder (coagulation disorders will be present in 20% of those presenting with 'unexplained' HMB)
History of PPH	
Excessive postoperative bleeding	
Excessive bleeding with dental extractions	
Family history of bleeding problems	
Unusual vaginal discharge	PID
Urinary symptoms, abdominal mass or abdominal fullness	Pressure from fibroids
Weight change, skin changes, fatigue	Thyroid disease

IMB, intermenstrual bleeding; PCB, postcoital bleeding; PID, pelvic inflammatory disease; PPH, postpartum haemorrhage.

After examining the patient for signs of anaemia, it is important to perform an abdominal and pelvic examination in all women complaining of HMB. This enables any pelvic masses to be palpated, the cervix to be visualized for polyps/carcinoma, swabs to be taken if pelvic infection is suspected or a cervical smear to be taken if one is due.

Investigations

The NICE guidelines for HMB indicate the following investigations and are useful guide for clinicians:

- Full blood count (FBC) should be performed in all women (but serum ferritin should not be performed).
- Coagulation screen only if coagulation HMB since menarche or family history of coagulation defects.
- Hormone testing should not be performed.
- Pelvic ultrasound scan if history suggests structural or histological abnormality such as PCB, IMB, pain/pressure symptoms, or enlarged uterus or vaginal mass is palpable on pelvic examination.
- High vaginal and endocervical swabs.
- EB should be considered if risk factors such as age over 45, treatment failure or risk factors for endometrial pathology. Sensitivity of EB increases when performed in addition to using the cut-off of 4 mm endometrial thickness on TVUSS.

- Thyroid function tests should only be carried out when the history is suggestive of a thyroid disorder.

An outpatient hysteroscopy (**Figure 4.2**) with guided biopsy may be indicated if:

- EB biopsy attempt fails.
- EB biopsy sample is insufficient for histopathology assessment.
- TVUSS is inconclusive, for example to establish the exact location of a submucosal or intramural fibroid.
- There is an abnormality on TVUSS amenable to treatment (e.g. suggested endometrial polyp or submucosal fibroid), if there are facilities to perform resections.

If the patient fails to tolerate an outpatient procedure, if the cervix needs to be dilated to enter the cavity, or for treatment of large polyps or submucosal fibroids, then a hysteroscopy proceeding to treatment under general anaesthetic may be required.

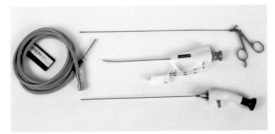

Figure 4.2 An outpatient hysteroscopy set.

Role of EB in HMB

An EB or outpatient hysteroscopy is indicated if there is:

- PMB and endometrial thickness on TVUSS >4 mm.
- HMB over 45 years.
- HMB associated with IMB.
- Treatment failure.
- Prior to ablative techniques.

Management

For some women, the demonstration that their blood loss is in fact 'normal' may be sufficient to reassure them and make further treatment unnecessary. For others, there are a number of different treatments for HMB. The effectiveness of medical treatments is often temporary, while surgical treatments are mostly incompatible with desired fertility.

When selecting appropriate management for the patient, it is important to consider and discuss:

- The patient's preference of treatment.
- Risks/benefits of each option.
- Contraceptive requirements:
  - family complete?
  - current contraception?
- Past medical history:
  - any contraindications to medical therapies for HMB?
  - suitability for an anaesthetic.
- Previous surgical history on uterus.

Management of HMB

- LNG-IUS.
- Transexmic acid/mefenamic acid or combined oral contraceptive pill (COCP).
- Progestogens.
- Endometrial ablation.
- Hysterectomy or umbilical artery embolization (UAE) for fibroids.

Medical

Initial management of HMB in the absence of structural or histological abnormality should be medical. The National Institute for Health and Care Excellence (NICE) guidelines (see Further reading) suggest the following order:

- Levonorgestrel intrauterine system (LNG-IUS, Mirena™), provided long-term use of at least 12 months is expected. LNG-IUS, Mirena™ (as further described in Chapter 6, Contraception and abortion) has revolutionized the treatment of HMB. Mean reductions in mean blood loss (MBL) of around 95% are achieved by 1 year after LNG-IUS insertion. It provides a highly effective alternative to surgical treatment, with few side-effects. Indeed, the Royal College of Obstetricians and Gynaecologists (RCOG) has suggested that the LNG-IUS should be considered in the majority of women as an alternative to surgical treatment. It is obviously not suitable for women wishing to conceive.
- Tranexamic acid, an antifibrinolytic that reduces blood loss by 50% and is taken during menstruation, or mefenamic acid, which inhibits prostaglandin synthesis and reduces blood loss by 30%, or COCP, which will induce slightly lighter periods.
- Norethisterone, taken 15 mg daily in a cyclical pattern from day 6 to day 26 of the menstrual cycle.
- Gonadotrophin-releasing hormone (GnRH) agonists: these drugs act on the pituitary to stop the production of oestrogen, which results in amenorrhoea. These are only used in the short term due to the resulting hypo-oestrogenic state that predisposes to osteoporosis. They may be used preoperatively to shrink fibroids or cause endometrial suppression to enhance visualization at hysteroscopy. In severe HMB they can allow the patient the opportunity to improve their haemoglobin by providing a respite from bleeding.

Surgical

Details of surgical interventions including preoperative assessment, consent and complications are covered in Chapter 17, Gynaecological surgery and therapeutics.

Surgical treatment is normally restricted to women for whom medical treatments have failed or where there are associated symptoms such as pressure symptoms from fibroids or prolapse. Women contemplating surgical treatment for HMB must be certain that their family is complete. While this caveat is obvious for women contemplating hysterectomy, in which the uterus will be removed, it also applies to women contemplating endometrial ablation. Therefore, women wishing to preserve their fertility for future attempts at childbearing should be advised to use medical methods of treatment. The risks of a pregnancy after an ablation procedure theoretically include prematurity and morbidly adherent placenta.

Endometrial ablation

All endometrial destructive procedures employ the principle that ablation of the endometrial lining of the uterus to sufficient depth prevents regeneration of the endometrium. Ablation is suitable for women with a uterus no bigger than 10 weeks' size and with fibroids less than 3 cm.

The first-generation techniques including transcervical resection of the endometrium with electrical diathermy or rollerball ablation have largely been replaced by newer second-generation techniques including:

- Impedance controlled endometrial ablation (Novosure™).
- Thermal uterine balloon therapy.
- Microwave ablation (Microsulis™) (**Figure 4.3**).

As a general rule, all women undergoing endometrial ablation should have access to a second-generation technique. After treatment, 40% will become amenorrhoeic, 40% will have markedly reduced menstrual loss and 20% will have no difference in their bleeding. Some authorities have suggested that endometrial ablation is so successful that all women

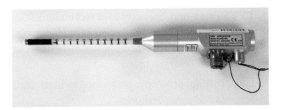

Figure 4.3 Microwave ablation (Microsulis™).

> ▶ **eResource 4.2**
>
> Endometrial ablation
> http://www.routledgetextbooks.com/textbooks/tenteachers/gynaecologyv4.2.php

with HMB should be encouraged to consider it before opting for hysterectomy. While there are merits to this argument, some women, after informed discussion, will still prefer hysterectomy and they should therefore be considered for this procedure instead.

Umbilical artery embolization

UAE is treatment useful for HMB associated with fibroids, as discussed in Chapter 12, Benign conditions of the uterus, cervix and endometrium.

Myomectomy

This may be a sensible option or women with HMB secondary to large fibroids with pressure symptoms who wish to conceive (and are at an age where this is realistic).

Transcervical resection of fibroid

As described in Chapter 12, Benign conditions of the uterus, cervix and endometrium and Chapter 17, Gynaecological surgery and therapeutics, transcervical resection of a large submucosal fibroid (TCRF) may reduce HMB and is appropriate in women wishing to conceive.

Hysterectomy

A hysterectomy is the surgical removal of the uterus as described in Chapter 17, Gynaecological surgery and therapeutics. It can be avoided in some women by medical and ablation procedures. However, it can be necessary to control HMB in women who have not responded. It may be a first-line treatment in women who have HMB associated with large fibroids who also have pressure symptoms, or who have a smaller uterus and associated uterine prolapse.

Acute HMB

Not infrequently women are admitted to hospital with AUB. They require stabilization, examination to exclude cervical abnormalities and pelvic masses, medication to arrest bleeding and correct anaemia, investigation and discharge with a long-term plan to avoid further admissions.

Management of acute HMB

- Admit.
- Pelvic examination.
- FBC, coagulopathy screen, biochemistry.
- Intravenous access and resuscitation or transfusion as required.
- Tranexamic acid oral or IV.
- TVUSS.
- High-dose progestogens to arrest bleeding.
- Consider suppression with GnRH or ulipristol acetate in the medium term.
- Longer-term plan when a diagnosis has been made.

Dysmenorrhoea

Dysmenorrhoea is defined as painful menstruation. It is experienced by 45–95% of women of reproductive age. Primary dysmenorrhoea describes painful periods since onset of menarche and is unlikely to be associated with pathology. There is some evidence to support the assertion that primary dysmenorrhoea improves after childbirth, and it also appears to decline with increasing age. Secondary dysmenorrhoea describes painful periods that have developed over time and usually have a secondary cause.

Aetiology of secondary dysmenorrhoea

Aetiology includes:

- Endometriosis and adenomyosis (Chapter 11, Benign conditions of the ovary and pelvis).
- Pelvic inflammatory disease (Chapter 9, Genitourinary problems).
- Cervical stenosis and haematometra (rarely).

History and examination

Patients will have different ideas as to what constitutes a painful period. For some patients reassurance that the pain may be normal for her will help.

For others the ability to alter the menstrual cycle to avoid having a period during key events, for example school examinations or holidays, will be helpful.

To ascertain the actual severity of the pain, the following questions may be useful:

- Do you need to take painkillers for this pain? Which tablets help?
- Have you needed to take any time off work/school due to the pain?

Some primary dysmenorrhoea is associated with flushing and nausea, which may be prostaglandin related. It is important to distinguish between menstrual pain that precedes the period (a vital clue in endometriosis) and pain that only occurs with bleeding. Other important clues about the aetiology include pain that occurs with passage of clots, in which case medication to reduce flow may be effective.

Secondary dysmenorrhoea may be associated with dyspareunia or AUB, which may point towards a pathological diagnosis.

An abdominal and pelvic examination should be performed (excepting adolescents). Certain signs associated with endometriosis include a pelvic mass (if an endometrioma is present), a fixed uterus (if adhesions are present) and endometriotic nodules (palpable in the pouch of Douglas or on the uterosacral ligaments). An enlarged uterus may be found with fibroids. Abnormal discharge and tenderness may be seen with PID.

'Red flags' in the expression of dymenorrhoea lead the clinician to suspect serious pathology and include an abnormal cervix on examination, persistent PCB or IMB, which may indicate endometrial or cervical pathology, or a pelvic mass that is not obviously the uterus.

Investigations

- High vaginal and endocervical swabs.
- TVUSS scan may be useful to detect endometriomas or appearances suggestive of adenomyosis (enlarged uterus with heterogeneous texture) or to image an enlarged uterus.
- Diagnostic laparoscopy: performed to investigate secondary dysmenorrhoea:
  - when the history is suggestive of endometriosis;

- when swabs and ultrasound scan are normal, yet symptoms persist;
- when the patient wants a definite diagnosis or wants reassurance that their pelvis is normal.

Discussion about laparoscopy should include risks and the possibility that this investigation may show no obvious causes for their symptoms.

If features in the history suggest cervical stenosis, ultrasound-guided hysteroscopy can be used to investigate further. However, this condition is an infrequent cause of dysmenorrhoea, and this investigation should not be routine. Laparoscopy for primary dysmenorrhoea should not usually be performed.

Management

- Non-steroidal anti-inflammatory drugs (NSAIDs): effective in a large proportion of women. Some examples are naproxen, ibuprofen and mefenamic acid.
- Hormonal contraceptives: COCP is widely used but, surprisingly, a recent review of randomized controlled trials provides little evidence supporting this treatment as being effective for primary dysmenorrhoea. Progestogens, either oral (desogestrol) or parenteral (medroxyprogesterone, etonogestrel) may be useful to cause anovulation and amenorrhoea.
- LNG-IUS: there is evidence that this is beneficial for dysmenorrhoea and indeed can be an effective treatment for underlying causes, such as endometriosis and adenomyosis. It is often used as a first-line treatment before laparoscopy.
- Lifestyle changes: there is some evidence to suggest that a low fat, vegetarian diet may improve dysmenorrhoea. There are suggestions that exercise may improve symptoms by improving blood flow to the pelvis.
- Heat: although this may seem a rather old-fashioned method for helping dysmenorrhoea, there is strong evidence to prove its benefit. It appears to be as effective as NSAIDs.

- GnRH analogues: this is not a first-line treatment nor an option for prolonged management due to the resulting hypo-oestrogenic state. These are best used to manage symptoms if awaiting hysterectomy or as a form of assessment as to the benefits of hysterectomy. If the pain does not settle with the GnRH analogue, it is unlikely to be resolved by hysterectomy.
- Surgery: signs or symptoms of pathology such as endometriosis may warrant surgical laparoscopy to perform adhesiolysis or treatment of endometriosis/drainage of endometriomas.

KEY LEARNING POINTS

- HMB is one of the most frequent causes for consultation in primary care and referral to secondary care.
- HMG may be associated with symptoms that may indicate pathology, such as fibroids.
- Medical treatment of HMB with LNG-IUS, NSAIDs or other hormonal treatments is first line.
- Women should have access to second-generation ablation techniques, which should be offered before hysterectomy for HMB.
- Women with associated pathology such as fibroids or prolapse may opt for hysterectomy.
- Primary dysmenorrhoea is rarely pathological.
- Secondary dysmenorrhoea may be associated with pathology such as endometriosis or PID.
- First-line treatment of dysmenorrhoea is medical with NSAIDs, COCP or progestogens.
- Women with secondary dysmenorrhoea and signs or symptoms of other pathology may need laparoscopy.

Further reading

Munro MG, Critchley HOD, Broder MS, Fraser IS, for the FIGO Working Group on Menstrual Disorders (2011). FIGO classification system (PALM-COEIN) for causes of abnormal uterine bleeding in nongravid women of reproductive age. *Int J Gynaecol Obstet* **113**(1):3–13.
National Institute for Health and Care Excellence. Heavy menstrual bleeding: assessment and management. https://www.nice.org.uk/guidance/cg44ICE guideline.

Self assessment

CLINICAL HISTORY

A 28-year-old woman has presented to her GP with HMB of 2 years' duration. She also complained of some dysmenorrhoea that was getting worse. On examination there is tenderness over the uterosacral ligaments.

A What additional features of the history are important?

B What are the initial investigations?

C What is your management plan?

ANSWERS

A When taking the history it is important to determine how much the woman's periods are interfering with her daily life. The relationship of the pain to the periods is particularly important. Her plans for children will influence your choice of treatment, as will any previous treatments and drug allergies or contraindications.

She tells you that she is needing analgesia and frequent sanitary changes. She is working as a nurse, and is finding some shifts difficult and has taken some sick days. The pain is worse before the period rather than with the menstrual bleed. Additionally, she has been wanting to conceive for the last year.

B Appropriate investigations include FBC, TVUSS, high vaginal swab (HVS) and endo-cervical swab.

C Treatment options are limited by the desire to conceive. It is appropriate to offer laparoscopy to diagnose/treat endometriosis. It may be appropriate to perform tubal insufflation at the same time as there has been a slight delay in conception.

SBA QUESTIONS

1 A 47-year-old woman presents to her GP with symptoms of HMB with flooding and clots. She is otherwise well. Examination reveals a non-tender uterus that is not enlarged. A FBC has shown signs of reduced haemoglobin.

What investigation is indicated next according to recent NICE guidelines? Choose the single best answer.

A Thyroid function tests.

B Hormonal profile.

C Serum ferritin.

D Outpatient hysteroscopy.

E EB.

ANSWER

E Thyroid function is not indicated unless there are symptoms compatible with abnormal thyroid function. Likewise, a hormonal profile is not likely to yield useful results in the absence of symptoms. Serum ferritin will not add useful information to the FBC showing anaemia, which indicates the need for iron replacement anyway. A TVUSS is not necessary unless the uterus is enlarged, as it will not alter treatment (although in fact will often be ordered pragmatically to present a diagnosis such as adenomysosis to the patients).

In women over the age of 45 EB is indicated as a small percentage will have an underlying malignancy or endometrial hyperplasia.

2 A 32-year-old woman presents to her GP with regular HMB. She has two children and does not want more at present. She is medically well and has no allergies. On examination she has a normal sized uterus that is not tender.

What is the first-line treatment for HMB according to recent NICE guidelines? Choose the single best answer.

A Endometrial ablation.

B The oral contraceptive pill.

C The oral contraceptive pill used back to back.

D Northisterone.

E LNG-IUS.

ANSWER

E In women who do not wish to conceive, the LNG-IUS is recommended as a first-line treatment for HMB. Endometrial ablation can be considered as a permanent solution in women where other treatments have failed. Northisterone used regularly on days 6–26 of the cycle is likely to improve symptoms but the side-effect profile is worse. The oral contraceptive pill may slightly reduce blood flow.

Implantation and early pregnancy

CHAPTER 5

ANDREW HORNE

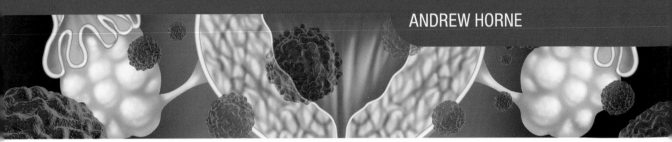

LEARNING OBJECTIVES

- Understand the social and emotional context of early pregnancy loss.
- Understand why a high suspicion of pregnancy is needed in all women of reproductive age with symptoms.
- Obtain a detailed knowledge of the clinical presentation and management of miscarriage and ectopic pregnancy.
- Obtain an awareness of less common early pregnancy conditions, including recurrent miscarriage, gestational trophoblastic disease and hyperemesis gravidarum.

Implantation and the establishment of pregnancy

After ovulation, the cells of the dominant follicle form the corpus luteum (CL) and the CL produces large amounts of progesterone. Progesterone prepares the endometrium to support a pregnancy. Successful implantation occurs when the oocyte is fertilized in the Fallopian tube and implants in the endometrium, around 7 days after ovulation (**Figure 5.1**). The implanted blastocyst secretes human chorionic gonadotrophin (hCG). Exponentially increasing hCG acts on the CL to rescue it from luteolysis to maintain progesterone secretion, prevent menstruation and support the early conceptus. The CL supports the pregnancy for approximately 8 weeks, after which the early placental tissue becomes the main source of progesterone support.

hCG can be detected in the urine in sensitive pregnancy tests 1 or 2 days before the expected date of menstruation. Most women delay taking a pregnancy test until after a missed period. However, it is relatively common for positive pregnancy tests to occur just prior to the time of the expected period, and for menstruation to occur as expected or 1 or 2 days later with a negative pregnancy test thereafter. This transiently positive hCG is a result of pregnancy failure during the early stages of implantation and it is known as a 'biochemical pregnancy'.

A transvaginal ultrasound scan (TVUSS) can detect an early intrauterine gestational sac, the first sign of a normal pregnancy, at around 5 weeks' gestation. A few days later a circular yolk sac can be seen within the gestational sac, and the embryonic f

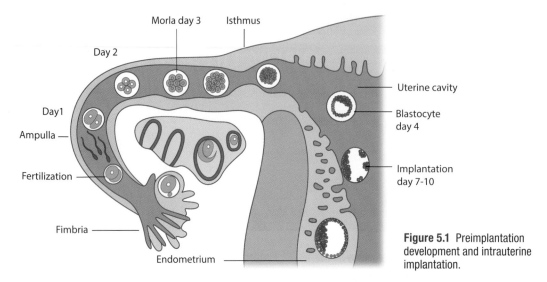

Figure 5.1 Preimplantation development and intrauterine implantation.

can usually be identified after 5.5 weeks' gestation (**Figure 5.2**). The fetal heartbeat may be visible as early as 6 weeks' gestation.

> ▶ **eResource 5.1**
>
> Pregnancy between 5 and 12 weeks' gestation
> http://www.routledgetextbooks.com/textbooks/tenteachers/gynaecologyv5.1.php

- The gestational age is calculated from the last menstrual period (LMP) rather than the time of conception. When someone is '6 weeks' pregnant', this means that they have conceived 4 weeks previously (assuming they have regular menstrual cycles). This is important as it sometimes causes the patient some confusion.
- In the early stages of a normally developing intrauterine pregnancy, serum concentrations of hCG will normally double every 48 hours.
- A normal pregnancy with serum hCG concentrations of >1,500 IU/l should be able to be confirmed as intrauterine on a TVUSS.

Miscarriage

Miscarriage is a pregnancy that ends spontaneously before 24 weeks' gestation.

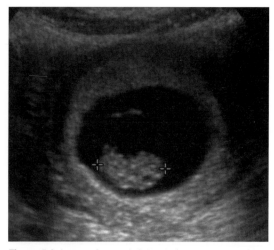

Figure 5.2 Image of an early intrauterine pregnancy with yolk sac and pole (~5–6 weeks).

Clinical presentation

The most common sign of miscarriage is vaginal bleeding.

Incidence and aetiology

Miscarriage is common, occurring in 10–20% of clinical pregnancies, with the risk increasing with maternal age. Clinically, miscarriages can be classified into different types based on the clinical presentation and investigation findings. *Table 5.1* illustrates the respective clinical presentation, examination findings and management of the different types of miscarriages.

Table 5.1 Types of miscarriages with the relevant ultrasound findings and clinical presentation

Type of miscarriage	Ultrasound scan (USS) findings	Clinical presentation	Management
Threatened miscarriage	Intrauterine pregnancy (with FH)	Vaginal bleeding and abdominal pain Speculum: cervical os closed	Supportive
Inevitable miscarriage	Intrauterine pregnancy (no FH)	Vaginal bleeding and abdominal pain Speculum: cervical os open	Expectant, medical or surgical
Incomplete miscarriage	Retained products of conception	Vaginal bleeding and abdominal pain Speculum: cervical os open, products of conception located in cervical os	Remove pregnancy tissue at time of speculum if possible Expectant, medical or surgical
Complete miscarriage	Empty uterus (need serum hCG to exclude ectopic pregnancy if no previous USS identifying intrauterine pregnancy)	Pain and bleeding has resolved Speculum: cervical os closed	Supportive
Missed miscarriage	Intrauterine pregnancy (no FH)	Asymptomatic Often diagnosed at booking USS	Expectant, medical or surgical

Note that a pelvic examination is not usually required if the patient has had an USS (so arrange a USS first if you possibly can). FH, fetal heart beat; hCG, human chorionic gonadotrophin.

Aetiological factors

- Chromosomal abnormalities.
- Medical/endocrine disorders.
- Uterine abnormalities.
- Infections.
- Drugs/chemicals.

Investigations

It is fundamentally important to assess the woman who is miscarrying clinically ('ABC', abdomino-pelvic examination) in conjunction with the results of investigations below. It goes without saying that your patient may be emotionally distraught, as well as distressed by her physical symptoms.

- Transabdominal/TVUSS: a single ultrasound scan can diagnose a miscarriage if there is a pregnancy within the uterine cavity and certain criteria are met.
- Haemoglobin and 'Group and Save' (or cross-match if patient is severely compromised):
  - measure to assess degree of vaginal loss and rhesus status.

Management

A miscarriage can be managed using an expectant (natural), medical or a surgical approach, depending on clinical presentation and patient choice.

Expectant management

Expectant management allows for the avoidance of surgery. After a spontaneous miscarriage where the pain and bleeding resolve, a repeat ultrasound scan is not required to confirm completion. Women may be advised to take a urinary pregnancy test after 3 weeks and attend if it is positive. Women undergoing expectant management may require unplanned surgery if they start to bleed heavily.

Medical management

Medical treatment is increasingly used in an outpatient setting to allow women to miscarry at home. It involves the administration of a single, or repeated, vaginal or sublingual dose of the prostaglandin E analogue misoprostol. Some centres use pretreatment with the progesterone antagonist mifepristone (if over 9 weeks' gestation). The side-effects include pain,

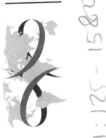
...omen are routinely ...iemetics. As with ... need for routine ...tment pregnancy ...rgoing medical ...understand that ...medical treat-...ed heavily.

...preferred if ...haemody-...is option. ...on under ιοcaι anaestnetic in an outpatient clinic setting if the woman is not compromised. More commonly it is done as a day case in theatre under general anaesthesia. Vaginal or sublingual misoprostol is frequently used to ripen the cervix to facilitate cervical dilatation for suction curette insertion and reduce the risk of trauma and haemorrhage. However, surgical evacuation has its drawbacks including risks such as uterine perforation, postoperative pelvic infection and cervical trauma and subsequent cervical incompetence (see Chapter 17, Gynaecological surgery and therapeutics).

Counselling

Miscarriage can be a very distressing experience and the psychological impact, sense of bereavement and feelings of depression and anxiety should not be underestimated. Patients who have suffered miscarriages should be counselled to ensure that they understand that most miscarriages are non-recurrent and that they are not to blame for their loss.

Recurrent miscarriage

Recurrent miscarriage is defined as the loss of three or more consecutive pregnancies and it affects 1% of couples. Risk factors for recurrent miscarriage include both advancing maternal and paternal age, obesity, balanced chromosomal translocations, uterine structural anomalies and antiphospholipid syndrome (APS). Investigation of recurrent miscarriage should involve testing for antiphospholipid antibodies and imaging of the uterus. Products of conception in subsequent miscarriages should be sent for cytogenetic analysis and, where testing reports an unbalanced structural chromosomal abnormality, parental peripheral blood karyotyping of both partners should be performed. Aspirin and low-dose heparin can reduce the miscarriage rate in women with APS by 50%. Balanced translocations may be overcome by preimplantation genetic diagnosis or gamete donation. Congenital uterine abnormalities, including uterine septum and cervical incompetence, may be amenable to surgery. Although treatment with progesterone, corticosteroids or metformin has been advocated, there is insufficient evidence to recommend their use at present. Most couples have normal investigations and the value of psychological support and serial ultrasound scans during pregnancy has been demonstrated in several non-randomized studies.

Ectopic pregnancy

Definition

An ectopic pregnancy (EP) is defined as the implantation of a pregnancy outside the normal uterine cavity. Over 98% implant in the Fallopian tube (**Figure 5.3**). Rarely, ectopic pregnancies can implant in the interstitium of the tube, ovary, cervix, abdominal cavity or in caesarean section scars. A heterotopic pregnancy is the simultaneous development of two pregnancies: one within and one outside the uterine cavity.

> ▶ **eResource 5.2**
>
> Ectopic pregnancy
> http://www.routledgetextbooks.com/textbooks/ tenteachers/gynaecologyv5.2.php

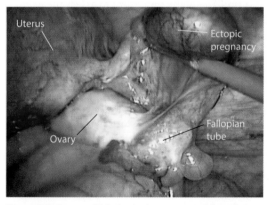

Figure 5.3 Image of tubal ectopic pregnancy taken at laparoscopy.

Incidence and aetiology

One in 80 pregnancies are ectopic. They account for 9–13% of maternal deaths in the Western world and 10–30% in low resource countries. The incidence of a heterotopic pregnancy in the general population is low (1:25,000–30,000), but significantly higher after in-vitro fertilization (IVF) treatment (1%) due to the transfer of two blastocysts.

Aetiological factors for ectopic pregnancy

- Fallopian tube damage due to pelvic infection (e.g. *Chlamydia/Gonorrhoea*), previous ectopic pregnancy and previous tubal surgery.
- Functional alterations in the Fallopian tube due to smoking and increased maternal age.
- Additional risk factors include previous abdominal surgery (e.g. appendicectomy, caesarean section), subfertility, IVF, use of intrauterine contraceptive devices, endometriosis, conception on oral contraceptive/morning after pill.

Clinical presentation

The majority of patients with an EP present with a subacute clinical picture of abdominal pain and/or vaginal bleeding in early pregnancy. Rarely, patients present very acutely with rupture of the EP and massive intraperitoneal bleeding. The free blood in the peritoneal cavity can cause diaphragmatic irritation and shoulder tip pain. The diagnosis of ruptured EP is usually clear as they present with signs of an acute abdomen and hypovolaemic shock with a positive PT. It is, however, important to be aware that it is common for women to experience bleeding or abdominal pain with a viable intrauterine pregnancy.

Investigations

The following are useful investigations for the diagnosis of EP. Nonetheless, again, it is fundamentally important to assess the woman clinically ('ABC', abdominopelvic examination) in conjunction with the results of investigations to manage the patient.

- TVUSS: identification of an intrauterine pregnancy (intrauterine gestation sac, yolk sac +/− fetal pole) on TVUSS effectively excludes the possibility of an EP in most patients except in those patients with rare heterotopic pregnancy. A TVUSS showing an empty uterus with an adnexal mass has a sensitivity of 90% and specificity of 95% in the diagnosis of EP. The presence of moderate to significant free fluid during TVUSS is suggestive of a ruptured EP.
- Serum hCG: the serum hCG level almost doubles every 48 hours in a normally developing intrauterine pregnancy. In patients with EP, the rise of hCG is often suboptimal. However, hCG levels can vary widely in individuals and thus consecutive measurements 48 hours apart are often required for comparison purposes.
- Haemoglobin and 'Group and Save' (or crossmatch if patient is severely compromised):
  - measure to assess degree of intra-abdominal bleeding and rhesus status.

Pregnancy of unknown location

- In up to 40% of women with an EP the diagnosis is not made on first attendance and they are labelled as having a 'pregnancy of unknown location' (PUL).
- A PUL is a working diagnosis defined as an empty uterus with no evidence of an adnexal mass on TVUSS (in a patient with a positive pregnancy test).
- The mainstay of investigation of a PUL is consecutive measurement of serum hCG concentrations. An endometrial biopsy can occasionally be helpful when hCG levels are static. All PUL must be investigated to determine the location of the pregnancy.

Management

An EP can be managed using an expectant, medical or a surgical approach, depending on clinical presentation and patient choice.

Expectant management

Expectant management is based on the assumption that a significant proportion of all EPs will resolve without any treatment. This option is suitable for patients who are haemodynamically stable and asymptomatic (and remain so). The patient requires serial hCG measurements until levels are undetectable.

Medical management

Intramuscular methotrexate is a treatment option for patients with minimal symptoms, an adnexal mass <40 mm in diameter and a current serum hCG concentration under 3,000 IU/l. Methotrexate is a folic acid antagonist that inhibits deoxyribonucleic acid (DNA) synthesis, particularly affecting trophoblastic cells. The dose of methotrexate is calculated based on the patient's body surface area and is 50 mg/m^2. After methotrexate treatment serum hCG is usually routinely measured on days 4, 7 and 11, then weekly thereafter until undetectable (levels need to fall by 15% between day 4 and 7, and continue to fall with treatment). Medical treatment should therefore only be offered if facilities are present for regular follow-up visits. The few contraindications to medical treatment include: (1) chronic liver, renal or haematological disorder; (2) active infection; (3) immunodeficiency; and (4) breastfeeding. There are also known side-effects such as stomatitis, conjunctivitis, gastrointestinal upset and photosensitive skin reaction, and about two-thirds of patients will suffer from non-specific abdominal pain. It is important to advise women to avoid sexual intercourse during treatment and to avoid conceiving for 3 months after methotrexate treatment because of the risk of teratogenicity. It is also important to advise them to avoid alcohol and prolonged exposure to sunlight during treatment.

Surgical management

The standard surgical treatment approach is laparoscopy (**Figure 5.3**). Laparotomy is reserved for severely compromised patients or where there are no endoscopic facilities. The operation of choice is removal of the Fallopian tube and the EP within (salpingectomy), or in some cases a small opening can be made over the site of the EP and the EP extracted via this opening (salpingostomy). Salpingostomy is recommended only if the contralateral tube is absent or visibly damaged, and it is associated with a higher rate of subsequent EP. Pregnancy rates subsequently remain high if the contralateral tube is normal because the oocyte can be picked up by the ipsilateral or contralateral tube.

Anti-D administration

- Rhesus isoimmunization can occur after early pregnancy problems and there are some circumstances where women who are rhesus negative require anti-D prophylaxis.

- All rhesus-negative women who have a surgical procedure to manage an EP or miscarriage should be offered anti-D immunoglobulin at a dose of 50 µg (250 IU) as soon as possible and within 72 hours of the surgery.

- A Kleihauer test is not needed to quantify fetomaternal haemorrhage in the first trimester of pregnancy.

- Anti-D is not required for threatened, incomplete or complete natural miscarriage.

- Anti-D may not be required after the medical management of miscarriage or EP but guidelines differ, and prophylaxis is often given.

Table 5.2 Summary of other early pregnancy disorders

Disorder	Definition	Risk factors	Clinical presentation	Management
Gestational trophoblastic disease (GTD) (abnormal trophoblast proliferation)	Spectrum of conditions that includes complete and partial hyatidiform mole, invasive mole and choriocarcinoma	Previous molar pregnancy High or low maternal age Asian origin	Ultrasound features of intrauterine vesicles ('cluster of grapes') Persistently raised hCG levels after miscarriage	Registration Uterine evacuation by suction curettage (without misoprostol) Serial hCG measurements Avoid oestrogens
Hyperemesis gravidarum		Multiple pregnancies GTD	Excessive nausea and vomiting, often accompanied by dehydration	Antiemetics Fluid and electrolyte replacement Multivitamins Thromboprophylaxis

hCG, human chorionic gonadotrophin.

Other early pregnancy problems

Table 5.2 summarizes other less common early pregnancy disorders. It is important to remember that non-gynaecological conditions, such as urinary tract infection and medical/surgical problems (e.g. appendicitis), can present in early pregnancy.

Further reading

National Institute for Health and Clinical Excellence. NICE Clinical Guideline 154: Ectopic pregnancy and miscarriage.
Royal College of Obstetricians and Gynaecologists. Green-top Guideline 38: The Management of Gestational Trophoblastic Disease.
Royal College of Obstetricians and Gynaecologists. Green-top Guideline 17: The Investigation and Treatment of Couples with Recurrent First-trimester and Second-trimester Miscarriage.

Self assessment

CASE HISTORY

Mrs M is a 32-year-old woman who presents after 6 weeks of amenorrhoea with abdominal pain and dizziness. Her observations on admission are blood pressure 90/50 mmHg, pulse 115/min, temperature 36.9°C. She has a positive urinary pregnancy test.

A What is your differential diagnosis?
B What are the key points in her history, examination and investigation?
C Discuss her management.

ANSWERS

A EP. The findings of cardiovascular instability, in the presence of pregnancy, are an ectopic until proven otherwise.

B An EP should be suspected in any woman of reproductive age who presents with symptoms. This patient has classical symptoms of ectopic pregnancy: pain and dizziness. She also has signs of hypovolaemic shock. She has a positive urinary pregnancy test.

C 'ABC'. The patient should have a large bore cannula inserted and be given IV fluids. Bloods should be taken for full blood count (FBC) and 'Group and Save'. She should remain nil by mouth. She requires an abdominopelvic examination. A senior colleague should be informed about her admission and the possibility of her requiring an urgent laparoscopy.

The patient had a laparoscopy and was discovered to have a large right ruptured EP in her Fallopian tube with 1.5 litres of blood in her pelvis. She had a salpingectomy and subsequently recovered well.

EMQ

A TVUSS.
B Serum hCG levels.
C Midstream urine collection (MSU).
D FBC.
E Suction currettage of uterus.

F Misoprostol.
G Methotrexate.
H Salpingectomy.
I Abdominal X-ray.
J Avoid oestrogens.

For each description below, choose the SINGLE most appropriate answer from the above list of options. Each option may be used once, more than once or not at all.

1 Investigation of pain in early pregnancy.
2 Management of EP.

3 Management of miscarriage.
4 Management of suspected hyatidiform mole.

ANSWERS

1 A, B, C, D. A TVUSS will establish the location of the pregnancy, but if the gestation sac cannot be seen, series hCG measurements will help. An MSU will diagnose a uterine tract infection, which is a common cause of pain in pregnancy

2 D, G, H. FBC is essential in management of an ectopic as a baseline. Depending on the size of the ectopic and the symptoms, medical management with methotrexate or surgical with salpingectomy may be indicated.

3 D, E, F. Baseline FBC is essential in management of a miscarriage in case there is excessive blood loss. The decision for suction curettage or misoprostol is made according to the preference of the patient.

4 E, J. Suction curettage is essential for histological diagnosis and maximal evacuation. Subsequently, oestrogens should be avoided to prevent risk of choriocarcinoma.

SBA QUESTIONS

1 A 25-year-old woman presents with vaginal bleeding and a positive pregnancy test. Her TVUSS shows a non-viable intrauterine pregnancy. What would it be reasonable to offer her? Choose the single best answer.

A Laparoscopy.
B Serum hCG measurement.
C Misoprostol.

D Methotrexate.
E Progesterone.

ANSWER

C The non-viable pregnancy should be removed with suction curettage or by administration of misoprostol. hCG has no role here as it is used only to help manage a PUL or monitor an ectopic. Laparoscopy is not relevant as there is no suggestion of an EP. Methotrexate is not used for an intrauterine pregnancy, and progesterone should not be used in the presence of a non-viable pregnancy, as it will only prolong the time to completion of miscarriage.

2 A 43-year-old woman undergoes a surgical curettage for miscarriage and the pathology report confirms a partial mole. What would you do? Choose the single best answer.

A   Register the patient at a nationally recognized centre for treatment of gestational trophoblastic disease.

B   Start the COCP.

C   Prescribe methotrexate.

D   Arrange an urgent TVUSS.

E   Start serial hCG monitoring.

F   Start antibiotics.

ANSWER

A   All moles, partial and full, are registered via the recognized centre, who perform hCG monitoring themselves. Oestrogens should be avoided in women with molar pregnancy. TVUSS will not be necessary as evacuation of the uterus has been performed. Antibiotics and methotrexate have no role in the monitoring of a molar pregnancy.

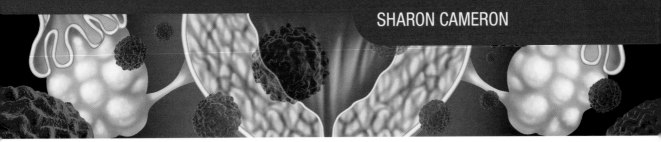

Contraception and abortion

CHAPTER

6

SHARON CAMERON

LEARNING OBJECTIVES

- Understand the mechanism of action of current contraceptive methods.
- Describe factors that affect contraceptive effectiveness.
- Understand the non-contraceptive benefits of methods.

- Remember the use of medical eligibility criteria for contraception.
- Understand the mechanism of action of modern medical methods of abortion.
- Describe common complications of abortion.
- Understand the importance of postabortal contraception.

Introduction

Correct and consistent use of effective methods of contraception can prevent most unintended pregnancies. Abortion is a major consequence of unintended pregnancy, and in many low- and middle-income countries that restrict abortion, abortions are often performed under unsafe conditions and result in women dying or suffering serious injuries. Unintended pregnancies can also lead to delayed or no antenatal care, which can pose health risks to both mothers and infants. It is estimated that there are 22 million unsafe abortions each year, approximately 47,000 deaths from unsafe abortion and 5 million women suffer injury/disability from unsafe abortion. These are preventable

through contraception and, as a back-up, access to safe abortion.

Global unmet need for contraception

- Over 200 million women worldwide would like to avoid a pregnancy, but are not using an effective method of contraception. This is due to a lack of supplies, cultural and political barriers and poor quality of services.
- Estimated 22 million unsafe abortions each year.
- Approximately 47,000 deaths from unsafe abortion.
- 5 million women suffer injury/disability from unsafe abortion.

Contraceptive targets in the female reproductive tract

In order to prevent pregnancy, contraceptive methods could be developed to target one or a number of key reproductive processes or sites in the male or female reproductive tract. None of the existing methods of contraception are 100% effective at preventing pregnancy. The effectiveness of a method depends on both mechanism of action and correct and consistent use. Compliance depends on acceptability of the method to the user and tolerability with any untoward effects that they experience related to use of the method. Even in high-income countries such as the UK, where contraception is free and a range of methods are readily available, unintended pregnancy rates remain high. Many women who present with an unintended pregnancy have used a method, but it is usually a method of low effectiveness (e.g. condom) or a method that has been used incorrectly or inconsistently (e.g. missed oral contraceptive pills). Uptake of existing methods is limited by their acceptability to women and for many methods discontinuation rates are high.

A woman's choice of contraception is just as likely to be based upon information from media, friends and family, as from a health care professional. The most effective methods of contraception are the long-acting reversible methods of contraception (LARC) – or so called 'fit and forget methods' such as the copper intrauterine device (Cu-IUD), levonorgestrel intrauterine system (LNG-IUS) and progestogen-only implant. Unfortunately, myths and misconceptions amongst both women and health care professionals surrounding use of LARC, are major factors that limit their uptake. Education, dispelling myths and promoting the significant non-contraceptive benefits of LARC methods could improve uptake and continuation, and have the potential to prevent many more unintended pregnancies for more women.

Mechanism of action

The current available methods of contraception work in the following ways:

- Prevent ovulation: this is the mechanism of action of the following methods: combined hormonal methods (pill, patch and vaginal ring), progestogen-only injectables, progestogen-only implant (Nexplanon®), oral emergency contraception, lactational amenorrhoea.
- Prevent sperm reaching the oocyte: female sterilization and male sterilization (vasectomy).
- Prevent an embryo implanting in the uterus: this is a mechanism of action of the Cu-IUD and LNG-IUS.
- Allow sperm into the vagina but poison them: mechanism of action of spermicides.
- Allow sperm into the vagina but block further passage: mechanism of action of diaphragm and cap. Also one of the mechanisms of action of progestogens.
- Prevent sperm entering the vagina:
  - male and female condoms;
  - avoid sex during the fertile time of the cycle;
  - fertility awareness-based methods (FAB).

Efficacy and effectiveness

The efficacy of a method depends on its mechanism of action. However, real-life effectiveness depends on compliance and continuation with the method. Compliance is influenced by the route of administration; some methods are easier to use than others. Continuation with a method depends on the acceptability to the user. The most effective method for a woman (or couple), therefore, is a method that will be used correctly and consistently.

Failure rates during perfect use show how effective methods can be, where perfect use is defined as following the directions for use. Failure rates during typical use show how effective the different methods are during actual use (including inconsistent or incorrect use).

Table 6.1 shows estimates of the probabilities of pregnancy during the first year of typical use of each method (based upon data from the USA). For some methods, such as implants and intrauterine contraceptives, the efficacy is high and proper and consistent use is nearly guaranteed once inserted, that extremely low pregnancy rates are found in all studies. For other methods, such as the oral contraceptive pill and progestogen-only injectable, efficacy is high, but they can potentially be misused (e.g. forgetting to take pills or failure to get repeat injections).

Table 6.1 Percentage of women experiencing an unintended pregnancy within the first year of use with typical use and perfect use

Method	Typical use %	Perfect use %
No method	85	85
Fertility awareness-based methods	24	0.4–0.5
Male condom	18	2
Female diaphragm	12	6
Progestogen-only pill	9	0.3
Combined hormonal contraception*	9	0.3
Progestogen-only injectable	6	0.2
Cu-IUD	0.8	0.6
LNG-IUS	0.2	0.2
Progestogen-only implant	0.05	0.05
Female sterilization	0.5	0.5
Vasectomy	0.15	0.1

Modified From Trussell *et al.* (2014). Cu-IUD, copper intra-uterine device; LNG-IUS, levonorgestrel intrauterine system; * includes combined oral contraceptive pill (COCP), patch and vaginal ring.

Characteristics of the user that determine risk of pregnancy include compliance, age (reducing fertility in late 30s) and frequency of intercourse.

LARC have been defined in the UK as a method that requires administration less than once per month (i.e injectable, implant, intrauterine device [IUD]), although in many other countries, the inject-able is not considered as LARC, but as a 'medium act-ing' method. LARC methods are the most effective as once inserted they do not require any action by the user until they need to be renewed (3 years for the implant Nexplanon® and 5–10 years or longer for IUDs). In contrast, the shorter-acting methods do require compliance by the user (e.g. to take a daily pill, change a weekly patch or use a condom for every act of sex). Unfortunately, reminders to the user such as daily SMS/text about when to take the next pill or letters/phone calls about when the next injectable is due, do not appear to improve compliance with these methods. Discontinuation rates of short-acting meth-ods (pill, patch and ring) and even the progestogen-only injectable, are all high, with approximately one-half of users stopping this method by 1 year. In contrast, discontinuation rates of LARC are lower, with studies reporting that 80% or more of women still use the implant/IUD at 1 year.

LARC methods have 'typical' failure rates within the first 12 months of use that are similar to those of 'perfect' failure rates. In contrast, for short-acting methods typical failure rates are much higher than perfect failure rates. Real life typical failure rates should be used when providing information to women about the effectiveness of a method. The use of simple diagrams can help put effectiveness of a method into context. Without contraception, approximately 85% of couples will conceive within 12 months.

Safety

Most women who use contraception are fit and healthy. However, some health conditions may be associated with real or theoretical risks if a particu-lar contraceptive method affects the health condi-tion. In an attempt to produce a set of international norms for providing contraception to individuals with a range of medical conditions that may contra-indicate a contraceptive method, the World Health Organization (WHO) developed a system address-ing medical eligibility criteria for contraceptive use. The WHO Medical eligibility criteria for contracep-tive use (MEC) is a guidance document that con-tains recommendations for whether or not women with given medical conditions are eligible to use a particular contraceptive method, based upon on evi-dence and also expert consensus opinion. The MEC categories are 1–4 and are shown in *Table 6.2A*. Category 1 includes conditions for which there is no restriction for the use of the method while category 4 includes conditions that represent an unaccept-able health risk if the contraceptive method is used (absolutely contraindicated). *Table 6.2B* shows some MEC 4 conditions for use of the combined hormonal contraception (CHC). For some conditions the MEC category may differ depending on whether the con-dition was pre-existing when the contraceptive was initiated or developed during use of the method. If a woman develops a condition while using a method

Table 6.2A Medical eligibility criteria (modified from WHO)

MEC category	Definition of category
1	A condition for which there is no restriction for the use of the contraceptive method
2	A condition where the advantages of the method generally outweigh the theoretical or proven risks
3	A condition where the theoretical or proven risks generally outweigh the advantages of using the method. The provision of a method requires expert clinical judgement and/or referral to a specialist contraceptive provider, since use of the method is not usually recommended unless other more appropriate methods are not available or not acceptable
4	A condition that represents an unacceptable health risk if the contraceptive method is used

Table 6.2B Examples of WHO medical eligibility criteria category 4 conditions and use of combined hormonal contraception

Age >35 and smoking

Blood pressure >160/100 mmHg

Hypertension with vascular disease

Deep vein thrombosis, current or past

Myocardial infarction, current or past

Cerebrovascular accident, current or past

Multiple serious risk factors for cardiovascular disease

Known thrombogenic mutations

Current breast cancer

Table 6.3 Drugs known to decrease efficacy of hormonal contraception through induction of liver enzymes (oral contraceptive pills, patch, ring and implant)

Type of drug	Liver enzyme induction
Anticonvulsant	Carbamazepine Eslicarbazepine Oxcarbazepine Phenobarbital Phenytoin Primidone Topiramate
Antibiotic	Rifampicin Rifabutin
Antifungal	Griseofulvin
Antiretroviral	**Protease inhibitors** Amprenavir Atazanavir Nelfinavir Lopinavir Saquinavir Ritonavir **Non-nucleoside reverse transcriptase inhibitors** Efavirenz Nevirapine

of contraception, then it is possible that the method contributed to the onset of the condition and she may need to stop using it. However, if a woman with a particular condition (which often makes pregnancy less safe) wishes to start a method of contraception, there may be less of an issue with safety.

Interaction with other medicines

There are a number of medicines (some anticonvulsants, antifungals, antiretrovirals and antibiotics) that induce liver enzymes cytochrome P450, and will reduce the efficacy of hormonal contraception such as CHC pills, patch or ring, progestogen-only implant and progestogen-only pill (POP) (*Table 6.3*). If a woman using enzyme-inducing medication wishes to use one of these hormonal methods, then the consistent use of condoms is also advised. Alternatively, she could consider use of the progestogen-only injectable, Cu-IUD or LNG-IUS, since efficacy of these methods is not affected by drugs that are enzyme inducers. Effectiveness of the combined oral contraceptive pill (COCP) (and all other methods) is not affected by administration of most broad-spectrum antibiotics.

Side-effects

Common side-effects that women report with all hormonal methods are unexpected bleeding, weight gain, headaches, mood swings and loss of libido. Concern about weight gain and women attributing weight gain to hormonal contraception have been shown to be one of the greatest perceived disadvantages of hormonal contraception. With the exception of the progestogen-only injectable in adolescents, there is no good evidence that hormonal methods cause weight gain. There is no evidence that intrauterine methods (Cu-IUD or LNG-IUS) cause weight gain. Furthermore, there is no good evidence that hormonal contraception has adverse effects upon either mood or libido.

Unexpected bleeding is common (15%) when women start a COCP and may settle with time. If not, there is some evidence that changing to a different contraceptive pill with a different dose of hormones may help. If bleeding problems persist for more than 3 months, then current guidelines from the UK would advise investigations to exclude other causes (e.g. cervical conditions such as polyps, chlamydial infection or intrauterine cavity lesions such as submucous fibroids or polyps).

If women using the COCP experience headaches in the pill-free week, then they may benefit from continuing packets of pills to avoid the hormone-free interval. If headaches develop during use of a hormonal method that are severe, frequent or migraine, then changing method of contraception is advisable.

Non-contraceptive health benefits

Hormonal contraceptives may be used for their beneficial side-effects, in which case the risk-benefit ratio changes(Table 6.4). Barrier methods, particularly condoms, protect against sexually transmitted infections.

Acceptability

This determines whether women choose to start a method and whether they continue to use that method. Determinants of method acceptability include: personal characteristics (e.g. age), fertility intentions (e.g. if planning a baby sooner, later or not at all), perceptions of effectiveness, perceptions of safety, fear of side-effects, familiarity with the method, experience of others (e.g. friends and family), ease of use, ease of access including whether or not they need to see a

Table 6.4 Non-contraceptive health benefits of hormonal contraception

Method	Benefit against
LNG-IUS (52 mg)	Heavy menstrual bleeding Endometriosis Adenomyosis Dysmenorrhoea Endometrial protection Simple hyperplasia
Combined hormonal contraception	Heavy menstrual bleeding Irregular menses Hirsutism Acne Premenstrual syndrome Reduces risk of ovarian cancer Reduces risk of endometrial cancer
Progestogen-only injectable (depot medroxyprogesterone acetate)	Heavy menstrual bleeding Endometriosis Dysmenorrhoea

health professional to obtain the method, perceived intrusiveness and non-contraceptive benefits of the method (e.g. reduction in menstrual flow or pain).

Determinants of contraceptive method acceptability

- Personal characteristics (e.g. age).
- Fertility intentions.
- Perceptions of effectiveness.
- Perceptions of safety.
- Fear of side-effects.
- Familiarity.
- Experience of others.
- Ease of use and of access.
- Need to see a health professional.
- Intrusiveness.
- Non-contraceptive benefits.

Practical prescribing

Women considering using a particular method of contraception require clear, accurate information, ideally backed up with written information. The information provided should cover the aspects shown in *Table 6.5*.

Table 6.5 What a woman needs to know before starting a method of contraception

- How to use the method (pill, patch or ring) and what to do when misused (e.g. missed pill)
- Typical failure rates
- Common side-effects
- Health benefits
- Fertility return on stopping
- When she requires review

Methods of contraception

Combined hormonal contraception

CHC methods contain two hormones: an oestrogen and a progestogen. They are available as oral pills, a transdermal patch and as a vaginal ring. They are similar in terms of effectiveness, safety and side-effects. These methods all work by inhibition of ovulation via negative feedback of oestrogen and progestogen on the pituitary, with suppression of follicle-stimulating hormone (FSH) and luteinizing hormone (LH).

Pills

Most of the commonly used COCPs are 'low dose' and contain ethinyl oestradiol in a dose of 15–35 µg (**Figure 6.1**). Some newer pills contain oestradiol valerate or oestradiol hemihydrate, which is more similar in structure to the 'naturally occurring' oestradiol, but confers no other proven benefits.

Most 'traditional' preparations contain 21 pills followed by a 7-day pill-free interval (or 7 placebo tablets in place of a 7-day pill-free interval). Some preparations contain 24 days of pills with a shorter pill-free interval. Preparations are commonly monophasic (i.e. same dose of hormones throughout), but some are phasic (dose varies). There is no advantage of phasic preparations over monophasic preparations. Although traditional 21 days on and 7 days off usually results in a withdrawal bleed during the pill-free interval, there is no reason why women cannot take the pill continuously. Women with dysmenorrhoea or headaches during the pill-free interval, are often advised to do so to avoid recurrence of symptoms during the hormone-free interval by tricycling (taking three packets without any break). Tailored pill use is also often recommended. This is where women continue to take the pill until they want to start a bleeding episode. They then have the pill-free interval at this time.

The progestogens that are used in currently available pills are often referred to as second-generation (levonorgestrel, norethisterone), third-generation (gestodene desogestrel) and fourth-generation progestogens (drospirenone and dienogest). Newer (third-and fourth-generation) progestogens were developed to have advantages due to less androgenic activity, but seem to be associated with a higher risk of venous thrombosis than pills containing second-generation progestogens. In view of this, COCPs containing second-generation progestogens are generally recommended as first choice.

Patch and ring

The combined hormonal transdermal patch releases 33.9 µg ethinyloestradiol/day and norelgestromin 203 µg/day. It is applied to the skin of the lower abdomen, buttock or arm for 7 days, although it can be applied to any skin covered area, except the breast (**Figure 6.2A**). The regimen usually involves application of patches for a total of 21 days followed by a 7-day hormone-free interval. Continued use (tricycling or tailored use) is also possible. Some women may experience problems with patch adherence or skin sensitivity to the patch.

The combined hormonal ring is a flexible ring of 54 mm diameter that releases 15 µg ethinyloestradiol and 120 µg etonorgestrel daily, and as such is the lowest dose combined hormonal method (**Figure 6.2B**). The ring is self inserted and worn in the vagina for 21 days, followed by a 7-day hormone-free interval, during which a withdrawal bleeding occurs. Women should not feel discomfort from the ring and it can be removed

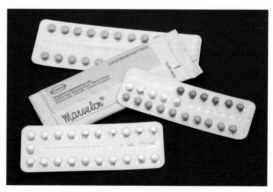

Figure 6.1 The oral contraceptive pill.

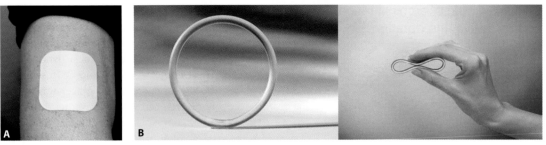

Figure 6.2 A: Combined hormonal patch. **B**: combined hormonal vaginal contraceptive ring.

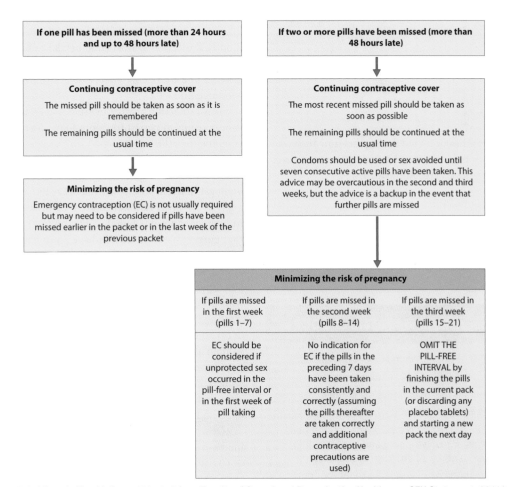

Figure 6.3 Missed pill guidelines. (Adapted from Faculty of Sexual and Reproductive Healthcare, CEU Statement, 2011.)

for a short time (less than 3 hours) and can be cleaned and replaced.

Missed pills, patches and rings

Missed pills are common and if two or more are missed, then this places a woman at risk of ovulation.

Additional contraceptive cover (condoms or abstinence) is required for most monophasic ethinyloestradiol-containing pills during the next 7 days of pill taking (**Figure 6.3**). Additional precautions are also required if a patch is not applied for 48 hours or a ring for more than 3 hours. If unprotected sexual

Table 6.6 Route of administration of contraceptive and duration

Route of currently available contraceptives	Duration
Oral CHC and progestogen	24 hours
Transdermal CHC	7 days
Vaginal ring CHC	21 days
Progestogen-only injectable	14 weeks
Progestogen-only implant	3 years
Cu- IUD	3 years, 5 years, 10 years or more
LNG-IUS	3 years or 5 years or more

CHC, combined hormonal contraception; Cu-IUD, copper intrauterine device; LNG-IUS, levonorgestrel intrauterine system.

intercourse has occurred during this time then there is a risk of pregnancy and so emergency contraception (see below) is recommended.

Length of action

The length of action has an influence on the acceptability and efficacy and is shown in *Table 6.6*.

Safety of CHC

Cancer

Cancer risks among users of COCPs

- A 12% reduction in the risk of any cancer.
- Reduced risk of colorectal cancer.
- Reduced risk of endometrial cancer.
- Reduced risk of ovarian cancer.
- Increased risk of breast cancer during use (decreases on stopping and similar risk to never used by 10 years after stopping).
- Increased risk of cervical cancer (but early changes detected by cervical cytology and human papillomavirus [HPV] vaccination).

Large observational studies have shown that women who are current or ever users of COCPs have a 12% reduction in their risk of death from any cancer. Ever use of oral contraception has been associated with a 46% reduced risk of ovarian cancer compared to never use, and with 10 years use of COCP there is a halving of the risk of ovarian cancer. This protection is also evident for women with a family history of breast cancer (who may be particularly at risk of ovarian cancer). In the same studies, the risk of endometrial cancer was almost halved amongst women who had ever used the contraceptive pill compared to never users. Reduction in the risk of colon cancer was also observed. The reason for this reduction in risk of cancers with contraceptive pill use is not known. Protection against ovarian cancer could be due to the suppression of follicular rupture from the surface of the ovary each month. Protection against endometrial cancer could be due to the progestogen content of the pill, which opposes the mitogenic effects of oestrogen on the endometrium.

This protection against ovarian and endometrial cancer seems to persist for more than 15 years after stopping the pill.

Most (but not all) observational studies have reported an increase in the risk of breast cancer amongst current users of the COCPs. A meta-analysis of observational studies of breast cancer in women and hormonal contraception suggests that current users of COCPs have an increased risk of breast cancer while taking the pill, but that soon after discontinuing this risk diminishes, so that their risk 10 years after stopping is the same as a women who never used the pill. It has been suggested that starting to use the pill may accelerate the appearance of breast cancer in susceptible women. Alternatively, women using the pill might have their tumours diagnosed earlier, although it is difficult to explain why a tendency to earlier diagnosis would persist for years after stopping. Nevertheless, a biological effect of CHC on the breast remains a possibility.

Observational studies have also reported an increase in the risk of cervical cancer amongst users of COCPs. While this may be due to confounding factors such as users being less likely to use condoms (that protect against HPV), a biological association cannot be excluded. However, women can be reassured that participating in a cervical screening programme can detect precancerous cells that can be effectively treated. Having HPV vaccination (against oncogenic HPV subtypes 16 and 18) before sexual activity commences, using condoms and not smoking also reduces the risk of cervical cancer.

Venous thromboembolism and arterial disease

CHC (pill, patch and ring) increases the tendency to thrombosis in both the venous and arterial circulation. The adverse effect on venous thrombosis is related to the dose of oestrogen and appears less with combined pills containing second-generation progestogens compared to those containing third- or fourth-generation progestogens. However, whichever progestogen is used, the absolute risk of venous thromboembolism (VTE) is very small and much less than that associated with pregnancy (see box highlighted below).

Risk of VTE in users and non-users of CHC

- 5 per 10,000 in non-pregnant non users.
- 10 per 10,0000 COCP users.
- 29–400 per 10,0000 in pregnant/postpartum.

The risk of VTE is greatest during the first year of use, possibly due to the unmasking of inherited thrombophilias. Screening for known thrombophilias is not cost effective, but women should be asked about a personal and family history of VTE if considering using this method, as these are contraindications to using a CHC method. Women who are using CHC and making long-distance travel (>3 h of immobility) should take appropriate exercise on the journey and consider wearing graduated compression socks.

Arterial disease is much less common but more serious. It is related to age, and the risk is strongly influenced by smoking. Women over 35 years old who smoke are not eligible to use a CHC method. The combined pill is also contraindicated in women who experience migraine with aura (homonymous hemianopia, unilateral paraesthesia, weakness, aphasia or unclassifiable speech disorder occurring before the headache), since this condition is associated with cerebral vasospasm and women may be at higher risk of stroke if they use a CHC.

Progestogen-only contraceptive methods

Progestogen-only methods are available as oral, injectable, implant and intrauterine system. The mechanism of action of the method and the bleeding pattern appear to depend on the dose of progestogen and also the route of administration.

The injectable, implant and desogestrel-containing POP inhibit ovulation. Lower-dose POP formulations inhibit ovulation only inconsistently. All progestogen-only contraceptive methods, regardless of the route of administration, thicken cervical mucus so reducing sperm penetrability and transport. The levonorgestrel intrauterine system (LNG-IUS) has little effect on ovarian activity but causes marked endometrial atrophy, which prevents implantation if ovulation and fertilization occur.

Progestogen-only pill

Unlike the COCP, the POP needs to be taken continuously. Medium-dose pills (e.g. containing desogestrel) inhibit ovulation in 99% of cycles, but lower-dose pills inhibit ovulation in less than one-half of cycles, relying on the cervical mucus effect for contraception. Side-effects of all POPs include possible irregular bleeding, persistent ovarian follicles (simple cysts) and acne.

If a POP is missed then the woman should continue taking the POP and use extra precautions (e.g. condoms) for the next 48 hours until the progestogen effect on the mucus is built up. If unprotected sex occurs during this time, then emergency contraception is required.

Implant

A single rod (Nexplanon®) containing the progestogen etonorgestrel is the currently available method in the UK. Nexplanon® contains 68 mg of 3-keto-desogestrel (a metabolite of desogestrel) providing contraception for 3 years. The initial release rate of 60–70 μg/day falls gradually to around 25–30 μg/day at the end of 3 years. Implants that are in use in other parts of the world include Uniplant® (single rod, nomegestrol, lasts 1 year) and Jadelle® (two rods, levonorgestrel, lasts 3–5 years).

Nexplanon® is a flexible rod, similar in size to a match stick (40 mm × 2 mm) and is inserted subdermally 8 cm above the medical epicondyle, usually of the non-dominant arm (**Figure 6.4**). Insertion is conducted under local anaesthesia using a specially designed insertion device. Nevertheless, poor insertion technique can still result in deep insertion with

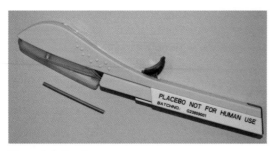

Figure 6.4 Nexplanon.

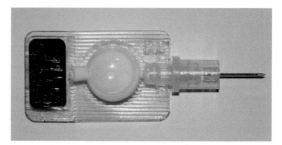

Figure 6.5 Sayana®-press single-dose container.

consequent difficult removal, so insertion should only be conducted by clinicians who have undertaken appropriate training. The implant is not usually visible, but should be easily palpable. Nexplanon® contains a small quantity of barium, which permits it to be visualized by X-ray. It can also be localized using low-frequency ultrasound probes, which can help aid removal of implants that are not easily palpable.

Once inserted, there is no need for any routine follow-up until the device is due for replacement or the user wishes it removed. Nexplanon® releases a steady low dose of progestogen (similar to levels of a POP). After removal, serum levels of etonorgestrel levels are undetectable within 1 week, and fertility is restored immediately after removal.

Progestogen-only injectable

The most commonly used injectable worldwide is a depot injection of medroxyprogesterone acetate, which can be administered intramuscularly (buttock, upper arm, lower abdomen) as the formulation Depoprovera® (150 mg) or subcutaneously as the micronized lower-dose formulation of Sayana press® (104 mg). Both intramuscular and subcutaneous preparations have similar features: same mode of action (inhibition of ovulation), same efficacy, similar injection interval (every 12–14 weeks) and similar bleeding pattern (over 50% amenorrhoea rates at 1 year). Since subcutaneous injections are easier to give, this preparation offers the possibility of training users to self administer, and also increases the range of health care professionals who can give the injection (e.g. trained pharmacists). This can increase access to this method for women, and may increase its acceptability (**Figure 6.5**).

The injectable is the only hormonal method that may delay return of fertility after discontinuation.

In some cases it may take up to 1 year after the last injection for ovulation to return. There is no permanent impairment of fertility but this delay makes the injectable an inappropriate method for women wishing short-term contraception.

Both the intramuscular and subcutaneous preparation may cause weight gain in a minority of women and loss of bone mineral density (BMD) (5% loss of BMD at lumbar spine) in the first few years of use. However, women should be advised that BMD loss seems to plateau, has not been associated with osteoporotic fractures and appears to be reversible on stopping.

There have been concerns over studies from countries of high human immunodeficiency virus (HIV) prevalence (such as sub-Saharan Africa) that have reported increased transmission and acquisition of HIV amongst users of Depoprovera®, compared to users of other hormonal methods. However, users of the injectable are less likely to use condoms that protect against HIV, and so at present, the expert opinion of the WHO is that the injectable can be safely used in women living with HIV or at high risk of HIV. Condom use in addition to the injectable should also be encouraged to protect against transmission or acquisition of HIV.

Progestogen-releasing intrauterine system

The currently available intrauterine systems release the progestogen levonorgestrel into the uterus. There are two LNG-IUS that are available in Europe and the USA. The 52 mg LNG-IUS (Mirena®) (Chapter 4, Disorders of menstrual bleeding, **Figure 4.3**) is licensed for 5 years for contraceptive use (but if inserted in women 45 years or older, may be used for contraception until the menopause) and the 13.5 mg LNG-IUS (known as Jaydess®

in Europe and Skyla® in the USA) is licensed for 3 years for contraceptive use. The 13.5 mg LNG-IUS has a slightly narrower insertion device and it has a shorter frame, which may make insertion easier in young or nulliparous women. The 13.5 mg LNG-IUS also has a silver band at the proximal end, which helps distinguish it from the 52 mg LNG-IUS on ultrasound.

The LNG-IUS works by exerting a potent hormonal effect on the endometrium, which prevents endometrial proliferation and implantation. Its progestogenic effect on thickening the cervical mucus also impedes entry of sperm.

The LNG-IUS does not prevent ovulation. In the first few months of use, many women experience unpredictable bleeding. Women should be advised that this usually improves with time and many women will eventually have lighter or absent periods. Provision of quality information about side-effects in advance of fitting a LNG-IUS is important to reduce unnecessary discontinuation rates. Reported side-effects of the LNG-IUS include acne, breast tenderness, mood disturbance and headaches.

The most notable non-contraceptive benefit of the 52 mg LNG-IUS is that of reducing HMB (reduced by 90% at 12 months). It is more effective than oral treatments, such as norethisterone, the COCP and tranexamic acid, at reducing menstrual blood (see Chapter 4, Disorders of menstrual bleeding). It is also effective for treating dysmenorrhoea, pain associated with endometriosis and adenomyosis and protecting the endometrium against hyperplasia.

Intrauterine contraceptives (Cu-IUD, LNG-IUS)

- Last 3–10 years (or more) depending on type, woman's age at insertion.
- Failure rate less than 1 in 100.
- Prevent fertilization.
- Impair cervical mucus.
- Inhibit implantation.

While the 13.5 mg LNG-IUS is not licensed for use as a treatment for HMB, it does reduce blood loss but is less likely to give amenorrhoea compared to the 52 mg LNG-IUS.

Intrauterine contraception

Intrauterine methods of contraception include the copper intrauterine device Cu-IUD and the LNG-IUS (above).

The Cu-IUD duration of use is between 3 and 10 years, depending on the device used and age of woman at insertion. If a woman has a Cu-IUD inserted at 40 years or above, it can be left *in situ* until the menopause. For women who have a 52 mg LNG-IUS inserted at 45 years or over, the device can be left for contraceptive purposes until the menopause.

There are a number of Cu-IUDs available and they vary in size, shape, copper content and duration of use. Most consist of a plastic frame with copper wire wound around the stem and some may have copper on the arms of the device. The LNG-IUS consists of an elastomere frame with a reservoir on the stem containing levonorgestrel. With both Cu-IUD and LNG-IUS, threads protrude through the cervical canal into the upper vagina to permit easy removal. Once inserted, the effectiveness of IUDs does not rely on the user and so typical failure rates are much lower than the shorter-acting methods of contraception. In addition to routine contraception the Cu-IUD can also be used for emergency contraception.

Research shows that women and health care professionals often lack accurate knowledge and often hold negative misconceptions about IUDs. Evidence suggests that the Cu-IUD and the LNG-IUS do not cause a delay in return to fertility or increase the risk of infertility and women should be advised of this.

Mode of action

IUDs stimulate an inflammatory reaction in the uterus. The concentration of macrophages and leucocytes, prostaglandins and various enzymes in both uterine and tubal fluid increase significantly. It is thought that these effects are toxic to both sperm and egg and interfere with sperm transport. If a healthy fertilized egg reaches the uterine cavity, implantation is inhibited.

Bleeding pattern with IUD

Although women with the LNG-IUS tend to experience lighter, less painful menses, women using the

Cu-IUD may experience more painful or heavier menses. The use of a non-steroidal anti-inflammatory drug at menses may help lessen the pain and blood loss. Tranexamic acid during menses may also reduce blood loss with a CU-IUD. Alternatively a woman could switch to a LNG-IUS.

Women using an IUD should be informed that their overall risk of ectopic pregnancy is much reduced compared with women who are using no contraception. However, if a pregnancy does occur with an IUD *in situ* then the 'relative' risk of that pregnancy being ectopic is higher. If women become pregnant with an IUD *in situ*, an ultrasound scan should be conducted to exclude ectopic pregnancy. It is generally advisable that IUDs should be removed before 12 weeks' gestation in view of the greater risk of miscarriage, preterm delivery, septic abortion and chorioamnionitis if the device is left *in situ*. Although there is a theroretical concern about teratogenicity if a pregnancy is exposed to the LNG-IUS, to date no birth defects have been reported in the small number of cases exposed.

Insertion of IUD

An IUD can be fitted at any point in the cycle provided there is no risk of pregnancy. Insertion is associated with the following risks:

- **Perforation**. Uterine perforation with insertion of an IUD is rare: approximately 1 in 1,000. Factors associated with an increased risk of perforation include relative inexperience of clinician, breastfeeding and being less than 6 months postpartum. Usually the woman presents with 'missing threads' and a history of severe pain following insertion. An ultrasound of the uterus confirms no IUD is seen in the uterus and an abdominal X-ray shows an IUD. Laparoscopic retrieval of the device from the pelvis (often attached to omentum) is possible in most cases, but laparotomy may rarely be required to remove the IUD.
- **Expulsion**. 1 in 20 IUD devices will be expelled in the first 3 months after insertion. After this, the risk of expulsion diminishes. Given that some expulsions are not always obvious to women, IUD users should be advised to perform regular self checks for the presence of threads in the upper vagina to ensure the device is still present.

- **Infection**. The overall risk of pelvic infection in the first 3 weeks following insertion of an IUD is low (1 in 100). Thereafter, the risk of infection is the same as women not using contraception. In most cases, the IUD can be left *in situ* and antibiotic therapy commenced. If the IUD is removed then the clinician should provide oral emergency contraception if required (i.e. due to recent unprotected sex). Actimomyces-like organisms (ALOs) are commonly identified on cervical smears in women with and without an IUD. The role of ALOs in infection in IUD users is not clear. If a woman with an IUD has ALOs but has no symptoms of infection, then the IUD can be left *in situ*. However, if ALOs are present and a woman with an IUD has symptoms of infection, then the device should be removed and penicillin-based antibiotics given. In addition, women with symptoms of pelvic infection with an IUD should be tested for sexually-transmitted infections (STIs). In order to minimize risk of pelvic infection, screening women at risk of STIs before insertion is advised. Prophylactic antibiotics (at least to cover chlamydia) can be given to women at high risk of infection if insertion needs to be done before results of tests are known (e.g. Cu-IUD insertion for emergency contraception).
- **'Missing' threads**. 'Missing' threads may indicate pregnancy, expulsion or perforation. However, it is often the case that the threads are merely sitting in the cervical canal or uterus. A pregnancy test should be performed and emergency contraception/alternative contraception provided until the IUD can be confirmed to be *in situ*, either by visualization of the threads on speculum examination or an ultrasound confirming presence of the IUD within the uterus.

Barrier contraception

Condoms

Male condoms are cheap and widely available. They protect against STIs including HIV. They are the only reversible male method. Typical failure rates are in the region of 24% since they rely on the user to put it on it correctly, before penetration and before every act of sex. The female condom is a lubricated polyurethane condom that is inserted into the vagina. It also protects against STIs (**Figure 6.6**).

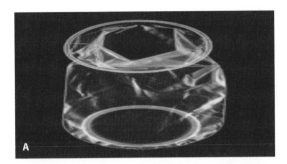

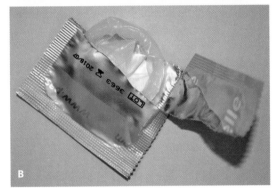

Figure 6.6 **A**: Female condom; **B**: male condom.

Diaphragm and cap

These are latex or non-latex devices that are inserted into the vagina to prevent passage of sperm to the cervix (**Figure 6.7**). They can be inserted in advance of sex. Caps fit over the cervix whereas diaphragms form a hammock between the post-fornix and the symphysis pubis. Caps and diaphragms are often used in conjunction with a spermicide. Disadvantages are that women need to be taught how to insert and remove the device and typical failure rates in the region of 18% are reported. In some women their use may be associated with increased vaginal discharge and urinary tract infections.

Spermicides

Spermicide alone is not recommended for prevention of pregnancy as it is of low effectiveness. Nonoxynol 9 (N-9) is a spermicidal product sold as a gel, cream, foam, sponge or pessary for use with diaphragms or caps. Some data have suggested that frequent use of N-9 might increase the risk of HIV transmission. It is therefore no longer recommended for women who are at high risk of HIV infection.

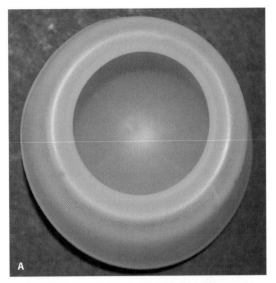

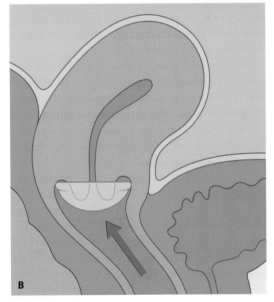

Figure 6.7 **A**: The cap; **B**: correct siting of a cap.

Female sterilization

This is a permanent method of contraception that prevents sperm reaching the oocyte in the Fallopian tube. It can be performed by (1) laparoscopy, (2) hysteroscopy or (3) laparotomy (e.g. at caesarean section).

Laparoscopic sterilization

Laparoscopic sterilization most commonly occludes the Fallopian tube with filshie clips (**Figure 6.8**). Effective contraception should be used until the next

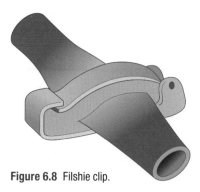

Figure 6.8 Filshie clip.

> ▶ **eResource 6.1**
>
> Laparoscopic sterilization
> http://www.routledgetextbooks.com/textbooks/
> tenteachers/gynaecologyv6.1.php

menses after the procedure, due to the risk of pregnancy from implantation of an early fertilized egg in the same cycle as sterilization.

Women who pose a higher surgical risk due to obesity or previous abdominal surgery, for example, may be better suited to the hysteroscopic approach.

Women who are requesting sterilization at the same time as having a caesarean section must be counselled and give consent for this well in advance of this procedure.

Since sterilization results in permanent loss of fertility and involves a surgical procedure, it is important that valid consent is obtained. Individuals would be deemed unable to consent if it is clear that having been provided with appropriate support and information they cannot comprehend, retain, assess or use the information provided to them to make a decision. In such cases, legal advice should be sought.

> **Advice to women considering sterilization**
>
> - Method is considered as irreversible.
> - Failure rate 1:200 for laparoscopic, 1:500 for hysteroscopic (comparable to long-acting reversible methods).
> - Risks and complications (laparoscopic 1:1,000 risk of trauma to bowel, bladder or blood vessels).
> - Vasectomy is safer, quicker, safer and with less morbidity.

- High proportion of women regret sterilization. Risk factors are age under 30 years, nulliparity, recent pregnancy (birth, abortion, miscarriage) and relational issues.
- Does not protect against STIs.
- Effective contraception is required until the menstrual period following laparoscopic procedure or 3 months following hysteroscopic procedure.
- Pregnancy following female sterilization is rare but if it does occur there is an increased risk of ectopic.
- Reversal of sterilization is a highly-skilled procedure to obtain tubal reanastomosis. It cannot be performed after hysteroscopic sterilization, and if it is successfully conducted after laparoscopic sterilization, then it is associated with an increased risk of ectopic pregnancy.

Hysteroscopic sterilization

This has the advantage that it can be performed as an outpatient procedure without general anaesthesia. Microinserts (Essure®), which are expanding springs (of 2 mm diameter and 4 cm in length) made of titanium, steel and nickel-containing Dacron fibres, are inserted into the tubal ostia via a hysteroscope (**Figure 6.9**). These induce fibrosis within the cornual section of each Fallopian tube over the following 3 months. Contraception is required during the 3 months and can only be discontinued once correct placement of the inserts are confirmed by X-ray imaging or ultrasound.

Vasectomy

This is the technique of interrupting the vas deferens to provide permanent occlusion. The so-called 'no scalpel' vasectomy involves a puncture wound in the skin of the scrotum under local anaesthesia to access and then divide and occlude the vas using cautery (**Figure 6.10**).

There is a small risk of a scrotal haematoma and infection with the procedure. Postvasectomy semen analysis should be conducted at 12 weeks to confirm the absence of spermatozoa in the ejaculate.

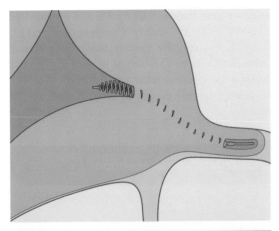

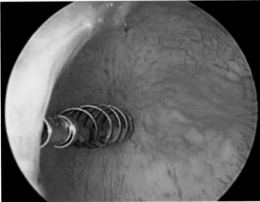

Figure 6.9 Essure® hysteroscopic sterilization. (Courtesy of Justin Clark.)

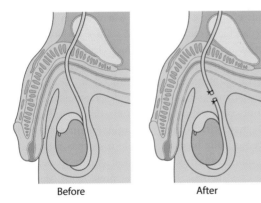

Before   After

Figure 6.10 Vasectomy.

Alternative contraception should be used until azoospermia is confirmed. The failure rate is significantly less than female sterilization at approximately 1 in 2,000.

Fertility awareness-based methods (FAB)

Formerly known as 'natural family planning', FAB rely on the signs and symptoms that reflect the physiological changes that occur during the menstrual cycle that define the fertile period, with avoidance of intercourse at that time. Use of FAB requires motivation and a regular menstrual cycle, and so cannot be used for women at extremes of reproductive age. Typical failure rates are high.

The method depends on the use of one or more of the following indicators to enable avoidance of intercourse during the fertile days.

Calendar or rhythm method

Fertile days are calculated based upon the cycle length recorded over at least six cycles. First fertile day = shortest cycle minus 20. Last fertile day = longest cycle minus 10. For women with a 28-day cycle this equates to abstinence for 10 days in each cycle (i.e. day 8–18).

Temperature method

This relies on the increase in basal body temperature (0.2–0.4C) produced by the rise in progesterone following ovulation. Daily temperatures must be measured using the same route. Infection, exercise and some medications can affect body temperature and interfere with this method.

Cervical mucus method

Mucus on toilet tissue after wiping the vulva can be examined for consistency. Midcycle 'fertile' mucus due to rising oestradiol levels is clear, watery and slippery rather like raw egg white. Following ovulation, progesterone renders it thick and opaque. Semen in the vagina may make it difficult to recognize the mucus.

Cervical palpation

At midcycle, the cervix rises 1–2 cm and feels softer and moist.

Personal fertility monitor

This hand-held monitor analyses diposable urine dipsticks that record the presence of metabolites of oestrogen and LH in the urine. It recognizes urinary oestrogen concentrations corresponding to the midfollicular phase of the cycle and the preovulatory LH peak, so that the beginning and end of the fertile phase can be identified. A red light indicates fertile phase (risk of conception) and green, infertile. Users need to perform urine dipstick tests on early morning urine. A red light is usually shown for 6–10 days in the cycle.

Lactational amenorrhoea

If a mother is within the first 6 months postpartum, is amenorrhoeic and is fully or nearly fully breastfeeding, then the risk of pregnancy is about 2%. After 6 months, or if menses occur or breastfeeding reduced, then another method of contraception must be used.

Emergency contraception

All women deserve a second chance to prevent an unintended pregnancy.

The Cu-IUD is the most effective method of emergency contraception (EC) available (failure rate 1 in 1,000) and should ideally be offered as first choice to women. When used for EC, its effect on the endometrium is thought to prevent implantation if fertilization has occurred. The Cu-IUD can be removed once pregnancy has been excluded or can be left in place for ongoing contraception. Since the blastocyst will implant between 6 and 10 days after fertilization, an emergency Cu-IUD can be inserted up to 5 days after the unprotected sex or 5 days after predicted ovulation (i.e. in a 28-day cycle, predicted ovulation day 14 plus 5 days = insert up to day 19 for EC) in order to avoid disrupting an implanted pregnancy. There is no evidence that the LNG-IUS is effective as EC and should therefore not be used for this purpose.

The two oral methods of EC that are licensed for use are levonorgestrel (LNG 1.5 mg) and the progesterone receptor modulator uliprstal acetate (30 mg). LNG appears effective up to 96 hours after unprotected sex and uliprstal acetate for up to 120 hours. Both methods work by delaying ovulation, so that any sperm present in the reproductive tract will have lost the ability to fertilize the oocyte once it is eventually released. Oral EC is much less

effective than the Cu-IUD for EC and is estimated to prevent only two-thirds of pregnancies. Oral EC is much less effective than regular contraception. Women should be encouraged to start an effective method of contraception immediately after EC, to protect against pregnancy from further acts of intercourse.

Emergency contraception

- The most effective method of EC is an IUD (about 99% effective).
- An IUD can be inserted up to 5 days after ovulation for EC.
- Uliprstal acetate (UPA) or levonorgestrel (LNG) are available as oral methods of EC.
- UPA can be given within 120 hours of unprotected intercourse.
- LNG can be used within 96 hours of unprotected intercourse.
- Effective ongoing contraception should be started after EC.

Opportunities to provide contraception

There are important opportunities to discuss and provide effective contraception when women present to gynaecology clinics (Table 6.7). These include presentation to a general gynaecology clinic, presentations for EC, presentation to request an induced abortion and also antenatally or after childbirth. The antenatal/postpartum period is a particularly important opportunity since 95% of postpartum women want to avoid pregnancy in the next 12 months, and in women who are not fully breastfeeding, fertility may return at 1 month postpartum. In addition, closely-spaced pregnancies increase the risks of preterm delivery, low birthweight and small for gestational age babies. The risk of child mortality is highest for very short birth to pregnancy intervals (<12 months). It is estimated that 30% of maternal and 10% of child deaths worldwide could be prevented if couples space pregnancies more than 2 years apart.

Table 6.7 Opportunities to provide contraception

Opportunity	Rationale
Gynaecology clinic	Gynaecological benefits of many hormonal methods of contraception
Emergency contraception	Two- to threefold higher risk of unintended pregnancy if women have further unprotected sex in same cycle Cu-IUD can be used for EC and provide ongoing contraception
Request for induced abortion	Most women ovulate in the month following an abortion Women who choose to start a LARC method at the time of abortion have a significantly reduced risk of a further abortion in the next few years
Antenatal/postpartum	50% of women resume sex by 6 weeks after childbirth Non-breastfeeding women may ovulate at day 21

Cu-IUD, copper intrauterine device; EC, emergency contraception; LARC, long-acting reversible methods of contraception.

The future

Given the wide range of existing contraceptive methods and delivery systems (pill, patch, ring, injectable, intrauterine) and hormonal methods with established safety, the question is often posed: Do we need new methods of contraception?

We should remember that even in high-income countries, unintended pregnancy rates remain high. Uptake of existing methods is limited by their acceptability to women, and for many methods discontinuation rates are high. As science advances our understanding of reproductive physiology, women should be able to benefit from more sophisticated methods of contraception that may be devoid of side-effects and offer more health benefits (such as protection against STIs or breast cancer). It is also important that male methods are developed, since they are currently limited to condoms or vasectomy.

KEY LEARNING POINTS

- In sexually active women, contraception is required until a woman reaches the menopause (or at the age of 55 years).
- The long-acting reversible methods of contraception (LARC) are currently the most effective methods, with typical failure rates close to perfect failure rates.
- Uptake of contraception and continuation is limited by acceptability to the user.
- If no contraceptive method is used, or a method fails, then women need easy access to EC.

Abortion

No method of contraception is perfect and so there will always be the need for safe abortion. Safe abortion saves mothers' lives and prevents the severe morbidity associated with unsafe abortion. Modern methods of inducing an abortion are safer than all common gynaecological operations, such as sterilization and hysterectomy, and there is a lower risk of dying than during childbirth. There is evidence that liberalization of abortion laws does NOT lead to more abortions. Restricting access to abortion simply leads to unsafe abortion, with consequent death of the women or severe morbidity.

UK abortion law

The 1967 Abortion Act states that abortion can be performed if two registered medical practitioners acting in good faith agree that the pregnancy should be terminated on one of the recognized legal grounds (*Table 6.8*). There is actually no medical need for two doctors to be involved, and the British Medical Association Ethics Committee have argued that the law should be changed to reflect this. Any medical practitioner who has an objection to abortion is not required to participate in

Table 6.8 UK legal grounds for termination of pregnancy

Ground A	Continuance of the pregnancy would involve risk to the life of the pregnant woman greater than if the pregnancy were terminated
B	Termination is necessary to prevent grave permanent injury to the physical or mental health of the pregnant woman
C	Pregnancy has not exceeded its 24th week and continuance of the pregnancy would involve risk, greater than if the pregnancy were terminated, of injury to the physical or mental health of the pregnant woman
D	Pregnancy has not exceeded its 24th week and continuance of the pregnancy would involve risk, greater than if the pregnancy were terminated, of injury to the physical or mental health of any existing child(ren) of the family of the pregnant woman
E	There is a substantial risk that if the child were born, it would suffer from such physical or mental abnormalities as to be seriously handicapped
F	To save the life of the pregnant woman
G	To prevent grave permanent injury to the physical or mental health of the pregnant woman

Table 6.9 Preabortion investigations

Recommended	Consider
Gestation assessment – ultrasound (or clinical assessment if unavailable)	STI testing – chlamydia, gonorrhoea, HIV, syphilis
Rhesus status – Anti-D required for non-immunized rhesus negative	Full blood count – determine if anaemic

HIV, human immunodeficiency virus; STI, sexually-transmitted infection.

abortion services, unless the treatment is necessary to save the life of the pregnant woman. However, a medical practitioner who conscientiously objects to abortion should still provide advice and refer a woman promptly to another doctor who does not hold such views.

The 1967 Abortion Act does not apply to Northern Ireland, where abortion is only legal in exceptional circumstances to save the life of the mother. There is continuing debate within Northern Ireland about introducing legislative change. However, at present women in Northern Ireland need to travel to other parts of the UK for abortion or continue an unintended pregnancy. This is also the situation for women living in the rest of Ireland. In recent years, women living in Ireland (and other parts of the world where abortion is not legal or access is severely restricted) have risked

imprisonment and have used the Internet to obtain medical advice from other countries and to purchase the medical abortion drugs needed to induce an early medical abortion.

The vast majority (>95%) of all abortions in the UK are carried out under Ground C (*Table 6.8*), with approximately 1% carried out for serious fetal abnormality (Ground E). With the exception of emergency abortion to save the mother's life or severe fetal abnormality, the upper legal limit for abortion is 24 weeks (23 completed weeks), which reflects fetal viability as a result of improvement in neonatal care. Delivery of abortion services varies between countries in the UK.

The Royal College of Obstetricians and Gynaecologists (RCOG) guideline on the care of women requesting an abortion recommends that services should be organized so as to minimize delay. At early gestations, medical methods can be used with greatest efficacy, and there is less pain and bleeding and lowest risk of complications. Most women requesting an abortion are certain of their decision and so routine counselling for decision making is not required. However, women who are uncertain should be offered sympathetic non-directional support in decision making. No woman should be subjected to compulsory counselling. The RCOG has also advised on the tests that are required as part of the preabortion work-up and of those that are not necessary but that can be offered (*Table 6.9*).

Methods of abortion

Neither medical nor surgical abortion is a complex procedure and both have a very low rate of complications. Indeed, the WHO advise that in the first trimester it can be safely performed by a range of health care providers, from a specialist obstetrician/gynaecologist to a non-specialist doctor or an appropriately trained nurse or midwife (if country legislation permits this). Both medical and surgical methods can be used to induce abortion throughout pregnancy. The choice of method used depends on factors such as the gestation, pre-existing medical conditions, preference of the woman and local availability of a skilled surgeon.

Medical abortion

The majority of women undergoing abortion in the UK (as in other countries where medical methods are available) choose to have abortion performed medically. This involves the combination of mifepristone (a progesterone receptor modulator) followed by a prostaglandin analogue, misoprostol.

Progesterone is necessary to maintain uterine quiescence, so administration of mifepristone (oral) brings about an increase in uterine contractility. It also sensitizes the uterus to exogenous prostaglandins. This permits lower doses of misoprostol to be used to bring about expulsion. The effect of mifepristone is maximal at 48 hours so that if misoprostol is administered at an interval of 24–48 hours later, then there is an increase in cramping pain, bleeding and expulsion of the fetus through the slightly dilated cervix. In the first 9 weeks of pregnancy, women can safely self-administer these medications at home (if the country legislation permits) and expel the pregnancy at home. Simple oral analgesia (e.g. ibuprofen, dihydrocodeine) is usually sufficient to provide pain relief. Women can be advised that at 9 weeks' gestation they will bleed for on average 2 weeks following the medical abortion.

After 9 weeks' gestation, the same combination of mifepristone and misoprostol is used, except that the regimen requires repeated doses of misoprostol to be administered every 3 hours until expulsion occurs. After 9 weeks' gestation, the discomfort, increased bleeding and passage of a larger fetus mean that women are managed in a clinical setting. In the second trimester, the average induction to abortion time (from first dose of misoprostol to expulsion) is 7 hours.

After 21 completed weeks (i.e. 21 weeks and 6 days) the RCOG recommends that for women undergoing medical abortion, feticide should be used to eliminate the possibility of the aborted fetus displaying any signs of life. This is usually conducted by intracardiac injection of potassium chloride or an intrafetal or intramniotic injection of digoxin. The neural pathways necessary to experience pain are not fully developed in the fetus until after 24 weeks.

Surgical methods

Vacuum aspiration

Vacuum aspiration is the method that should be used to conduct a surgical termination of pregnancy up to 14 weeks. The procedure involves gently dilating the cervix with graduated dilators (usually to the size in mm that the uterus is in weeks' gestation) and then evacuating the cavity with gentle suction. This usually takes less than 10 minutes to perform. Sharp curettage should never be performed (increased risk of perforation and intrauterine adhesions). Vacuum aspiration can be performed either using a manual handheld aspirator (manual vacuum aspiration, MVA) or using electrical vacuum aspiration (EVA). There is little to choose between MVA and EVA. The MVA may be more practical and portable for use in the outpatient setting. The EVA gives a more constant suction.

Surgical termination can be performed under either local or general anaesthesia. Local anaesthesia in the first trimester is preferred as it minimizes any small risk of anaesthestic drugs. It is important to consider pretreatment of the cervix with misoprostol for all women undergoing surgical abortion. The use of misoprostol has been shown to bring about cervical dilation and so makes instrumental cervical easier and minimizes the risk of incomplete abortion. As a minimum, pretreatment should always be used after 12 weeks' gestation or in women in whom cervical dilation may be anticipated to be more difficult (e.g. nulliparous, adolescent, previous cervical surgery). The optimal regimen for cervical pretreatment is 400 µg misoprostol given sublingually 1 hour prior to the surgical procedure.

It is recommended that prophylactic antibiotics should be given (periabortal) with surgical abortion, since this has been shown to significantly reduce the risk of postabortal infection following this procedure. Prophylactic antibiotics are not considered necessary following medical abortion, since the overall incidence of postabortal infection is lower after medical than after surgical abortion.

Dilation and evacuation

After 14 weeks, the surgical technique of choice is dilation and evacuation. In skilled hands, this procedure has a low complication rate and is highly acceptable to women. It is widely used in North America, but is less common in Europe. It is necessary to achieve good cervical dilation before the procedure (up to 20 mm) in order to remove larger fetal parts. This is achieved using one or a combination of either osmotic dilators (hygroscopic sticks placed in the cervix several hours preprocedure that absorb fluid from surrounding tissues, causing them to swell and bring about cervical dilation), or misoprostol (vaginal or sublingual) or mifepristone (oral). At surgery, the cervix is then further dilated using graduated dilators and the contents of the uterus removed by a combination of aspiration and extraction of fetal tissue using appropriate instruments; ultrasound is performed to confirm complete evacuation.

Sequelae of abortion

Both medical and surgical abortion are safe with a low incidence of complications. Complications when they do occur include failure to end the pregnancy (ongoing pregnancy), incomplete abortion requiring evacuation, infection and haemorrhage. In the absence of a serious complication (such as operative complication or severe infection), there is no impact on future reductive potential. There is no association with future infertility or ectopic pregnancy. While several studies have suggested an increased risk of preterm delivery following abortion, findings of recent studies have suggested that modern medical and surgical methods of inducing abortion are not associated with this risk.

There is no association with breast cancer. There is no adverse effect on mental health, although women with an existing history of mental health are at increased risk of exacerbation postabortion, as they are postpartum. Women for whom the pregnancy was originally intended, women who are unsupported, women who are ambivalent about the decision to terminate or who belong to a group that feels that abortion is morally wrong, are at higher risk of ongoing distress or regret following the procedure. Women should be given information on how to seek help under such circumstances.

Follow-up after abortion

There is no medical need for a follow-up after an uncomplicated abortion. Rather, women should be provided with good verbal and written advice about signs and symptoms that might indicate the need to seek medical attention, together with access to a 24-hour emergency care. Women should also be provided with their chosen method of ongoing contraception at the time of the abortion procedure. For women who have had an early medical abortion at home, there should be an effective method of confirming success of the abortion. This could be a scheduled ultrasound (to exclude ongoing pregnancy) or a self-performed urine pregnancy test at home in combination with/without a telephone call from the provider to determine the result of the pregnancy test and confirm that the woman has had expected duration of bleeding and that symptoms of pregnancy have disappeared.

Postabortal contraception

Most women ovulate in the first month after the abortion, and more than one-half of women will have resumed sex by 2 weeks postabortion. Effective contraception should therefore be commenced immediately if women want to avoid another unintended pregnancy.

There is evidence that women who choose to use the most effective LARC postabortion (and start these immediately after the abortion) have a significantly reduced risk of having a subsequent unintended pregnancy, compared to women choosing other methods. There has been much effort in recent years in ensuring abortion services provide high-quality information about contraception and are able to provide all methods at the time of discharge following the procedure (including provision of LARC). All methods (including hormonal and intrauterine) can be safely commenced at the time of abortion. Intrauterine methods can be inserted at the time of surgical abortion, and following expulsion of the fetus at medical abortion.

Further reading

Faculty of Sexual and Reproductive Healthcare, Clinical Effectiveness Unit Guideline (2015). Problematic bleeding with hormonal contraception. www.fsrh.org.

Trussell J (2014). Contraceptive efficacy. *Glob Libr Womens Med* [last accessed 06.05.14], ISSN: 1756-2228, http://dx.doi.org/10.3843/GLOWM10375. This chapter was last updated, http://www.glowm.com/section_view/item/374; 2014.
World Health Organization (2015). *Medical Eligibility Criteria for Contraceptive Use*, 5th edn. Geneva: WHO; www.WHO.org.

Self assessment

CASE HISTORY

A 44-year-old woman requests sterilization as she does not want any more children. She has three children. Her partner will not consider a vasectomy. She has regular but heavy menses. She is currently using no method of contraception. She smokes and suffers from migraine.

A What are the key points to cover in the counselling on sterilization?
B What alternative methods of contraception might be appropriate for this woman?
C What methods of contraception is she not medically eligible for?

ANSWERS

A Important points to cover are that sterilization should be considered as irreversible, that it has a failure rate of approx 1:200 and that it is a surgical procedure with associated risks and complications. It is no more effective than long-acting reversible methods. Also, pregnancy following female sterilization is rare but if it does occur there is an increased risk of ectopic, and reversal of sterilization is a highly-skilled procedure to obtain tubal reanastomosis. It cannot be performed after hysteroscopic sterilization and if it is successfully conducted after laparoscopic sterilization, then it is associated with an increased risk of ectopic pregnancy.

B The LNG-IUS provides comparable contraceptive effectiveness, and also has the non-contraceptive benefit of reduced menstrual blood loss. Other progestogen-only methods such as POP or implant may also be appropriate, but irregular bleeding is common and POP has higher typical failure rates. The injectable could also be considered.

C CHCis contraindicated since the woman is a smoker who is over 35 years and also has migraine. The Cu-IUD is not ideal since this may exacerbate the existing heavy menses.

EMQ

Characteristics of contraceptive methods

A UPA.
B Progestogen-only injectable.
C COCP.
D Cu-IUD.

E LNG-IUS.
F Progestogen-only implant.
G Lactational amenorrhoea.
H Diaphragm.

For each description below choose the SINGLE most appropriate answer from the above list of options. Each option may be used once, more than once or not at all.

1 Which is the most effective emergency contraceptive available?

2 Can delay return to fertility on discontinuation.

3 Is associated with typical failure rates of 12 per 100 in the first 12 months.

4 Main mode of action is prevention of fertilization.

ANSWERS

1D Cu-IUD. But must be used within 5 days of predicted ovulation.

2B Progestogen-only injectable. Irregular bleeding and involution can persist for several months.

3C COCP. This figure should be known as the COCP is frequently prescribed and patients need to know the risk of failure.

4D Cu-IUD. Through the effect of spermicide as well as thickened cervical mucus.

SBA QUESTIONS

1 A 19-year-old woman who previously had a medical abortion attends a clinic requesting contraception. She is overweight and has acne but has no other medical history of note. Her mother had a deep vein thrombosis (DVT) after childbirth.

Which of the following is not a suitable method for her? Choose the single best answer.

A Depoprovera.

B POP.

C CHC patch.

D LNG-IUS.

E Progestogen-only implant.

ANSWER

C The family history of DVT in a first-degree relative is a contraindication to all CHC methods.

2 A 29-year-old female presents requesting contraception. She is known to have polycystic ovary syndrome and struggles with acne and hirsutism. She would like to have a baby in 12 months time. She has no other medical conditions and is fit and healthy.

What would be the best contraceptive option for her? Choose the single best answer.

A IUD.

B Progestogen-only implant.

C COCP.

D Progestogen-only injectable.

E IUS.

ANSWER

C COCP will provide non-contraceptive benefit for acne and hirsutism because it causes an increase in sex hormone-binding globulin (SHBG), which reduces free testosterone. There is no delay of return to fertility.

The other choices would provide good contraception but no improvement in PCOS symptoms.

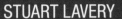

CHAPTER

Subfertility | 7

STUART LAVERY

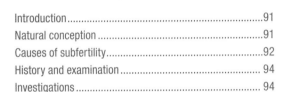

LEARNING OBJECTIVES

- Understand the definition and causes of subfertility.
- Describe the concept of ovarian reserve.
- Understand the history, examination and investigations relevant to subfertility.
- Understand the provision and regulation of fertility treatment.
- Explain the processes and procedures involved in assisted reproductive treatment (ART).
- Understand the outcomes and success rates of ART.

Introduction

A delay in conception is one of the commonest reasons that a woman will consult her doctor. There is no one universal definition of subfertility, but the commonest accepted definition is a failure to conceive after 12 months of regular unprotected intercourse. The incidence of subfertility is thought to affect about one in seven heterosexual couples. There has been a small increase in the prevalence of reported infertility, and a larger number of couples accessing treatment services over the last 10 years in the UK. This may be related to an increased acceptance of fertility treatments and a reduction in couples resigning themselves to childlessness. The diagnosis of subfertility in a couple may be primary in couples that have never conceived together, or secondary in couples that have previously conceived together (although either partner may have conceived in a different relationship, which requires further elucidation). The approach to fertility investigation and management should always be couple-centred. Specialist teams should be available to offer evidence-based advice and treatment to couples, supported by counselling services and accurate information.

Natural conception

A healthy couple having frequent intercourse have about an 18–20% chance of conceiving in a single menstrual cycle. As a species this makes us relatively infertile. There is of course a cumulative increase in pregnancy rates over time as couples try for conception. Within 6 months 70% of couples will have conceived, after 12 months 80% and after 24 months 90% of couples will achieve a pregnancy (**Figure 7.1**). The most important factor affecting fertility is female age, which is related to a decline in the quality and quantity of eggs. Female fertility tends to fall sharply over the age of 36, with a further dip after the age of 40. However, there is a considerable variation and biological age (or ovarian reserve) does not always precisely correlate with chronological age. Male age is also an important factor; semen quality tends to fall in men over the age of 50, while frequency of intercourse tends to fall in men over the age of 40.

Both frequency and timing of sexual intercourse impact strongly on the chance of conceiving naturally. Couples having intercourse three times a week are three times more likely to conceive than couples having intercourse once a week. Maximum 'efficiency' is probably intercourse at least every alternate day. There should, however, be awareness among physicians and patients of the added stress and anxiety that 'overmedicalizing' this advice can bring to couples. Increased frequency of intercourse should be encouraged in the periovulatory period. Eggs are thought to be fertilizable for about 12–24 hours postovulation, while sperm can survive in the female reproductive tract for up to 72 hours. Ovulation usually occurs about 14 days prior to menstruation, with the luteal phase being relatively stable at this length. The 'fertile window' for women will, therefore, be different depending on the average length of their menstrual cycle (e.g. for a woman with a 28-day menstrual cycle, her optimal fertile window will be between days 12 and 15).

External factors may influence the chance of conception. There is now strong evidence that smoking can decrease the quality and quantity of eggs and sperm. The role of alcohol and caffeine remains controversial, and there is no compelling evidence to totally abstain from these while trying to conceive, but moderation is probably sensible. Body mass index (BMI) exerts a strong influence on fertility, with male and female BMI at both the high and low extremes associated with a reduced chance of conceiving. However, there is little evidence for so-called fertility diets to improve natural fertility. Stress can have a direct influence on the hypothalamic–pituitary–ovarian (HPO) axis, interfering with regular ovulation, and may indirectly reduce conception by reducing libido and frequency of intercourse.

All women trying to conceive should commence taking folic acid to reduce fetal neural tube defects.

Causes of subfertility

The main causes of subfertility will vary in different countries. In the UK around 30% of subfertility is caused by male factor, 30% female factor, 25% unexplained and 15% both male and female or other causes. This can be further broken down into causes (some of which are male, some female) as shown in **Figure 7.2**.

Female subfertility

Ovulatory disorders, tubal damage and uterine disorders (e.g. fibroids) are the most common causes with endometrial pathology, specific gamete or embryo defects and endometriosis contributory. Cigarette smoking reduces fertility. General medical conditions such as diabetes, epilepsy, thyroid disorders and bowel disease can also reduce the chance of conception. Decreased ovarian reserve and age are major factors in reduced female fertility.

Ovulatory disorders

The commonest cause of problems with ovulation is polycystic ovary syndrome (PCOS) (see Chapter 3, Hormonal control of the menstrual cycle and hormonal disorders). Women with PCOS who suffer from oligomenorrhoea due to anovulation may require treatment. However, the hormonal treatments taken by women to regulate their periods or help hirsutism may be incompatible with getting pregnant (e.g. the combined oral contraceptive pill).

Hypothalamic disorders (e.g. hypothalamic hypogonadism), pituitary disease (e.g. hyperprolactinaemia) and endocrine abnormalities (thyroid disease) are less common causes due to anovulation.

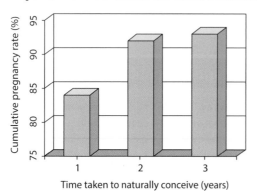

Figure 7.1 The natural conception rate over a 3-year period.

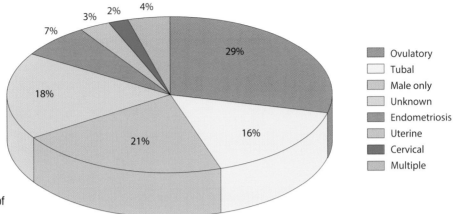

Figure 7.2 Causes of subfertility.

Tubal problems

Tubal blockage is usually associated with inflammatory processes in the pelvis such as pelvic inflammatory disease (PID) or endometriosis. Chlamydial infections in particular can produce significant degrees of tubal damage, often resulting in a hydrosalpinx – a blocked Fallopian tube, often with a thickened wall, flattened epithelial mucosa and peritubal adhesions.

Previous pelvic or abdominal surgery can result in postoperative scar tissue or adhesions that can also compromise tubal patency and function. The Fallopian tube is not a passive conduit – normal tubal function requires both patency and a healthy anatomy and physiology for gamete and embryo transport.

> ▶ **eResource 7.1**
>
> Tubal blockage
> http://www.routledgetextbooks.com/textbooks/tenteachers/gynaecologyv7.1.php

Uterine problems

Uterine factors such as fibroids can interfere with fertility, but their impact depends on their size and location. There is good evidence that submucosal fibroids have a direct impact on embryo implantation and intramural fibroids may reduce fertility if they are large (>5 cm). Subserosal fibroids have very little impact if present in isolation. Endometrial polyps can reduce the chance of implantation, although this tends not to be absolute. Endometrial scarring (Asherman's syndrome) from surgery or infection can be associated with lighter periods and a significantly reduced chance of conception.

Male factor

Compromised sperm number or quality is an important contributor to subfertility. There is some evidence that sperm counts are falling, and there are various theories that try to explain this, including environmental and dietary issues. Spermatogonial cells that produce the sperm can be damaged by inflammation (orchitis) or the epididymis that stores mature sperm can also be damaged. Certain iatrogenic influences such as pelvic radiotherapy or surgery for undescended or torted testes can reduce sperm production or damage or block the male reproductive tract. Medical conditions such as diabetes and certain occupations involving contact with chemicals or radiation are associated with male factor subfertility. Occasionally, sperm production may be normal but there are erectile difficulties or problems with ejaculation.

Genetic causes of male factor infertility include aneuploidy of sex chromosomes (Klinefelter XXY most commonly) or structural abnormalities of the autosomes, such as inversions, deletions or balanced translocations. Microdeletions of the azoospermic factor (AZF) regions of the Y chromosome are associated with low sperm counts and motility.

> ▶ **eResource 7.2**
>
> Normal and abnormal sperm
> http://www.routledgetextbooks.com/textbooks/tenteachers/gynaecologyv7.2.php

Table 7.1 Key points to cover in history and examination of patients presenting with subfertility

History	
Female	**Male**
Age	Age
Length of time spent trying for pregnancy	Length of time spent trying for pregnancy
Any previous pregnancies	Fathered any previous pregnancies
Coital frequency	History of mumps or measles
Occupation	History of testicular trauma, surgery to testis
General gynaecological history	Occupation
Previous history of pelvic inflammatory disease	Medical and surgical history
Previous medical and surgical history	
Previous fertility treatment	
Cervical smear history	
General health – screen for history of thyroid disorders	
Examination	
Pelvic examination – any uterine pathology such as fibroids and adnexal masses or tenderness General blood pressure, pulse, height and weight	Testicular examination – testicular volume, consistency, masses, absence of vas deferens, varicocele, evidence of surgical scars

History and examination

A thorough and detailed history must be taken from patients presenting with subfertility. As this is a couple-centred issue it is advisable for both partners to be present at the consultation. Key features are presented in *Table 7.1*. In many clinics a template is employed to ensure all these features are covered.

Investigations

It is usually preferable to diagnose a cause of subfertility so that an appropriate treatment can be targeted to a specific pathology. However, even with a detailed series of investigations, a significant delay in conception for a significant number of couples will remain unexplained. There is some debate as to when investigations should be started; considerations such as age and the level of anxiety in the couple are important. Most authorities suggest that investigations are sensible in a couple that have not conceived after 1 year of regular unprotected intercourse.

Investigations can be justifiably commenced earlier if the couple have a history of predisposing factors such as amenorrhoea, oligomenorrhoea, PID, women with low ovarian reserve or known male factor subfertility.

Female investigations

Blood hormone profile. In a woman with a regular menstrual cycle this should include early follicular phase follicular-stimulating hormone (FSH), oestradiol and luteinizing hormone (LH). Anti-Müllerian hormone (AMH) (see below) is proving particularly helpful in the assessment of ovarian reserve and is independent of the menstrual cycle, which is practical. A midluteal progesterone measurement should be taken to confirm ovulation. In women with an irregular menstrual cycle, thyroid function, prolactin and testosterone can also prove useful.

Chlamydia testing should be offered prior to any uterine instrumentation. If ART is to be offered, viral screening for human immunodeficiency virus (HIV) and hepatitis B and C should be offered.

Transvaginal ultrasound (TVUSS) should be performed where possible. This provides an accurate assessment of pelvic anatomy, including uterine size and shape, the presence of any fibroids, ovarian size, position and morphology, with antral follicle count (AFC) an important parameter of ovarian reserve. Pathology such as hydrosalpinges and endometriotic cysts can be detected, and access to the ovaries for ART can be assessed. Tubal potency testing may be necessary as described below.

Tubal assessment

Tubal patency and an assessment of the uterine cavity are traditionally investigated by hysterosalpingography (HSG) using X-ray, hysterocontrast synography (HyCoSy) using ultrasound or, more recently, 3D hysterocontrast synography (**Figure 7.3**). There is some evidence that patients deemed at high risk of pelvic pathology could benefit from a more invasive laparoscopy and hysteroscopy as a dual diagnostic and potentially therapeutic procedure. It is crucial to remember that tubal patency is not equivalent to tubal function. Currently, there is as yet no effective test to check for tubal function.

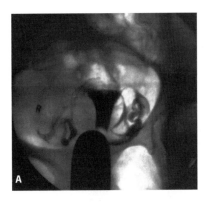

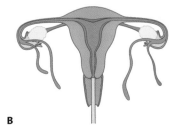

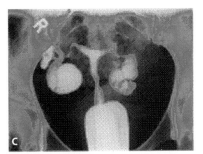

Figure 7.3 A: Hysterosalpingogram (HSG) showing normal patency of the Fallopian tubes; **B**: pictorial illustration of a normal HSG; **C**: abnormal HSG with pocketed areas suggesting blocked tubes.

Measurement of ovarian reserve

- Female reproductive potential is directly proportionate to the remaining number of oocytes in the ovaries, which is called ovarian reserve.

- Ovarian reserve declines after the age of 35 in an average healthy woman, or at an earlier age due to genetic predisposition, surgery or following exposure to toxins, such as chemotherapy.

- The ovarian reserve can help to predict the response to ovarian stimulation in ART.

- The AFC seen on TVUSS is a good indicator of ovarian reserve (<4 predicting low response, >16 high response).

- AMH is produced in the granulosa cells of ovarian follicles and does not change in response to gonadotrophins during the menstrual cycle. As a result, it can be measured and compared from any point in the cycle and, at present, is the most successful biochemical marker.

- Neither AMH nor AFC are perfect indicators and most clinics utilize both to assess ovarian reserve.

Male investigations

The only routine investigation on the male side is a semen fluid analysis (SFA). Most centres recommend between a 2- and 4-day abstinence from ejaculation before providing the semen sample. The new WHO criteria (2010) for semen analysis are presented in *Table 7.2*. These are not average or median measurements, but represent lower reference limits (5th centile). If the initial SFA is abnormal it should be repeated 3 months later, to allow adequate time for spermatogenesis, because occasionally an abnormal SFA will result from insults such as viral infections.

Some clinics will also assess total motile count, the presence of round cells or leucocytes to assess for inflammation and the presence of sperm antibodies. For men with a very low sperm count or azoospermia, a hormone profile including FSH, LH and testosterone should be performed. This may have later importance in male health as testicular failure may be associated with symptomatic low testosterone. We also recommend a karyotype and a cystic fibrosis screen.

Microdeletions of the AZFa and AZFb regions of the Y chromosome are not tested for routinely, because they are not ameliorable to treatment. However, they carry a poor prognosis for surgical sperm retrieval procedures and may be tested for in this context in the presence of azoospermia.

Table 7.2 World Health Organization parameters for semen analysis – 5th centile

Parameter	Lower and reference limit
Semen volume (ml)	1.5 (1.4–1.7)
Sperm concentration (million/ml)	15 (12–16)
Total sperm number (million per ejaculate)	39 (33–46)
Progressive motility (%)	32 (31–34)
Morphology normal forms (%)	4 (3–4)
Vitality – live sperm (%)	58 (55–63)
pH	>7.2

Less evidence-based tests include measuring deoxyribonucleic acid (DNA) fragmentation levels in the sperm.

Management

The management of the couple's subfertility should be evidence based and relies on an accurate diagnostic evaluation of the history, clinical examination and investigations. Management may be expectant, medical, surgical or a combination of these. Fertility treatment should be individualized to optimize the treatment result (*Table 7.3*).

Ovulation induction

For patients with PCOS ovulatory problems, ovulation induction (OI) is usually the first line of management so long as there is tubal patency and normal semen analysis. The most common ovulation induction agent used is the antioestrogen clomiphene citrate. Clomiphene binds to oestrogen receptors in the hypothalamus and pituitary. This blocks the normal feedback loops of oestrogen and results in a surge of gonadotrophin release, stimulating the ovary to recruit more follicles for maturation. Approximately 70% of women on clomiphene will ovulate and approximately one-half of these will be pregnant within 6 months of trying. There is a risk of multiple pregnancies (12%) and therefore women on clomiphene should be monitored by ultrasound scans to track the growth of their follicles, identify the time of ovulation and reduce the risk of multiple pregnancy. In clomiphene-resistant women, alternative strategies include augmentation with metformin, use of aromatase inhibitors (although not licensed for this indication in some countries) and injectable gonadotrophins. OI can also be induced by laparoscopic ovarian drilling (LOD) in PCOS. For unknown reasons, passing electrical energy through polycystic ovaries can result in the induction of ovulation. However, as LOD is a surgical procedure with the attached risks associated with surgery and anaesthesia, it is only appropriate to offer such treatment to women who have not responded to clomiphene treatment.

In women with anovulation of hypothalamic origin, OI using injectable gonadotrophins is more effective.

Table 7.3 Summary of the medical and surgical management of subfertility

Medical	Treatment criteria
Ovulation induction (OI) – clomifene or FSH	Anovulation – PCOS, idiopathic
Intrauterine insemination – with or without stimulation with FSH	Unexplained subfertility, mild male factor
Anovulation unresponsive to OI	
Mild male factor	
Minimal to mild endometriosis	
Donor insemination – with or without stimulation with FSH	Presence of azospermia
Single women	
Same sex couples	
In vitro fertilization (IVF)	Patients with tubal pathology
Patients who underwent above treatment with no success in pregnancy	
Donor egg with IVF	Women whose egg quality is poor (e.g. older women, premature ovarian failure)
Previous surgery/chemo-radiotherapy where ovarian function was adversely affected	
Surgical	**Treatment criteria**
Operative laparoscopy to treat disease and restore anatomy	Adhesions
Endometriosis	
Ovarian cyst	
Myomectomy – hysteroscopy, laparoscopy, laparotomy, fibroid embolization	Fibroid uterus
Tubal surgery	Blocked Fallopian tubes amenable to repair
Laparoscopic ovarian drilling	PCOS unresponsive to medical treatment

PCOS: polycystic ovary syndrome.

Surgery

Surgery to treat subfertility can be helpful in a variety of different scenarios. Most fertility surgery is currently performed using minimal access techniques such as laparoscopy of hysteroscopy. Investigation of infertility and tubal potency testing by minimal access surgery (MAS) is undertaken if the patient is symptomatic or if specific therapeutic treatment is planned. There is good evidence that laparoscopic ablation of endometriosis can help improve natural conception rates. Often surgery may be used as an adjunct to ART. For example, the surgical disconnection from the uterus or removal of hydrosalpinges is associated with a significant improvement in in-vitro fertilization (IVF) success rates (**Figure 7.4**). Some practitioners still recommend a more traditional open laparotomy approach for the use of myomectomy for very large uterine fibroids or for the use of tubal microsurgery in reversal of sterilization, proximal or distal tubal microsurgery. Submucosal fibroids, endometrial polyps, Asherman syndrome and some congenital uterine anomalies, such as a septum, are usually managed hysteroscopically.

Intrauterine insemination

Intrauterine insemination (IUI) is performed by introducing a small sample of prepared sperm into the uterine cavity with a fine uterine catheter. IUI may be helpful in cases of mild endometriosis, mild male

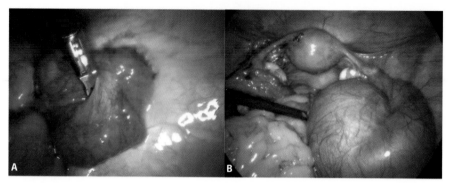

Figure 7.4 **A**: Photograph of the normal fimbrial end of Fallopian tube; **B**: photograph of right hydrosalpinx.

factor subfertility, in couples who do not have intercourse or in single women or same sex couples using donor sperm. The success rate of this procedure ranges between 10% and 20% per treatment cycle. This process may be preceded by several days of mild stimulation with subcutaneous injections daily of exogenous FSH, with the aim of stimulating the ovaries to produce 2–3 mature follicles (this is termed stimulated IUI). Follicular tracking with ultrasound is essential to avoid over- or understimulation. Triggering of ovulation (and therefore the timing of the insemination) is achieved with a subcutaneous injection of human chorionic gonadotrophin (hCG). This mimics the endogenous LH surge, due to cross-over of the alpha-subunits of the two hormones.

In-vitro fertilization

IVF was originally designed for couples with tubal factor subfertility. Steptoe and Edwards performed the first successful case in 1978. There are now over 5 million babies worldwide as a result of IVF. IVF is now used for almost all cases of subfertility including tubal disease, endometriosis, failed ovulation induction, failed IUI or where donor eggs are needed.

Originally, IVF was performed in the natural menstrual cycle, but the use of gonadotrophin-controlled ovarian stimulation made IVF a much more efficient process. ART in the UK is regulated by the Human Fertilisation and Embryo Authority (HFEA), who provide guidelines and statistics for patients and clinicians, as well as inspecting clinics to ensure adherence to mutually agreed quality standards. IVF can be performed with many different protocols and medications, but the principal steps of IVF are shown in **Figure 7.5** and are as follows.

Pituitary down-regulation

In the most commonly used IVF cycle the pituitary gland is down-regulated to prevent endogenous LH surges and premature ovulation. A gonadotrophin-releasing hormone (GnRH) agonist is used to block the FSH and LF release from the pituitary. Newer approaches involving the use of GnRH antagonists can shorten treatment time and reduce the incidence of ovarian hyperstimulation syndrome.

Controlled ovarian stimulation

This is achieved using daily subcutaneous doses of gonadotrophin medications, which cause multiple follicle recruitment. Close monitoring with TVUSS predicts the number of follicles and the timing of the egg collection. Ideally, around 15 follicles are recruited. Blood levels may be taken to measure oestradiol levels, and are used by some to measure ovarian response to stimulation. Ultrasound measurement of endometrial thickness is also performed.

Inhibition of premature ovulation

Feedback from rising oestradiol associated with follicular development should lead to an LH surge from the pituitary, resulting in final oocyte maturation and ovulation. In IVF this is blocked to allow scheduling of egg collection. This is traditionally done by the administration of GnRH agonists, or with a newer shorter GnRH antagonist protocol.

hCG trigger

hCG is used as a surrogate for the endogenous LH surge. It causes final maturation of the egg and allows scheduling of the egg collection procedure.

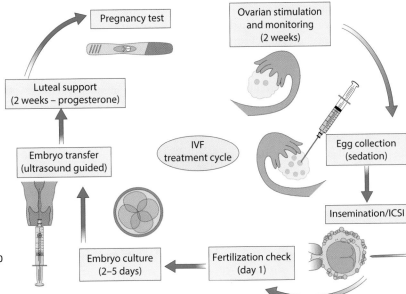

Figure 7.5 Pictorial in-vitro fertilization (IVF) cycle. (ICSI, intracytoplasmic sperm injection.)

Egg collection

This procedure is usually performed about 37 hours post hCG trigger. Under anaesthesia a needle is inserted into the ovaries under TVUSS control, and follicular fluid is aspirated from each follicle that contains an oocyte, which is collected by the embryologist into the laboratory.

> ▶ **eResource 7.3**
>
> Egg collection using TVUSS
> http://www.routledgetextbooks.com/textbooks/tenteachers/gynaecologyv7.3.php

Fertilization

Fertilization is performed using prepared sperm. Conventional IVF fertilization involves the insemination of around 100,000 sperm in a petri-dish with an egg. In cases of poor sperm parameters or in cases of previous poor fertilization, individual sperm can be isolated and directly injected into the cytoplasm of the oocyte (intracytoplasmic sperm injection, ICSI) (**Figure 7.6**). Fertilization is checked the next morning and is usually in the region of 60% for IVF and 70% for ICSI.

Embryo culture

Embryos are incubated under strict conditions of temperature, pH, humidity and oxygen concentration.

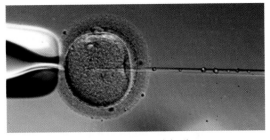

Figure 7.6 Intracytoplasmic sperm injection.

They may be transferred back into the uterus after 2, 3 or 5 days of development. Embryos reaching the blastocyst stage on day 5 of development usually exhibit the best chance of implantation. A variety of different protocols are available for embryo selection, including a morphological and a morpho-kinetic assessment.

Embryo transfer

Embryos are transferred into the uterus using a soft plastic catheter. The choice of how many embryos to transfer is the decision of the couple following expert medical and embryological advice; this

> ▶ **eResource 7.4**
>
> TVUSS-guided embryo transfer
> http://www.routledgetextbooks.com/textbooks/tenteachers/gynaecologyv7.4.php

may be constrained by local regulatory or funding parameters. Embryo transfer is usually performed under transabdominal ultrasound control to ensure correct placement of the embryos. In the UK and Europe there are recommendations regarding the transfer of single embryos to reduce the incidence of multiple pregnancies and their associated risks.

Embryo cryopreservation

Spare embryos of good quality may be cryopreserved for future use. Vitrification techniques now allow for success rates from frozen embryos to approximate success rates in fresh treatment cycles. This makes the transfer of fresh single embryos with the vitrification of spare embryos more appealing to couples.

Luteal phase support

The use of gonadotrophin agonists or antagonists to prevent a premature LH surge will lead to a reduction in the ability of the corpus luteum to produce progesterone. Patients are therefore supplemented with progesterone following the egg collection. There is no consensus on the ideal dose, route or duration of progesterone supplementation. A pregnancy test is performed around 14 days after embryo transfer.

ART success rates

IVF success rates are exquisitely sensitive to female age. In young patients under the age of 35 success rates can be as high as 40–45% from a single cycle, while in women over the age of 40 they will fall below 15%. Undergoing IVF does not preclude the patient from the normal complications of pregnancy, such as miscarriage or ectopic pregnancies. The most significant risk of IVF treatment is ovarian hyperstimulation syndrome (OHSS), occurring in 1–3% of cases. Patients with severe OHSS present with ascites, enlarged multifollicular ovaries, pulmonary oedema and coagulopathy. These patients need to be admitted to hospital and managed under strict protocols under the care of specialist teams. The use of low-dose stimulation, ultrasound monitoring, GnRH antagonist protocols, GnRH agonist triggers and a more liberal freezing policy have significantly reduced the incidence of this very serious condition.

Donor gametes

Donor sperm can be used to treat patients where the male partner is azoospermic or in the case of single women or female same sex couples. Both IUI and IVF treatments are possible. Donor eggs may be used if the female has undergone early menopause or if IVF treatments have been unsuccessful and associated with a reduced ovarian reserve and low egg number and quality. Gamete donation requires careful and thorough counselling and most countries have legislation to regulate its use.

Surgical sperm retrieval

Where the sperm quality or quantity is low but sperm are present, ICSI is required to help achieve a pregnancy. However, in the absence of naturally ejaculated sperm (termed azoospermia – which may relate to blockage of the vas deferens or testicular problems), patients may undergo surgical sperm retrieval (SSR). SSR can be performed under sedation or general anaesthesia. A fine needle is inserted into the epididymis or the testicular tissue to obtain sperm or testicular tissue with sperm, respectively. The retrieved sperm can then be cryopreserved or injected into the oocyte as part of a fresh IVF/ICSI cycle.

Preimplantation genetic diagnosis

Couples who carry a genetic disease (but who are fertile) may choose to use IVF and preimplantation genetic diagnosis (PGD) to avoid an affected pregnancy. These patients may previously have had affected children or terminations for an affected fetus. IVF will create multiple embryos. These embryos can then be genetically tested for the relevant disease, by the removal of several cells at the blastocyst stage that are tested and taken to reflect the genotype of the remaining embryo. Only embryos free of the disease are transferred into the uterus. PGD has now been used worldwide for most monogenic diseases, as well as for translocations. The use of PGD for social sex selection is illegal in the UK but available controversially in many other countries.

There is a large attrition rate in PGD treatment from the number of eggs to embryos to unaffected embryos available for transfer. In some cycles none

 eResource 7.5

Embryo biopsy for PGD
http://www.routledgetextbooks.com/textbooks/tenteachers/gynaecologyv7.5.php

of the embryos will be unaffected and no embryo transfer will result. Success rates therefore reflect this, and vary according to the inheritance pattern of the disorder.

Similar genetic analysis of embryos has been used to detect chromosomal aneuploidy in embryos in patients having IVF treatment, in an attempt to select the embryos with the greatest implantation potential and reduce the time to a pregnancy. This remains controversial and subject to research trials.

Fertility preservation

Patients may face treatments such as chemotherapy, radiotherapy or surgery that could significantly damage their gonads and reduce their reproductive potential. For many years men have been able to 'bank' sperm ahead of these treatments. Couples can now undergo rapid IVF procedures and cryopreserve embryos for use later on when health is regained.

KEY LEARNING POINTS

- A careful history, appropriate clinical examination, correct investigation and advice on evidence-based treatments underpin successful fertility treatment. The approach should always be couple-centred with counselling when necessary.
- The couple should be given information on the chances of conceiving naturally and how to optimize this. This should include the impact of advancing age and advice on lifestyle issues relating to diet, smoking, weight and alcohol consumption.

- Ovarian reserve decreases significantly with age, with the gradient increasing over the age of 36 and again at 40.
- Fertility treatment is a combination of expectant, surgical and medical treatments that are complementary to each other.
- Treatments should be tailored to an individual couple's needs, and can include ovulation induction, surgery, IUI and IVF.
- Fertility preservation and PGD are new and effective treatment options for selected patient groups.

Recent advances in vitrification have now also allowed young, healthy, single women to go through IVF and freeze their oocytes.

There is very promising evidence, and some successful reports of live births, on the role of laparoscopic ovarian cortex collection and cryopreservation. Tissue could be auto-transplanted back into the patient's pelvis once health is regained.

Further reading

Human Fertilisation and Embryology Authority. www.hfea.gov.uk.
National Institute for Clinical Excellence. Fertility assessment and treatment for people with fertility problems. Clinical guidelines (CG11) https://www.nice.org.uk/guidance/cg156.
Van Voorlis BJ (2007). Clinical practice. In vitro fertilisation. *New Engl J Med* **356**:379–86.

Self assessment

CLINICAL HISTORY

A 36-year-old woman, Jane, and her 39-year-old partner, David, have come to the fertility clinic after trying for a baby for 3 years. The referral letter notes that Jane has irregular periods and David had a hernia repair as a child. Neither have any children.

A *What important parts of the history must you ask?*

B *What investigations will you request?*

C *What treatment will they need?*

ANSWERS

A   In the fertility clinic a general gynaecological history must first be obtained, and then

more specific questions will follow. You must determine how long exactly they have been having unprotected intercourse and what 'irregular periods' means by enquiring about frequency of bleeds, length of bleeds, any other abnormal uterine bleeding. Irregular periods must prompt questions about hirsutism, weight and acne, as these will support the diagnosis of PCOS, a common cause of anovulation. You must ask for how long the irregular bleeds have happened, as you may be mindful of a diagnosis of decreasing ovarian reserve, a cause that may be associated with hot sweats. Do not forget to ask about smear tests and STIs. Confirm that Jane has never been pregnant before, including miscarriages and ectopic pregnancies. Also check that none of David's previous partners have become pregnant.

Ask about frequency of intercourse and any problems with intercourse, because fertility problems are strongly associated with psychosexual problems, both female and male. On the male side you need to ask more about the hernia repair: was it one side or both, and at what age?

You find that Jane has always had irregular periods except when she was on the OCP. She usually has a period every 2–3 months and they vary from very heavy to normal. She has struggled with androgenic symptoms, except when on the OCP. She manages to keep her weight down with difficulty, and keeps her BMI below 30 with a combination of diet and exercise.

David had a unilateral uncomplicated hernia repair aged 4 years. He had a sperm count measured about 2 years ago by the GP, which was 'borderline', so they felt it was worth continuing to try naturally for a while. Intercourse is every few days; they no longer try to work out when ovulation has occurred.

B   The investigations required are a hormone profile for Jane, a TVUSS to look for PCOS and other abnormalities and SFA for David. Tubal testing at this point is not indicated.

On review Jane has a hormone profile indicating PCOS, with LH slightly higher than FSH, and high AMH. Her TVUSS confirms PCOS, with a corpus luteum suggesting recent ovulation. David's SFA shows a sperm count of 10 million/ml with reduced total motility and morphology.

C   On review you should explain that there are two problems: infrequent ovulation and abnormal sperm count. Together with the length of infertility, these problems mean that IVF and ICSI are indicated. There is no need to check for tubal patency as it is irrelevant. Treatment of ovulation induction or IUI will not give good pregnancy rates because the sperm count is low.

SBA QUESTIONS

1   A 32-year-old woman and her partner are assessed for 2 years' subfertility. The SFA has been checked and is normal, and the woman has a normal hormone profile and normal markers for ovarian reserve. The TVUSS is normal. She has a 3-year history of premenstrual pain for 3 days before each period, constant right iliac fossa pain and dyspareunia.

What is the most suitable test for tubal potency? Choose the single best answer.

A   Hysteroscopy.
B   HyCoSy.
C   HSG.
D   Laparoscopy and dye insufflation.
E   MRI.

ANSWER

D   The symptoms raise the concern of endometriosis. Hysteroscopy alone will not determine tubal potency. HyCoSy should be used for low-risk women. HSG is suitable and will show tubal potency and would be appropriate for someone who declined surgery or was at high risk. MRI will sometimes diagnose endometriotic implants and rectovaginal nodules. However, laparoscoy and dye is the best choice as it will enable simultaneous diagnosis of tubal potency, pelvic causes of pain such as endometriosis and adhesions, and will permit treatment of endometriosis, which may be causing the symptoms.

2 A woman aged 34 years and her 32-year-old partner have had 8 years' infertility and have attended a fertility clinic. The woman has been shown to have a normal hormone profile with normal ovarian reserve and the TVUSS is normal. A HyCoSy has demonstrated tubal patency. The SFA has shown a sperm count of 6 million/ml and motility of 20%.

What should they be advised is the most suitable treatment? Choose the single best answer.

A   IVF and ICSI.

B   IUI.

C   PGD.

D   Ovulation induction.

E   IVF alone.

ANSWER

A   The sperm count and motility is very low and IUI will have very low pregnancy rates. In IVF alone the fertilization rate of eggs will be low, resulting in few embryos to transfer, hence a low pregnancy rate. Ovulation induction is not a suitable treatment as there is no ovulation problem. PGD is not required unless there is a diagnosed inheritable genetic disease. If the sperm count was below 1 million/ml, further male genetic testing for sex chromosome abnormalities and balanced translocations would be indicated. Absence of one vas deferens would indicate the need for cystic fibrosis testing. IVF and ICSI will give good fertilization rates and a good chance of pregnancy for this couple.

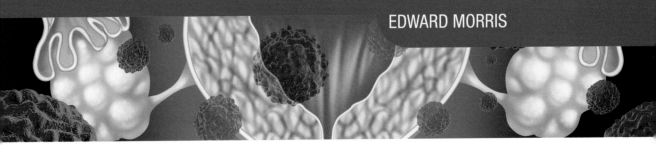

The menopause and postreproductive health

CHAPTER

8

EDWARD MORRIS

Physiological menopause 106

Non-physiological menopause.....................................107

Postmenopausal reproductive health............................108

Assessment of the menopausal woman 112

Hormonal replacement therapy.......................................114

Further reading..118

Self assessment..118

LEARNING OBJECTIVES

- Know the definition of menopause.
- Understand physiological and non-physiological menopause.
- Understand the effect of menopause on women.
- Understand the modifiable and non-modifiable aspects of menopausal health.
- Explain the main forms of treatment of the menopause.
- Know the side-effects and the relative and absolute contraindications of hormonal replacement therapy (HRT).
- Describe the benefits of hormonal and non-hormonal HRT.

Definitions

The menopause is defined as the woman's final menstrual period and the accepted confirmation of this is made retrospectively after 1 year of amenorrhoea. The cause of the menopause is cessation of regular ovarian function. There is great heterogeneity in the experiences of different women as they go through the menopausal transition and several descriptive phrases exist, which can cause confusion amongst practitioners and women alike.

Descriptive terms for menopause

- Menopause: the last menstrual period (LMP).
- Perimenopause: time of life from the onset of ovarian dysfunction until 1 year after the last period and the diagnosis of menopause is made. This time is also known as the climacteric.
- Postmenopause: all women who have been 1 year since their last period are deemed postmenopausal.
- The 'change': a colloquial description of perimenopause and postmenopause.

Physiological menopause

Timing of the menopause

The average age of the menopause worldwide has not changed for decades (**Figure 8.1**) remaining at a median age of between 51 and 52 years, with 95% of women attaining menopause between the age of 45 and 55 years. Menopause occurring outside these ages is relatively rare and premature ovarian failure is discussed later.

Endocrine changes

Current understanding is that menopause occurs at the time of the depletion of oocytes from the ovary and is irreversible. Groundbreaking and yet to be widely accepted research challenges this assumption, with the finding of oogonial stem cells from primordial follicles in the ovary. This might radically affect our understanding of the menopause and offer the remote possibility of being able to influence the timing of menopause.

Unsurprisingly, the endocrinology is not as simple as the ovaries just running out of eggs and the capacity to produce hormones at a particular age. As discussed in Chapter 3, Hormonal control of the menstrual cycle and hormonal disorders, reproductive function is maintained by a subtle interplay of the hypothalamic production of gonadotrophin-releasing hormone (GnRH), the pituitary hormones luteinizing hormone (LH) and follicle-stimulating hormone (FSH), the ovarian peptide hormone inhibin B and the steroid hormones oestrogen, progesterone and testosterone. These hormones not only change during the menstrual cycle but also throughout a woman's reproductive life, with their production changing at differing times and rates according to the age of the woman (*Table 8.1*).

Inhibin B is produced by follicles within the ovary, so as the number of follicles decline the production of inhibin decreases. In the perimenopausal years small declines in inhibin drive an overall increase in the pulsatility of GnRH secretion and overall serum FSH and LH levels, which results in an increased drive to the remaining follicles in an attempt to maintain follicle production and oestrogen levels.

Androgenic hormone production comes from ovaries, peripheral adipose tissue and the adrenal glands, with the ovaries producing approximately 30–50% of total circulating levels. A decline in ovarian testosterone and other androgens accompanies the process of ageing in women, although these changes are less dependent on the neuroendocrine axis and the processes involved in ovulation. This is shown by the fact that overall androgen concentrations in a woman in her 20s are approximately double those at 40 years old and then slowly decline over the rest of her life, with very low levels maintained from about 70 years.

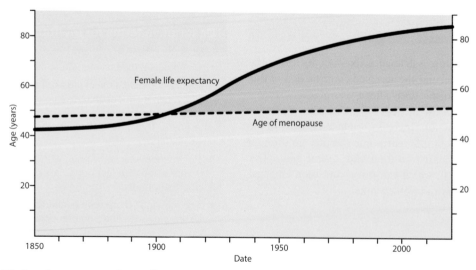

Figure 8.1 Age of menopause and mean life expectancy in the UK since 1850.

Table 8.1 Female hormone production and changes around the menopausal years

Hormones	Perimenopause	Early postmenopause	Late postmenopause and elderly
GnRH	Increased pulsatility	Progressive decrease in pulsatility	Reduction in overall levels
LH & FSH	Increased	Increased	Progressive decline
Oestrogen	Slight declines	Rapid decline in levels	Sustained very low levels
Progesterone	Moderate falls	Unpredictable	Undetectable
Inhibin	Slight decline	Significant decline	Undetectable
Testosterone	Progressive decline	Progressive decline	Sustained low levels

FSH, follicle-stimulating hormone; GnRH, gonadotrophin-releasing hormone; LH, luteinizing hormone.

Diagnosis

The diagnosis of menopause is a largely clinical diagnosis that is made according to symptoms experienced, such as menstrual irregularities and amenorrhoea, and oestrogen deficiency symptoms, such as vasomotor symptoms.

The use of serum endocrine tests such as hormone levels are of little value in the perimenopausal years as they are unpredictable due to the hormonal variations that frequently occur in association with episodic and irregular ovulatory cycles at this time of life. An elevated serum FSH in association with a low serum oestradiol may be suggestive of menopause, but as this combination of levels can occur during a normal menstrual cycle this test can therefore be misleading.

In all women in whom a diagnosis of menopause is being considered, the possibility of pregnancy should also be considered. The special circumstance of diagnosis of menopause in a woman who has undergone hysterectomy can be difficult due to the lack of signalling from the bleeding that accompanies the menstrual cycle. However, in these circumstances the use of other symptoms of the menopause as biological indicators is usually enough to make a confident diagnosis.

Non-physiological menopause

Premature ovarian insufficiency

If menopause occurs before the age of 40 years it is defined as premature ovarian insufficiency (POI), also sometimes called premature ovarian failure (POF),
or premature menopause. It is thought to occur in approximately 1% of women under 40 years and 0.1% under 30 years. It is a distressing diagnosis for a woman to receive, especially if it occurs prior to the completion of her family. For young women who wish to conceive, gamete donation is the only option.

POI is usually diagnosed following either primary or secondary amenorrhoea. Women who have a diagnosis of POI can experience unpredictable spontaneous ovarian activity, resulting in irregular vaginal bleeding and the small risk of pregnancy.

While no cause is found in most cases of primary POI, a suspected case should be investigated where possible for causes that are associated with issues that require separate treatment, as detailed in *Table 8.2*.

All women with POI should be offered supportive care and counselling delivered by a specialist unit to ensure that they fully understand their condition, the specifics of their reproductive needs and that they receive an individualized package of care with

Table 8.2 Principal causes of premature ovarian insufficiency

Primary	Chromosome anomalies (e.g. Turner's, fragile X) Autoimmune disease (e.g. hypothyroidism, Addison's, myasthenia gravis) Enzyme deficiencies (e.g. galactosaemia, 17a-hydroxylase deficiency)
Secondary	Chemotherapy or radiotherapy Infections (e.g. tuberculosis, mumps, malaria, varicella)

close attention to both short-term and long-term management of their health.

Iatrogenic menopause – medical treatments and menopause after cancer treatment

There is an increasing array of non-surgical treatments that result in an iatrogenic temporary or permanent menopause and there is an increasing number of women living long lives but with permanent menopause, often from an early age. Modern screening programmes, technologies to achieve early diagnoses in suspected malignancy and early radical treatment of female reproductive tract malignancy have contributed to this. Such women, especially those under the age of 40 years, must be carefully counselled as to what to expect prior to definitive irreversible treatment, and then managed as someone with POI thereafter. Special consideration should be given to women whose lifelong treatment demands a hormone-free environment, as these women will need to manage on regimes that avoid hormone replacement.

If GnRH is given in a constant high dose, it desensitizes the GnRH receptor and reduces LH and FSH release. Drugs that are GnRH agonists (e.g. buserelin and goserelin) can be used as treatments for endometriosis and other gynaecological problems. Although they mimic the GnRH hormone, when administered continuously they will down-regulate the pituitary and consequently decrease LH and FSH secretion. This will induce a temporary menopause with a relatively rapid onset, which can be managed with the introduction of hormone therapies and other drugs to relieve some of the unwanted menopausal symptoms – known as add-back therapy.

Iatrogenic menopause – surgical menopause

Women may be placed into surgical menopause aiming to permanently treat benign gynaecological conditions such as menstrual disorders, fibroids and endometriosis. Bilateral salpingo-oophorectomy (BSO) may also be performed prophylactically for women at high risk of inherited malignancies such as breast and ovarian cancer, with BRCA 1 and 2 gene mutation screening. Good clinical practice in these women should ensure that before making the irreversible decision to have a

BSO for these diseases they consider the correct time in their life for the procedure and that they are given plans for how they can manage the sudden hormone deficits that they will have to endure. It is important during preparation that they are aware that as well as losing oestrogen they will also lose the effect of testosterone.

Postmenopausal reproductive health

Overview

As the UK population expands it is clear from data predictions from the Office for National Statistics Projection that longevity is also going to increase. The whole UK female population is projected to increase in the 25 years between 2012 and 2037 from 32.4 to 36.8 million girls and women. The vast majority of this 4.4 million increase is accounted for by the over 50 year age group, increasing from 11.9 to 15.8 million women over the same time period (**Figure 8.2**).

This means that the population of women who are likely to experience problems during their postreproductive years will expand by one-third over the next 25 years. Given that we already understand that the ageing population places a significant strain on the health care system of any country, it makes it more important than ever to try to improve the health of these women in a preventative fashion.

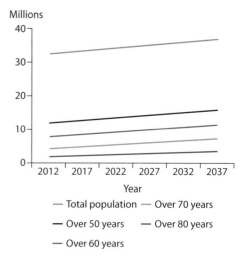

Figure 8.2 Population projections. Females over 50 years in the UK. Office for National Statistics Projection data 2012–2037, extracted and plotted by Author.

Medicine traditionally delivers health care in system- and condition-specific silos, such as cardiology, urogynaecology, bone medicine, surgical site-specific cancers, etc. This is sensible when it comes to delivery of specialist expertise, but when designing strategies to prevent diseases it makes much more sense to look at the various stages in a woman's life and what measures can be taken at different ages to reduce the risk of disease later in life. This may be described as a continuum of care. A good example of this approach is the management of obesity in postmenopausal women. While it is well understood that obesity increases the risk of cardiovascular disease and type 2 diabetes, it is less well known that obesity in the postmenopausal woman increases the risk of hot flushes, breast cancer and endometrial cancer. In addition, as the woman gets older obesity increases the risk of falls, fractures and stroke, all of which attract a high mortality rate.

Bringing all of these items together in primary care to make a health improvement plan in the early menopause could significantly improve a woman's health and on a population basis could mean significant reductions in health care resource use.

How women are affected by the menopause

The hormonal changes during and after the menopause have radical changes on the woman. The timing of when each system is affected not only varies dramatically between women, but also the degree of how the changes influence each woman is remarkably unpredictable. The reasons for these variations are not clearly understood but there is some evidence that genetic influences play a part.

While most effects of the menopause have long-term implications, the effects of menopause are commonly categorized as having an early onset or an onset in the medium to long term (*Table 8.3*).

Central nervous system

Vasomotor symptoms

Some of the earliest changes during the menopause are the onset of vasomotor symptoms that often appear during the perimenopausal years. The colloquial term applied to vasomotor symptoms is 'hot flush', and when a hot flush occurs at night it is termed 'night sweat'.

Table 8.3 Effects of the menopause by time of onset

Immediate (0–5 years)	Vasomotor symptoms, (e.g. hot flushes, night sweats) Psychological symptoms (e.g. labile mood, anxiety, tearfulness) Loss of concentration, poor memory Joint aches and pains Dry and itchy skin Hair changes Decreased sexual desire
Intermediate (3–10 years)	Vaginal dryness, soreness Dyspareunia Urgency of urine Recurrent urinary tract infections Urogenital prolapse
Long term (>10 years)	Osteoporosis Cardiovascular disease Dementia

The exact aetiology of a vasomotor symptom is unknown but is thought to be loss of the modulating effect of oestrogen on serotinergic receptors within the thermoregulatory centre in the brain, resulting in exaggerated peripheral vasodilatory responses to minor atmospheric changes in temperature.

Hot flushes occur in up to 80% of women, with less than 30% seeking help. Perhaps the most distressing effect of vasomotor symptoms is through the occurrence of night sweats. The woman may be asleep at the time of the sweat, but during the episode she can be fully woken or her level of sleep can be converted from deep rapid eye movement (REM) sleep to a shallower sleep that is less refreshing. Such disturbances lead to tiredness, exhaustion, poor performance during the day and impaired quality of life.

While hot flushes tend to appear unpredictably, additional triggers include alcohol, caffeine and smoking. Women with a high body mass index (BMI) tend to get worse vasomotor symptoms.

Psychological symptoms

While there is little evidence to support a direct effect of the menopause as a cause for depression, it is clear that menopause is associated with low mood, irritability, lack of energy, tiredness and impaired quality of life from the early perimenopausal period.

Some of these symptoms may be attributed to hormonal changes but it is also important to consider

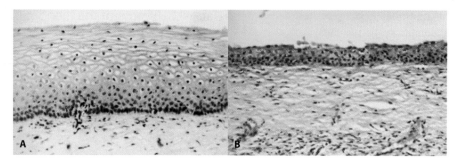

Figure 8.3 Vaginal epithelium in a (**A**) premenopausal woman and (**B**) a postmenopausal woman showing atrophic changes. Note the loss of epithelial structure and architecture. (Reproduced with permission, Whitehead MI, Whitcroft SIJ, Hillard TC (1993). *An Atlas Of The Menopause.* Carnforth, Lancs, UK: Parthenon.)

other external influences on mood such as relationship and family changes, financial issues, previous history of depression and anxiety and the woman's attitude to ageing.

Cognitive function

At present there is no clear evidence that menopause is associated with an acceleration of the onset or incidence of dementia. Most women, however, complain of some change in memory and global cognitive function around the time of the menopause. It is likely that these changes can partly be explained by the impact of vasomotor symptoms and other symptoms on patterns of sleep.

The genital tract

Changes in menstrual bleeding are amongst the key symptoms and signs that herald the effects of the onset of the menopause on the endometrium. They occur relatively soon during the process of menopausal transition. However, it is important to consider that other areas within the genital tract such as the vulva, vagina and urinary tract may also be affected.

Endometrial effects

The initial irregular or scanty vaginal bleeding is due to the reduction in oestrogenic endometrial stimulation with failing ovarian function, ultimately resulting in periods completely stopping when the endometrium is no longer stimulated.

Episodic and infrequent ovulation with fluctuations in oestrogen levels leads to unpredictable progestogenic levels, which usually has the effect of inadequate regular endometrial shedding. This can

then lead to some women experiencing irregular heavy bleeding.

The urogenital tract and vulvovaginal atrophy

Once oestrogen levels start to fall in the perimenopausal years, many women, particularly those who are sexually active, may become aware of vaginal dryness, irritation, burning, soreness and dyspareunia. Loss of the oestrogenic support to the vaginal epithelium leads to reduced cellular turnover and reduced glandular activity, leading to a vaginal epithelium that is less elastic and more easily traumatized (**Figure 8.3**). Other conditions that frequently worsen during the menopause, including incontinence and prolapse, are covered in Chapter 10, Urogynaecology and pelvic floor problems.

The inherent resistance of the urogenital system to infection is also impaired, considered to be due to an increase in pH of the normally mildly acidic environment within the vagina. The incidence of urinary tract infections is also increased, as is the incidence of episodes of minor cystitis that can accompany sexual activity.

Examination of women with postmenopausal urogenital atrophy normally demonstrates dryness affecting most of the surfaces of the vagina along with pallor and, in extreme cases, small petechial haemorrhages. Older women may also have shrinkage and fusion of the labia along with narrowing of the vaginal introitus.

All women experience these changes in the lower genital tract to some degree. It is an intimate area that many women may have difficulty raising in conversation, even though they may be experiencing severe symptoms, so it is therefore essential that health care professionals looking after these women proactively ask about and manage these issues.

Bone health

One of the best understood areas of long-term postreproductive health is the changes in bone that occur on loss of the oestrogenic support of skeletal metabolism. To fully understand this area it is important to be aware of the fact that the skeleton is maintained by a constant process of remodelling, with bone being laid down by osteoblasts and resorbed by osteoclasts (**Figure 8.4**). The balance of the rates of resorption vs. deposition is affected by many different factors, one of which is oestrogen. An important consideration is the attainment of peak bone mass (**Figure 8.5**). Bone density naturally increases during childhood, reaching a peak between 20 and 30 years of age. Males generally achieve a greater peak bone density in comparison to females. After peak bone mass attainment in women there is a steady decline until the menopause, then an accelerated phase of bone loss until 60 years, followed by further steady decline until death. After the age of 60 in women, the likelihood of osteoporotic fractures of the hip and spine increases.

Osteoporosis is defined as 'a skeletal disorder characterized by compromised bone strength predisposing to an increased risk of fracture'. It is more frequent in women than men with an approximate ratio of 4:1.

Risk factors for osteoporosis

- Family history of osteoporosis or hip fracture.
- Smoking.
- Alcoholism.
- Long-term steroid use.
- POI and hypogonadism.
- Medical treatment of gynaecological conditions with induced menopause.
- Disorders of thyroid and parathyroid metabolism.
- Immobility.
- Disorders of gut absorption, malnutrition, liver disease.

Cardiovascular system

Approximately 30% of all deaths occur as a result of ischaemic heart disease and stroke. This makes cardiovascular disease (CVD) a condition that significantly burdens the global health system. While management of CVD is not usually within the realms of the gynaecologist, it is important to recognize that because many women seek the help of a gynaecologist during their life there may be significant opportunities for identification of, and improvement in, modifiable risk factors for CVD.

During the menopausal transition there are several changes in the female physiology that can influence individual risk of CVD. These include lifestyle issues such as nutrition and exercise, changes in the distribution in fat from a more gynaecoid (fat on breasts and hips) to android (abdominal fat deposition) and changes in serum lipid levels that include increases in triglycerides, total cholesterol and low-density lipoprotein (LDL) cholesterol with reduction in high-density lipoprotein (HDL) cholesterol.

Oestrogen also has a supportive effect on the vessel wall that favours vasodilatation and prevents atherogenesis; effects that are reduced after the menopause.

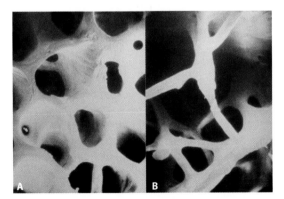

Figure 8.4 Electron micrograph of trabecular bone showing (**A**) normal structure and (**B**) osteoporotic bone. Note the loss of architecture and density in (**B**) making the bone weaker and more prone to fracture. (Reproduced with permission, Whitehead Malcolm I, Whitcroft SIJ, Hillard TC (1993). *An Atlas Of The Menopause.* Carnforth, Lancs, UK: Parthenon.)

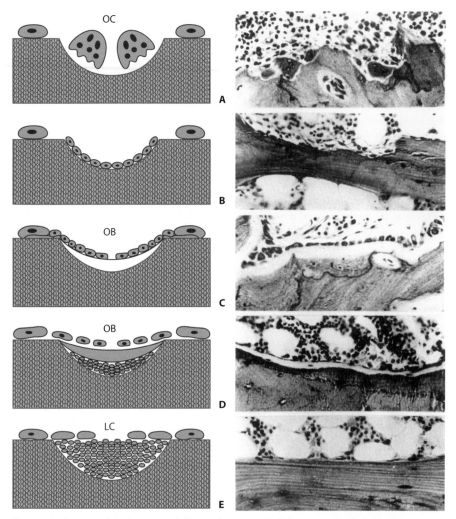

Figure 8.5 The principal stages of the bone remodelling cycle represented diagrammatically (left) with corresponding light micrographs of iliac crest biopsies (right). **A**: Resorption by osteoclasts (OC); **B**: reversal with disappearance of OC; **C**: OC formation with the deposition of osteoid by osteoblasts (OB); **D**: mineralization of the osteoid; **E**: completion of the cycle with bone lining cells on the surface (LC). (Light micrographs reproduced with permission, Dempster DW [1992]. *Disorders of the Bone and Mineral Metabolism*. New York: Raven Press.)

Assessment of the menopausal woman

Key to any consultation around the menopause is not only to assess the impact of the menopause on the systems discussed above, but also to take the opportunity to appraise the presence of other risk factors, both modifiable and non-modifiable, that may affect health and longevity.

Modifiable and non-modifiable risk factors affecting health and longevity

Relevant symptoms

- Vasomotor.
- Urogenital tract, including sexual concerns.
- Cognition.
- Joint pains.
- Vaginal bleeding (if relevant).

Signs

- Blood pressure.
- BMI.
- Vaginal assessment including cervical smear.
- Breast examination if indicated.

Lifestyle

- Exercise levels.
- Nutrition.
- Smoking and alcohol intake.
- Relationship and sexual history.
- Contraceptive needs.

Personal medical/gynaecological history

- Obstetric history.
- Administration of drugs that influence oestrogen levels.
- Age of menopause.
- History of cancer and cancer treatment.
- Chronic disease and treatment.
- Corticosteroid administration.
- Fracture history.

Family history

- CVD.
- Osteoporosis.
- Thromboembolic disease.

There is rarely a need for investigations to confirm menopause. While a serum FSH level more than 30 IU/l is highly suspicious of menopause, the diagnosis can be confidently made in most women based on history alone; the key features being oligo/amenorrhoea and the typical symptoms of vasomotor symptoms, joint aches and minor cognitive changes.

The moment a perimenopausal woman presents for an assessment as to whether she is menopausal or not gives an important opportunity for preventative health care. It is important to address her reasons for presentation, but also to appraise her compliance with various national screening programmes, her general health and opportunities for improvement in health. Nationally, it is recognized that not all women spontaneously present for such advice and there are currently national campaigns to lobby for funding for at least one such 'health check' to occur at or around the menopause.

Management

Key to the management of the postmenopausal woman is, as discussed above, to embrace the main message of prevention of long-term health problems in the context of managing any menopause-related symptoms.

Diet and lifestyle

Extensive evidence exists to support improved longevity with regular exercise, stopping smoking and reducing alcohol consumption. Most will be aware of the beneficial effects of the above measures, which are well publicized, including reduced heart disease and the prevention of lung cancer and liver disease. However, few will be aware of the additional benefits of these actions, which should be emphasized in the menopausal consultation (*Table 8.4*).

Table 8.4 Beneficial effects of various lifestyle changes in postmenopausal women

Stopping smoking	Prevention of lung cancer Reduction of CVD Beneficial effects on bone loss
Reducing alcohol consumption	Reduction of calorie intake Fewer, less severe vasomotor symptoms Beneficial effects on bone loss Prevention of alcohol-related liver damage Reduction in incidence of breast cancer Reduction of CVD
Normal BMI	Reduction of calorie intake Fewer, less severe vasomotor symptoms Beneficial effects on bone loss Reduction in incidence of breast cancer Reduction in incidence of endometrial cancer Reduction of CVD

BMI, body mass index; CVD, cardiovascular disease.

One of the more challenging messages to communicate to women after the menopause is that on average body weight increases by approximately 1 kg per year and this, along with a more android fat distribution, contributes to a greater sensation of being overweight. Often women who start HRT early in the menopause erroneously blame this weight gain on HRT. They should be informed that there is no evidence from extensive research to support the belief that hormone therapy causes weight gain.

Non-hormonal approaches

Most women on experiencing the early symptoms of the menopause will seek out a solution from the wide range of alternative and 'natural' solutions available in reputable pharmacies, supermarkets, health food shops, high street herbalists, clinics and on-line suppliers with various levels of reliability. Usually a woman will present for medical input after she has tried or discounted some of the above measures. She should be informed of the beneficial effects of lifestyle measures before exploring appropriate non-hormonal measures.

Alternative and complementary treatments

These groups of treatments are widely available (*Table 8.5*) but very poorly researched in the scientific manner that the medical profession requires to make evidenced-based clinical decisions. This can make it difficult to fully counsel a woman as to how effective the treatment is, how long any effect will last and, most importantly, how safe the therapy is. Efficacy is usually limited and of a short duration, with the potential for interactions with other pharmaceutical agents.

When counselling a woman about taking 'natural' hormones, it is important to make her aware that these are essentially weak HRT and that if they are taking a high-dose therapy there is a possibility they could be exposing themselves to the known risks of HRT.

Non-hormonal prescription treatments

This group of therapies (*Table 8.6*) is increasingly important to consider in the management of women to reduce symptoms of hot flushes when hormones are not wanted or contraindicated, for example previous diagnoses of hormone-sensitive cancers such as breast cancer.

Other issues specific to the menopause can also be treated without hormones using prescribable

Table 8.5 Alternative and complementary treatments

Complementary drug-free therapies (delivered by a practitioner)	Acupuncture Reflexology Magnetism Reiki Hypnotism
Herbal/natural preparations (designed to be ingested)	Black cohosh (*Actaea racemosa*) Dong quai (*Angelica sinensis*) Evening primrose oil (*Oenothera biennis*) Gingko (*Gingko biloba*) Ginseng (*Panax ginseng*) Kava kava (*Piper methysticum*) St John's wort (*Hypericum perforatum*)
'Natural' hormones (designed to be ingested or applied to the skin)	Phytoestrogens such as isoflavones and red clover Natural progesterone gel Dehydroepiandrosterone (DHEA)

Table 8.6 Non-hormonal treatments for vasomotor symptoms

Alpha-adrenergic agonists	Clonidine
Beta-blockers	Propanolol
Modulators of central neurotransmission	Venlafaxine Fluoxetine Paroxetine Citalopram Gabapentin

preparations. These include vaginal moisturizers and lubricants for vaginal dryness and some of the many therapies for treating osteoporosis, which include bisphosphonates, raloxifene denosumab and teriparatide.

Hormonal replacement therapy

HRT has been the mainstay of the treatment of menopausal symptoms for decades. Its use has always attracted controversy, initially in its promotion as a drug with rejuvenating abilities, and then during a period where long-term benefits on osteoporosis and CVD prevention from large cohort studies were appearing. In 2002 a large randomized trial highlighted a series of potential risks from HRT use. This attracted so much media attention that many women either stopped treatment themselves or their prescribers stopped prescribing.

Since the initial publication of this study there have been significant changes in the data presented from the study. These new data, along with subsequent studies, have either significantly reduced or removed the risks initially described. It is important when digesting the risks of hormone therapy that recent publications (preferably after 2010) are considered.

Types of hormones contained in HRT

Oestrogens

There is a group of hormones with oestrogenic activity. If oestrogen is given without progestogenic opposition, there is a risk that in time endometrial hyperplasia and cancer may develop. Systemic oestrogen-only HRT is suitable for women who no longer have a uterus following a hysterectomy.

Oestrogen with progestogen

The administration of progestogen is necessary to protect the endometrium in women who have not had a hysterectomy. It is normally given cyclically in preparations over a 28-day cycle, of which 16–18 days will provide oestrogen alone and 10–12 days will provide oestrogen and progesterone combined (cyclical HRT). This results in regular monthly menstruation and is suitable for women during the perimenopause or early postmenopausal years.

Oestrogen and progesterone may be given continuously (continuous combined HRT) to women who are known to be postmenopausal or over the age of 54 years. These are usually preparations with the same dose of daily oestrogen combined with a smaller dose of progestogen taken every day. These regimes normally result in about 90% of women not experiencing vaginal bleeding.

Several types of progestogens are used in HRT by different manufacturers. A change of type, dose or route of progestogen is occasionally required to reduce unwanted side-effects of the drug.

Hormones used in HRT

- Oestrogens:
  - oestradiol (the main physiological oestrogen);
  - oestrone sulphate;
  - oestriol;
  - conjugated equine oestrogen.
- Progestogens:
  - norethisterone;
  - levonorgestrel;
  - dydrogesterone;
  - medroxyprogesterone acetate;
  - drospirenone;
  - micronized progesterone.

Testosterone

Testosterone has traditionally been given to women with disorders of sexual desire and energy levels who have failed to respond to normal HRT. These beneficial effects of testosterone are well documented; however, few long-term studies into the adverse effects of testosterone exist.

Over the past years manufacturers have stopped making testosterone drugs for women to the point that the only available preparations available now are those licensed for use in men. This usually means that testosterone needs to be instigated under the care of a doctor with specialist menopause knowledge.

Routes of hormone therapy administration

The two main routes of HRT delivery are oral and transdermal. The oral route is normally a daily tablet that contains the appropriate mix of oestrogen and progestogen, depending on the preparation. The oral route is convenient and cheap but does influence lipid metabolism and the coagulation system through its effects on the liver during first-pass metabolism.

The transdermal route, either given as patches applied to the skin on the trunk or as measured amounts of gel, is also effective, with the advantage of delivery of oestradiol directly into the circulation, avoiding the above potentially adverse effects on the liver and the coagulation system. Oestradiol is also available as small vaginal tablets and a vaginal ring, and oestriol as measured dose vaginal creams that are important in the management of lower genital tract symptoms.

Progestogen in the form of levonorgestrel may be administered as an intrauterine releasing system (IUS), Mirena®. This device not only provides contraception and control of troublesome bleeding, but also provides endometrial protection for up to 5 years (see Chapter 17, Gynaecological surgery and therapeutics).

Beneficial effects of hormone therapy

Vasomotor symptoms

The principal reason for taking HRT is vasomotor symptom improvement. Well over 90% of women note a significant improvement within 6 weeks, with reductions in frequency and severity of hot flushes and night sweats and consequent improvements in sleep and daytime energy levels as well as concentration.

The skeleton

The protective effects of HRT on the skeleton include prevention of bone loss and the prevention of osteoporotic fractures of the hip and spine. The use of HRT is strongly recommended for women after POF as they are at a much greater risk of osteoporosis. Most postmenopausal women should consider HRT as a means to prevent bone loss, especially if they require HRT for other symptomatology.

Key benefits of HRT

- Symptoms improved:
  - vasomotor symptoms;
  - sleep patterns;
  - performance during the day.
- Prevention of osteoporosis:
  - increased bone mineral density;
  - reduced incidence of fragility fractures.
- Lower genital tract:
  - dryness;
  - soreness;
  - dyspareunia;
  - CVD: preventative effect if started early in menopause.

The lower genital tract

Both systemic and locally administered HRT have significant beneficial effects on the lower genital tract. There is good evidence that its administration improves vulvovaginal dryness, irritation, soreness and dyspareunia. There is also an improvement in symptoms of cystitis and occasionally dysuria. Local hormone therapy is unlikely to cure prolapse but may improve some of the symptoms of prolapse. There is no evidence that local HRT improves incontinence. Many women considering local HRT are dissuaded from its use due to concerns about the published risks. They can often be reassured that were they to use the form of local hormone therapy as a 10 μg twice weekly dose vaginal tablet, they would only be administering approximately the equivalent of a 1 mg oral tablet over a whole year.

The cardiovascular system

The cardiovascular benefits of HRT were first demonstrated in large observational cohort studies. The principal benefits were reduction in ischaemic heart disease and overall mortality. However the large randomized Women's Health Initiative (WHI) study demonstrated reductions in survival from CVD in women taking HRT. This study has been widely criticized due to the overweight and generally older population studied, a population probably at greater risk of CVD. The current understanding is that there is a 'window of opportunity' in the perimenopausal or early postmenopausal years during which the administration of HRT may reduce the morbidity and mortality from CVD by prevention of atheroma formation.

While the prevention of CVD is not currently a licensed indication for HRT, the data are sufficient to include a discussion with women that they should consider these benefits.

The colon

While the WHI study demonstrated a clear benefit of HRT on the incidence and mortality of colon cancer, the use of HRT to prevent this malignancy is not indicated.

Prescribing and side-effects of hormone therapy

Prior to prescribing HRT it is important to weigh up the indications, proposed benefits and potential risks for each patient individually. For example, hormone therapy may be contraindicated in a patient with a prior history of breast cancer or thromboembolic disease.

In general, side-effects with HRT are few and minor. It is therefore important before starting HRT to ensure that the woman has no contraindications to HRT and to ensure that she has had no serious effects in the past when on the contraceptive pill, such as venous thrombosis or migraine with aura.

Contraindications and potential side-effects

- Absolute contraindications:
  - suspected pregnancy;
  - breast cancer;
  - endometrial cancer;
  - active liver disease;
  - uncontrolled hypertension;
  - known current venous thromboembolism (VTE);
  - known thrombophilia (e.g. Factor V leiden);
  - otosclerosis.
- Relative contraindications:
  - uninvestigated abnormal bleeding;
  - large uterine fibroids;
  - past history of benign breast disease;
  - unconfirmed personal history or a strong family history of VTE;
  - chronic stable liver disease;
  - migraine with aura.
- Side-effects associated with oestrogen:
  - breast tenderness or swelling;
  - nausea;
  - leg cramps;
  - headaches.
- Side-effects associated with progestogen:
  - fluid retention;
  - breast tenderness;
  - headaches;
  - mood swings;
  - depression;
  - acne.

Most side-effects can be managed with a change in dose of oestrogen or a change in type of progestogen. Some patients can also benefit from a switch of route. Many women find the IUS a useful device as it delivers much less progestogen into the circulation, thus reducing progestogenic side-effects.

The duration for which a woman should take HRT is frequently debated. There is little clear evidence to support how long, but it is recommended that there should be no exact maximum age at which a woman should stop HRT, rather employing regular assessment of the woman and her needs along with review of the type and dose of HRT she is taking.

Risks of hormone therapy

The risks attributed to HRT have attracted much media attention. At present, due to a combination of reanalysis of the data, new studies and a better understanding of the communication of risk, many more women are considering HRT in the management of their menopause.

Cancer

Breast cancer is without doubt the cancer that attracts most concern from patients and most attention from the world's media. The studies performed still do not fully inform patients of the additional risks they expose themselves to by using HRT. Useful figures to quote are that the background risk of breast cancer in the 50–59 year age group is 22.5 per 1,000 women for 7.5 years use of HRT and there may be an additional 2–6 cancers with combined HRT use, which reduces after stopping HRT. It is important to be aware that recent data with oestradiol HRT suggest that mortality from breast cancer is not increased and that certain types of HRT may promote the growth of pre-existing malignant cells rather than initiate tumours.

Endometrial cancer and ovarian cancer are not considered significant risks with HRT use. Endometrial malignancy risk is largely eliminated if women are given progestogens. Incidence of ovarian cancer has not been shown to significantly increase with HRT use.

Cardiovascular disease and stroke

As discussed above, most of the effects of HRT on the cardiovascular system when given to younger women are beneficial. However, when given to older women the effects may become deleterious. The degree to which this happens is unclear but is likely to be higher in women taking combined HRT.

Stroke incidence has a similar age effect, with the increased incidence greater in the older woman. The effect is small and is only on the incidence of ischaemic stroke, thought to be an increase of an additional 2 women per 10,000 women per year when on HRT.

Venous thromboembolism

The influence of HRT on the clotting system is similar to that of the oral contraceptive. The background incidence of all VTE in women over 50 is low (approximately 15–20 per 10,000) and HRT doubles this risk. There is evidence to suggest that transdermal HRT, through its avoidance of effects on the liver, may not have such a great effect on VTE incidence.

Using such an approach can address many elements of health, improving longevity and quality of life.

- HRT exists in a variety of forms and is effective in improving menopausal symptoms and bone mineral density.
- The potential use of HRT in prevention of disease, while considering the small additional risks its use attracts, means that over the coming years it may become a cost-effective means of improving the lives of the expanding numbers of the global population of menopausal women.

KEY LEARNING POINTS

- The menopause is a key time in the life of a woman.
- The physiological changes that occur have significant effects on the woman as a whole, affecting numerous body systems.
- Care of women during the postreproductive years should be managed in a holistic fashion that addresses lifestyle and general health issues first.

Further reading

Lobo RA1, Davis SR, De Villiers TJ, *et al.* (2014). Prevention of diseases after menopause. *Climacteric* **17**(5):540–56.

Panay N, Hamoda H, Arya R, Savvas M; British Menopause Society and Women's Health Concern (2013). The 2013 British Menopause Society & Women's Health Concern recommendations on hormone replacement therapy. *Menopause Int* **19**(2):59–68.

Rees M, Stevenson J, Hope S, Rozenberg S, Palacios S (2009). *Management of the Menopause*, 5th Edition. London: Royal Society of Medicine Press and British Menopause Society Publications.

Self assessment

CASE HISTORY

Mrs A is a 36-year-old woman. She has had one child delivered normally 6 years previously after a brief period of subfertility. Following delivery of that child she had 4 years of infrequent periods and over the last 2 years she has been amenorrhoeic and has had difficulty sleeping, often waking up feeling hot.

A What is the likely diagnosis?

B How would the diagnosis be confirmed?

C Following diagnosis Mrs A asks what the immediate and long-term issues are and how they might be managed. Outline the key issues.

ANSWERS

A POI.

B A combination of the clinical picture and serum FSH levels are usually adequate to confirm the diagnosis. On receipt of one elevated FSH level it is recommended that a repeat test no sooner than 6 weeks after the first is performed to confirm the diagnosis.

C One of the first issues on diagnosis of POI is to inform Mrs A that there is still an appreciable risk of unpredictable ovulation and as such her contraceptive needs should be discussed.

The issue of bone protection should be explained to her. With her prolonged entry into POI she could have osteoporosis or osteopaenia. Consideration of bone densitometry and management with HRT or bisphosphonates should be considered.

The benefits of HRT should be explained to her. It is often helpful to highlight that because she has lost her endogenous oestrogen at an early age in comparison to her peers, if she were to take HRT she would not be exposing herself to any appreciable excess risks from HRT until the age of approximately 51.

SBA QUESTIONS

1 A 68-year-old woman presents with recurrent episodes of postmenopausal bleeding. The volume of blood loss is only very small amounts of spotting that often, but not exclusively, follow intercourse. Her previous gynaecological history is unremarkable, with a lifetime of normal cervical smears. She is not on any drugs, including HRT. Pelvic ultrasound and endometrial biopsy are normal. Vaginal examination demonstrates vaginal dryness, small petechiae and loss of rugae.

What is the most appropriate next step in her management? Choose the single best answer.

A   Outpatient hysteroscopic assessment of the endometrium.

B   Transdermal continuous combined HRT.

C   Water-based vaginal lubricants.

D   Oestrogen-containing vaginal pessaries.

E   Flexible cystourethroscopy.

ANSWER

D   The normal ultrasound and endometrium indicate that there is no concern about endometrial pathology including malignancy. Therefore, outpatient hysteroscopy or examination of the bladder with flexible cystourethroscopy is unnecessary. Vaginal lubricants are useful for painful intercourse but local oestrogen will induce a return of the vagina to premenopausal flexibility and lubrication. Transdermal oestrogen therapy is not necessary unless there are systemic symptoms of hypoestrogenism.

2 With regard to the hormone changes that accompany the menopause, which of the following is true? Choose the single best answer.

A   As ovarian function fails, serum FSH levels increase.

B   12 months after the LMP serum levels of testosterone are close to zero.

C   Secretion of GnRH from the hypothalamus increases significantly in the late menopause to drive ovarian activity.

D   Progesterone levels are undetectable in the perimenopause.

E   High levels of peripherally-produced oestrogens reduce the frequency and severity of hot flushes in obese women.

ANSWER

A   FSH rises in response to increasing pulsatility of GnRH, itself responding to falling inhibin as the follicles become depleted in the perimenopause. Subsequently, there is a progressive decline in GnRH pulsatility and GnRH levels overall fall.

Only 30–50% of testosterone production is ovarian, and levels fall slowly after menopause because its production is mainly independent of the neuroendocrine axis. Although adipose tissue produces oestrogen, it is an insulator interfering with heat dissipation; hot flushes are worse in obese women.

There is a only a slow decline in progesterone during the perimenopause, and so levels remain detectable.

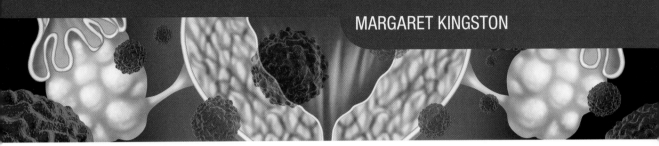

Genitourinary problems

CHAPTER

9

MARGARET KINGSTON

LEARNING OUTCOMES

- Understand the importance of sexually transmitted infections (STIs) in gynaecology.
- Describe the testing, diagnosis and transmission of common STIs and blood-borne viruses (BBVs).
- Understand that support is needed for patients to enable them to undertake screening.

- Appreciate that human immunodeficiency virus (HIV) has changed from life limiting into a chronic, manageable condition.
- Learn how to take a sexual history.
- Understand the diagnosis of and screening for HIV.
- Describe the care for the HIV-positive mother and child.

Introduction

An understanding of STIs and their complications is crucially important in gynaecological practice. The subject is frequently misunderstood and the impact on affected women, their partners and at times their children may be considerable. STIs are often asymptomatic, but can still be transmitted to others and cause significant problems at the time of infection or in the future; for example, human papillomavirus (HPV) infection and cervical cancer. STIs disproportionately affect younger people, but increasingly they are identified in older people, in whom the diagnosis is often not considered and so can be missed. STIs often coexist and when one is found, screening for others is required.

Tests for STIs have hugely improved in recent years, with the advent of highly sensitive and accurate molecular tests that are very easy to use and can detect several infections on a single swab or urine sample. In addition, serological tests for BBVs and syphilis have also increased in accuracy, and can be performed sooner after possible exposure than in the past. Women are often diagnosed first when they have young families and they attend for reproductive health care and are offered screening. They require support to inform present (and where necessary) previous partners, so they can also receive testing and treatment for their own health to prevent reinfection and/or on-going transmission within the community. Children may also require testing and treatment if they have been exposed during pregnancy, birth or breastfeeding. This aspect of managing STIs can be

121

very challenging but is crucially important. The consultation may lead to a consideration of safeguarding of women and girls who may be exposed to sexual or domestic violence, abuse, coercion or exploitation, which may only become apparent in this context.

The treatment and management of HIV infection has been transformed, and the disease has changed from life limiting into a chronic manageable condition. In addition, effective treatment also prevents transmission to sexual partners and children. The treatments are simpler with less toxicity and the widespread availability of cheaper, generic medicines has resulted in therapies that are acceptable, affordable and manageable, requiring less monitoring than before.

Unfortunately, STIs and HIV remain stigmatizing conditions for many women, who find informing partners or sharing news of any diagnosis with friends or family very difficult. Consequently they can feel isolated and may need additional support from their health care professionals. Respecting and maintaining patient confidentiality is vital when managing women with an STI or HIV diagnosis.

Taking a sexual history

This is the first step to identifying and treating STIs. It allows the health care professional to quantify risk, decide which tests are required and whether they need to be repeated later, and gather information needed for treatment. In addition, it provides an opportunity for patients to express concerns and ask questions. Raising the issue of STIs may be unexpected and it is important to start by ensuring privacy and then explaining why the subject is being broached, to ask permission to proceed and to reassure the patient about confidentiality. Important points to cover are summarized in *Table 9.1*. Abuse, exploitation or coercion can happen to anyone, but younger women and sexually active children

Table 9.1 Points to cover in a sexual history and screening questions for sexual exploitation

Rationale for questions	Points to cover in the questions
Assessment of clinical need and symptoms	Why the patient is attending If symptoms are present explore their specific features History of past or current STIs including HIV status
Sexual and other exposures to guide testing decisions	Sexual exposure: how many sex partners in the last 3 months and when, what sort of sexual exposure occurred in each case, were condoms used Partner details: what is the gender of each partner, what is their country of origin, are they contactable, did they have symptoms or are they known to have any STIs, what was the nature of the relationship, is it ongoing Other exposures: intravenous drug use, high risk tattoos or piercings or medical procedures
Contraception needs and pregnancy risk assessment	Last menstrual period, any current pregnancy risk and need for a pregnancy test Opportunity to provide contraception
Other sexual health needs	Cervical cytology; opportunity to provide if needed Vaccination: HPV or hepatitis B, opportunity to provide if appropriate Others usually as raised by the patient (e.g. sexual function and satisfaction)
Assessment of risk behaviours open to health promotion	Alcohol, smoking, recreational drug use assessment, brief interventions or signpost to services
Assessment of exploitation/ violence/abuse	Any forced sex or violence or other abuse from sex partners Any coercive sex; is the woman in a vulnerable position from her sex partner or on occasion their family or friends For younger people and all under 16 years, what is the age of their sex partner, do they receive presents for sex, do they attend school and do they have supportive family members and friends who know their partner(s), are there other vulnerability concerns

HIV, human immunodeficiency virus; HPV, human papillomavirus; STI, sexually-transmitted infection.

especially so, and screening questions for this are also included in *Table 9.1*.

Testing for STIs and associated conditions

Technological advances have facilitated accurate, non-invasive testing for most STIs. Point of care tests (POCTs) are available for many infections including HIV, but may have suboptimal sensitivity and/or specificity, and it is important to be aware of these limitations. Close liaison with local laboratory staff is crucial to ensure the best available tests are used, appropriately interpreted and communicated in a timely fashion. *Table 9.2* summarizes appropriate screening and diagnostic tests.

Infective causes of vaginal discharge (Figure 9.1)

Bacterial vaginosis

The commonest cause of abnormal vaginal discharge, bacterial vaginosis (BV) has been reported in 5–50% of female cohorts worldwide. While a definitive cause is not determined, depletion of the lactobacilli dominant in the healthy vaginal flora is observed, together with an elevation of vaginal pH to above 4.5. The existence of a vaginal epithelial biofilm consisting of *Gardnerella vaginalis* and other species has been more recently described. Other risk factors include douching, black race, smoking, having a new sexual partner and receiving oral sex.

Symptoms include an offensive vaginal discharge that is often reported as having a 'fishy' malodour, and on examination a homogenous off-white vaginal discharge with a high pH is observed. Diagnosis is made by evaluating a Gram stain of the vaginal discharge using a validated method, such as the Hay-Ison or Nugent criteria, or, less frequently in modern practice, by using Amsels criteria (3 of 4 are required: homogenous discharge, high pH, 'clue cells' on microscopy and a fishy odour when 10% potassium hydroxide is added to a sample of discharge). BV is associated with a number of pathologies including pelvic inflammatory disease (PID), posthysterectomy vaginal cuff cellulitis and, in pregnancy, preterm birth and rupture of membranes and miscarriage. An increased risk of HIV acquisition is observed in women at risk with BV.

Oral or intravaginal treatments with metronidazole or clindamycin are indicated in women with symptoms or those in whom it is diagnosed and

Table 9.2 Tests for STIs and related conditions in women

Bacterial vaginosis	Microscopy of vaginal discharge or Amsel's criteria Not required if asymptomatic
Candidiasis	Microscopy of vaginal discharge +/– culture, not required if asymptomatic
Trichomoniasis	NAAT test from vulvovaginal swab Culture or wet mount microscopy of vaginal discharge alternative Not required if asymptomatic
Chlamydia	NAAT test from vulvovaginal swab If history of receptive oral or anal sex, swab from those sites
Gonorrhoea	NAAT test from vulvovaginal swab Culture required if test positive before treatment, or as alternative test If history of receptive oral or anal sex, swab those sites
HIV	Serology for combined and HIV 1+2 antibodies, preferably in combination with HIV p24 antigen Tests also available on dried blood spot and saliva samples, some as near patient tests
Syphilis	Serology for treponemal test (usually EIA), if positive non-treponemal test titre
Hepatitis B and C	Serology for hepatitis B core antibody or surface antigen or both, hepatitis C antibody These tests to be done in a woman from a high prevalence area or at additional risk of infection (e.g. known or likely exposure, intravenous drug use, sex work)

EIA, enzyme-linked immunoassay; HIV, human immunodeficiency virus; NAAT, nucleic acid amplification test.

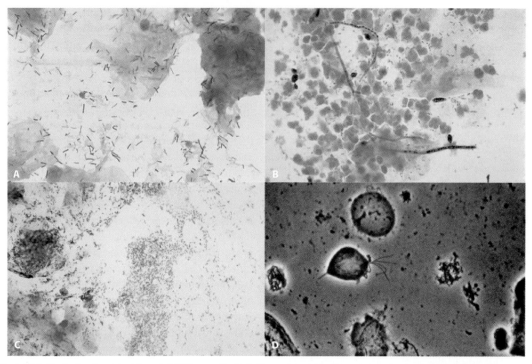

Figure 9.1 Vaginal and cervical flora (×1,000 magnified). **A**: Normal: lactobacilli – seen as large gram-positive rods – predominate. Squamous epithelial cells are gram-negative. with a large aount of cytoplasm. **B**: Candidiasis: there are speckled gram-positive spores and long pseudohyphae visible. There are numerous polymorphs present and the bacterial flora is abnormal, resembling bacterial vaginosis. **C**: Bacterial vaginosis: there is an overgrowth of anaerobic organisms, including *Gardnerella vaginalis* (small gram-variable cocci), and a decrease in the numbers of lactobacilli. A 'clue cell' is seen. This is an epithelial cell covered with small bacteria so the edge of the cell is obscured. **D**: Trichomoniasis: an unstained 'wet mount' of vaginal fluid from a woman with *Trichomonas vaginalis* infection. There is a cone-shaped, flagellated organism in the centre, with a terminal spike and four flagella visible. In practice, the organism is identified under the microscope by movement, with amoeboid motion and its flagella waving.

elect for treatment – especially prior to gynaecological surgical procedures. Women with BV should be advised that vaginal douching or excessive genital washing should be avoided.

Vulvovaginal candidiasis

This condition occurs when yeast of the *Candida* species, most frequently *C. albicans*, cause vulval and vaginal inflammation. The vagina is colonized with *Candida* sp. in up to 20% of women in their reproductive years, rising to 40% in pregnancy, and is most often asymptomatic. When symptoms occur they include itching, irritation and a typically white, curdy vaginal discharge. On examination, signs of inflammation, including erythema, oedema and fissuring of the vulva and vagina, together with the discharge may be observed. Symptoms may be more frequent and persistent when the woman is

diabetic, immunocompromised and in pregnancy. The diagnosis is made by taking a bacterial swab for microscopy and culture and treatment with topical intravaginal pessaries or oral imidazoles are effective. Topical vulval antifungals and the use of aqueous cream as an emollient and cleansing agent provide symptomatic relief. This is not an STI and partners without symptoms do not require treatment.

Trichomoniasis

Vaginal and urethral infection with the flagellate protozoan *Trichomonas vaginalis* (TV) results in symptoms of vaginal discharge with a variable appearance and symptoms and/or signs of vulvovaginitis. Asymptomatic infection is observed in up to 50% of women and most of their male sexual partners. TV is sexually transmitted and simultaneous treatment of current and recent sexual partners is required. There is some evidence of an association with pregnancy outcome: preterm birth, low birthweight and maternal postpartum sepsis, although further research is required. Testing is indicated in symptomatic women, and the gold standard is a nucleic acid amplification test (NAAT) preferably on a vaginal or endocervical swab or on urine, with sensitivities and specificities reaching over 95%, depending on the specimen and the test. Some NAATs also detect *Neisseria gonorrhoea* and *Chlamydia trachomatis* on the same sample; for these the optimal test is a vulvovaginal swab. Microscopy and culture of a sample of the vaginal discharge and POCT using different techniques are also used but are limited by reduced sensitivity. Treatment is with a systemic metronidazole regime.

Cervicitis and pelvic inflammatory disease

Gonorrhoea (Figure 9.2)

This condition is caused by infection with the bacteria *Neisseria gonorrhoea*. Infection occurs through sexual contact and simultaneous treatment of current and recent sexual partners is required. Endocervical infection is asymptomatic in up to 50% of cases, with altered vaginal discharge the most common symptom and lower abdominal pain in up to 25%. Rectal infection occurs through transmucosal spread and

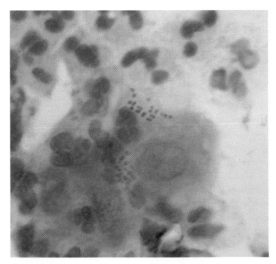

Figure 9.2 Gram-stained smear of cervical secretions showing polymorths and gram-negative intracellular diplococci (×1,000). This appearance is highly suggestive of gonorrhoea.

receptive anal sex, and pharyngeal infection through receptive oral sex; the latter is nearly always asymptomatic. Examination is often normal, although cervicitis with or without a mucopurulent discharge may be seen. Ascending infection may result in PID and, rarely, haematogenous spread can cause disseminated gonococcal infection with a purpuric non-blanching rash and/or an arthralgia or arthritis that is typically monoarticular in a weight-bearing joint. Ophthalmic infection occurs due to inoculation from infected genital secretions, and neonatal infection occurs when the mother has endocervical infection at the time of delivery.

Testing is indicated in symptomatic women or those who have another STI. NAAT tests are highly sensitive and specific, and if *N. gonorrhoea* is identified it is important to obtain a sample for culture and sensitivity testing as there has been a development of widespread antimicrobiological resistance that requires careful surveillance. Screening for other STIs is crucial, particularly for *C. trachomatis*, as dual infection is common. Dual treatment of uncomplicated infection is presently with a parenteral third-generation cephalosporin plus azithromycin; the recent addition of azithromycin to treatment regimens is an attempt to delay the emergence of further drug resistance.

Chlamydia

Chlamydial infection is the most common bacterial STI, with women under 25 years of age most frequently affected. Infection with *C. trachomatis* is often asymptomatic but can still result in subclinical PID and subsequent complications. For this reason screening programmes for this age group have been developed and there is some evidence that they reduce the rates of PID. Testing is also indicated in women with other risk factors, including a new sexual partner, or those with symptoms that include altered vaginal discharge, intermenstrual or postcoital bleeding or abdominal pain. Examination is often normal, but cervicitis with mucopurulent discharge may be present. Infection at other mucosal sites occurs as in gonorrhoea (although it is thought to a lesser extent) and similarly neonates born to mothers with cervical infection may develop conjunctivitis. A reactive arthritis that is typically monoarticular affecting the weight-bearing joints may occur, but is more common in men.

NAAT tests are widely available for *C. trachomatis*, and some test simultaneously for *N. gonorrhoea* with the option to add on testing for TV in women with indicative symptoms. These tests offer high levels of sensitivity and specificity, and in women the optimal genital specimen is a vulvovaginal swab that may be self-taken by the woman without compromising diagnostic accuracy. For uncomplicated genital chlamydia, equally effective treatment regimens include azithromycin or doxycycline; the benefit of the former is that it is single dose and well tolerated. Simultaneous treatment of current and recent sexual partners is required.

Pelvic inflammatory disease

This occurs when there is ascending infection from the endocervix to the higher reproductive tract. It is a recognized complication of chlamydia and less frequently of gonorrhoea, but they are often not isolated and other implicated organisms include *Mycoplasma genitalium* as well as those in the vaginal microflora. The diagnosis of PID is usually made clinically and symptoms typically include lower bilateral abdominal pain, dyspareunia, altered vaginal discharge and IMB or PCB. Systemic symptoms of infection may be present. Characteristic clinical findings include lower abdominal and cervical motion tenderness and cervicitis. Testing for all STIs is required, as is exclusion of pregnancy. Where PID is suspected empirical treatment should be started immediately, as delay increases the risk of complications. These include the sequelae of endometrial and Fallopian tube inflammation and damage such as subfertility, ectopic pregnancy and chronic pelvic pain. Right upper quadrant pain due to perihepatitis is an unusual complication called Fitz-Hugh–Curtis syndrome (**Figure 9.3**).

Laparoscopy in women with PID may reveal scarring and adhesion formation between the structures of the pelvis and the development of hydrosalpinges of the tubes. There is a predisposition to ectopic pregnancy (**Figure 9.4**). If an intrauterine device (IUD) is *in situ* it is advisable to consider removing this, although the risk of pregnancy if there has been unprotected sex in the last week should be considered. Treatment regimes should cover all common pathogens and are 2 weeks in duration; they usually include a macrolide or tetracycline plus metronidazole with a parenteral third-generation cephalosporin at the start. Sexual partners require simultaneous screening and empirical treatment, usually with azithromycin. Women require clear information regarding possible sequelae from their infection.

Viral STIs and systemic manifestations

Genital herpes

There are two types of herpes virus that cause this condition; herpes simplex virus (HSV) type 1 and type 2. HSV-1 causes orolabial herpes also and is often acquired in childhood, although it is also a common cause of genital herpes alongside HSV-2. Following acquisition the virus establishes latency in the local sensory ganglia and may reactivate, resulting in shedding of the virus, with or without symptoms. Primary infection is the first infection of either HSV-1 or -2; non-primary infection is subsequent infection with the other type. The majority of initial infections are asymptomatic, although the individual may still be infectious, and subsequent recurrences may be symptomatic. Recurrence rates are significantly higher with HSV-2 and reduce in frequency with time.

Symptoms include genital pain and dysuria, and on examination there are typically multiple superficial tender ulcers with regional lymphadenopathy (although this may be limited to the initial infection). Diagnosis is by detection of the virus from the genital lesions by gently taking a swab. The test of choice is a polymerase chain reaction (PCR) test

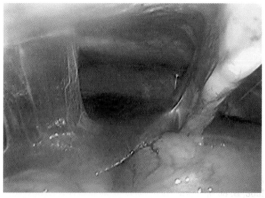

Figure 9.3 Fitz-Hugh–Curtis syndrome showing perihepatic adhesions (typical violin string appearance).

that types the virus, although less sensitive culture methods are still used in some centres. Type-specific serology, testing for immunoglobulin (Ig) G and IgM to HSV-1 and -2, can be helpful in establishing whether or not an individual is at risk of infection or if the infection is primary, non-primary or a recurrence. In clinical practice this is useful when assessing women and their sexual partners in pregnancy.

Neonatal herpes is a devastating infection with a mortality rate of up to 30% and consequent lifelong neurological morbidity in up to 70%. It is most often acquired during delivery if the mother has primary or non-primary initial infection within the third trimester and especially the last 6 weeks, when reported neonatal infection rates are as high as 41%. IgG to the virus in the serum crosses the placenta and provides neonatal protection from infection, and the risk of neonatal herpes when the mother has lesions of recurrent infection present at delivery is less than 3%. For this reason the recommended mode of delivery for women with first-acquisition genital herpes in the third trimester is prelabour caesarean section, and in those with proven recurrent lesions, vaginal delivery may be anticipated if other obstetric factors allow.

Treatment of the symptoms of genital herpes is a course of aciclovir, which is very safe and effective, including in pregnancy, or a related compound (such as valaciclovir). These medicines are most effective when given as soon as possible after symptoms develop, and episodic and suppressive regimens are effective in managing symptoms from repeated recurrences. Information for patients, including the lifelong nature of the infection, asymptomatic shedding and therefore risk to sexual partners and the need for disclosure, the effectiveness of condoms (up to 50%) and antivirals in limiting transmission, are important.

Genital warts

These are benign epithelial tumours caused by HPV infection. There are over 100 genotypes of HPV and types 6 and 11 cause over 90% of genital warts. Infection with HPV in the genital epithelium via sexual transmission is extremely common, with the vast majority of cases being subclinical. Infection with the oncogenic genotypes including types 16 and 18 is also through sex, but these cause anogenital dysplasia and cancer, not warts. HPV vaccination

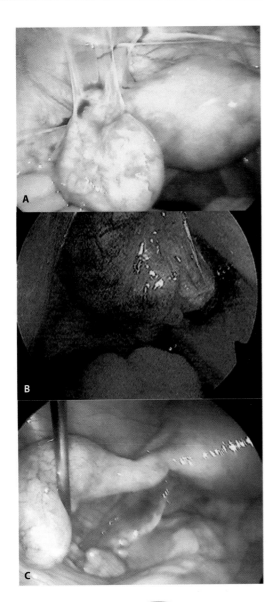

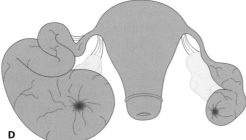

Figure 9.4 A: Peritubal adhesions of the left Fallopian tube; **B**: ectopic pregnancy within hydrosalpinx; **C**: left Fallopian tube hydrosalpinx; **D**: large hydrosalpinx of the left Fallopian tube with a smaller hydrosalpinx on the right side.

is available as a bivalent (against types 16 and 18) or quadrivalent (types 6, 11, 16 and 18) vaccine, and in cohorts where the latter has been introduced (such as in girls in Australia), a dramatic drop in the cases of genital warts has been observed.

Diagnosis is by clinical examination and treatments include ablative therapies such as application of liquid nitrogen or surgical techniques or patient-applied topical therapies, including podophyllotoxin-containing preparations or the local immune modulator imiquimod. As these are benign lesions treatment is optional. When genital warts are present in pregnancy treatment is limited to ablative options. Rarely, warts may become very large and obstruct the birth canal, necessitating caesarean delivery. Very rarely the neonate can develop respiratory papillomatosis, but the risk is extremely small and the benefit of caesarean delivery in preventing this unproven. Screening for other STIs is required and screening for cervical cancer is as usual.

Syphilis

Syphilis is caused by infection with the bacterium *Treponema pallidum* subspecies *pallidum*, which occurs through direct contact with secretions from an infective lesion or via transplacental passage of the bacteria during pregnancy. This infection is multisystem and has many clinical features that may mimic other conditions. Untreated it can relapse and remit and late complications can present many years after the original infection. Infectivity declines with time and treatment with penicillin-based regimens are curative, although reinfection may occur. Those living in African and Asian countries and Eastern Europe are more often affected, and in the last two decades there have been resurgences of infection observed in homosexual men in Western countries.

The infection is classified as congenital or acquired, and each of these as late or early. In acquired early syphilis the initial manifestation is the 'chancre', which develops at the site of exposure. This is usually a single, genital lesion but is increasingly seen at other sites such as the oral cavity and may be multiple. Typically the lesion is painless, indurated and exudes serous fluid containing *T. pallidum*, and there is regional lymphadenopathy. This resolves within a few weeks and following this as the bacteria

disseminate a plethora of variable clinical symptoms and signs may be apparent. These include a widespread erythematous rash typically including the palms and soles and that can result in alopecia, oral and genital mucous lesions and raised lesions, usually in the anogenital area, termed 'condylomata lata'.

Complications include neurological involvement, resulting in meningitis, an eighth nerve palsy and consequent deafness or tinnitus and ophthalmic involvement, most often uveitis. This stage also spontaneously resolves as the host immune response is effective in controlling the infection, although relapse may occur for up to 2 years, the accepted time limit of early infection, and approximately two-thirds of infected individuals suffer no further ill effects.

Late complications include:

- Gummatous lesions: granulomatous, locally destructive lesions typically affecting skin and bone.
- Cardiovascular involvement: usually affecting the ascending aorta, resulting in aortic valve incompetence.
- Neurological involvement: classified as meningovascular disease, tabes dorsalis and a progressive dementing illness, general paresis.

Congenital infection also consists of many symptoms and signs that are summarized in *Table 9.3*. The riskiest time for congenital infection is when syphilis is acquired either very soon before or during pregnancy. Screening for syphilis in pregnancy is well established, allowing effective treatment of most women, although infection may occur in pregnancy after this.

Diagnosis is by serology and/or directly detecting *T. pallidum* in infectious lesions, usually by dark field microscopy or, more recently, by PCR testing, although availability of this is limited. Non-treponemal serological tests include the rapid plasma reagin (RPR) and Venereal Disease Reference Laboratory (VDRL), which demonstrate rising titres during acute, active infection that drop with time and following treatment, and so can be used to monitor treatment. They may be negative in early infection, falsely positive in other physiological (such as pregnancy) or disease (including several rheumatological conditions) states, and so require confirmation by non-treponemal tests such as enzyme or

Table 9.3 Clinical feature of congenital syphilis

Early (within 2 years)	Late
Common manifestations (one of these is noted in 40–60% of infants): Rash Haemorrhagic rhinitis (bloody snuffles) Generalized lymphadenopathy/hepatosplenomegaly Skeletal abnormalities Other manifestations: Condylomata lata Vesiculobullous lesions, osteochondritis Periostitis Pseudoparalysis Mucous patches Perioral fissures Non-immune hydrops Glomerulonephritis neurological +/− ocular involvement Haemolysis and thrombocytopenia	These are termed the 'stigmata of congenital infection': Interstitial keratitis Clutton's joints Dental abnormalities including 'Hutchinson's incisors' and 'mulberry molars' High palatal arch Rhagades Sensineural deafness Fontal bossing Short maxilla Protuberance of mandible saddlenose deformity, sternoclavicular thickening, paroxysmal cold haemoglobinuria Neurological involvement including intellectual disability, cranial nerve palsies

chemiluminescence immunoassays (EIA/CLIA) or *T. pallidum* particle or haemagglutination assays (TPPA/TPHA). These treponemal tests may also be negative in the very early stages of disease, and should be repeated if negative 4–6 weeks later if this is suspected. Serological tests for syphilis may be positive for life, although reinfection results in the non-treponemal titre rising rapidly. Different testing algorithms are applied according to locally available tests and expertise is required together with a full clinical history to interpret their results adequately. Treatment is curative and involves depot preparations of penicillin; different regimes for differing stages of infection are the treatment of choice. Simultaneous treatment of current sexual partners is required, certainly in early disease. When the time of infection is not known, tracing and testing of previous partners, and where applicable children, is required.

Human immunodeficiency virus

Natural history, epidemiology, testing and treatment

Infection with HIV results in an initial acute viral illness followed by a chronic decline in cellular immunity due to progressive depletion of CD4-positive T-lymphocytes, and eventually resulting in one or more illnesses defined as the acquired immune deficiency syndrome (AIDS). These are listed in *Table 9.4* and, importantly in gynaecological practice, include cervical cancer, cervical intraepithelial neoplasia (CIN) grade 2/high-grade squamous intraepithelial lesion (HSIL) or above and vaginal intraepithelial neoplasia. HIV infection disproportionately affects those living in or originating from sub-Saharan Africa and their partners, homosexual men and intravenous drug users without access to clean injecting equipment. The global burden of HIV infection is depicted in **Figure 9.5**. Highly active retroviral therapy (HAART) has transformed the lives of HIV-positive people and their families, making early diagnosis and treatment crucial to allow maintenance of that individual's own health and to protect their partners and children from infection. For this reason USA guidelines recommend offering HIV testing to all those aged 13–64 accessing medical care and antiretroviral therapy to all those found to be HIV positive. The notification of present and previous partners, and if applicable children, is crucial as treatment in the earlier asymptomatic stages improves outcomes and prevents onward transmission.

Gynaecological complications in HIV-positive women

Women with HIV infection are more likely to have infection with HPV 16 or 18 and have a higher

Table 9.4 AIDS-defining illnesses

Bacterial infections, multiple or recurrent*	Lymphoid interstitial pneumonia or pulmonary lymphoid hyperplasia complex*†
Candidiasis of bronchi, trachea or lungs	
Candidiasis of oesophagus†	Lymphoma, Burkitt (or equivalent term)
Cervical cancer, invasive§	Lymphoma, immunoblastic (or equivalent term)
Coccidioidomycosis, disseminated or extrapulmonary	Lymphoma, primary, of brain
Cryptococcosis, extrapulmonary	*Mycobacterium avium* complex or *Mycobacterium kansasii*, disseminated or extrapulmonary†
Cryptosporidiosis, chronic intestinal (>1 month's duration)	
	Mycobacterium tuberculosis of any site, pulmonary,†§ disseminated,† or extrapulmonary†
Cytomegalovirus disease (other than liver, spleen or nodes), onset at age >1 month	
	Mycobacterium, other species or unidentified species, disseminated† or extrapulmonary†
Cytomegalovirus retinitis (with loss of vision)†	
Encephalopathy, HIV related	*Pneumocystis jirovecii* pneumonia†
Herpes simplex: chronic ulcers (>1 month's duration) or bronchitis, pneumonitis or oesophagitis (onset at age >1 month)	Pneumonia, recurrent†§
	Progressive multifocal leucoencephalopathy
	Salmonella septicaemia, recurrent
Histoplasmosis, disseminated or extrapulmonary	Toxoplasmosis of brain, onset at age >1 month†
Isosporiasis, chronic intestinal (>1 month's duration)	Wasting syndrome attributed to HIV
Kaposi sarcoma†	

Source: http://www.cdc.gov/mmwr/preview/mmwrhtml/rr5710a2.htm

* Only among children aged <13 years. (CDC. 1994 Revised classification system for human immunodeficiency virus infection in children less than 13 years of age. *MMWR* 1994;43[No. RR-12].)

† Condition that might be diagnosed presumptively.

§ Only among adults and adolescents aged >13 years. (CDC. 1993 Revised classification system for HIV infection and expanded surveillance case definition for AIDS among adolescents and adults. *MMWR* 1992;41[No. RR-17].

HIV, human immunodeficiency virus.

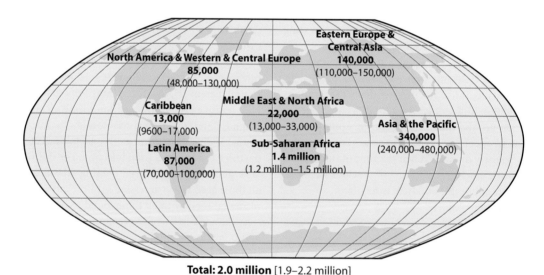

Total: 2.0 million [1.9–2.2 million]

Figure 9.5 Global burden of human infection. (Adapted from UNAIDS data, 2014.)

prevalence and incidence of CIN/HSIL. For this reason annual cervical cytology is recommended, with most guidelines recommending subsequent management as in HIV-negative women. It is worth noting that other anogenital malignancies resulting from oncogenic HPV infection also occur more frequently and at a younger age in HIV-positive people.

Contraception and preconception management

Many antiretrovirals interact with hormonal contraceptives, resulting in reduced contraceptive efficacy. However, this is dependent on the combination of specific medicines, and a holistic assessment is required assessing the woman's suitability for, and the availability of, both treatments. The dynamic HIV drug interaction website from the University of Liverpool (see Further reading) provides accurate information on specific drug interactions. Non-hormonal contraception such as condoms and IUDs are appropriate in most circumstances where they would otherwise be offered.

Prior to attempting pregnancy, the health of a HIV-positive woman and her partner should be optimized. This includes standard health promotion and for serodiscordant couples advice regarding prevention of HIV transmission. This is achieved by optimal HIV control as transmission between sexual partners is extremely low when the positive partner has undetectable HIV ribonucleic acid (RNA) levels (termed the 'viral load') in the serum. In addition, screening for and treating coexistent STIs and, where resources

permit, fertility assessment of both partners is good practice. It is appropriate to offer fertility treatment when this is indicated to couples where one or both are HIV positive, within regulatory frameworks.

Management of the HIV-positive mother and her child

All pregnant women must know their current HIV status, and those who are positive require access to high-quality medical and obstetric care. Effective antiretroviral therapy, ensuring an undetectable viral load in serum towards the end of pregnancy, provides excellent protection of the neonate. **Figure 9.6** presents information from the UK national study of HIV in pregnancy and childhood, which clearly demonstrates this. Most mother-to-child transmission (MTCT) occurs during birth or breastfeeding. Intrauterine infection is unusual and the risk of this is increased by an intervention that disrupts the placenta (for example, amniocentesis). Delivery by prelabour caesarean section further reduces MTCT rates when the HIV viral load is detectable. Obstetric risk factors that increase the risk of transmission include prolonged rupture of membranes, procedures that breach the infant's

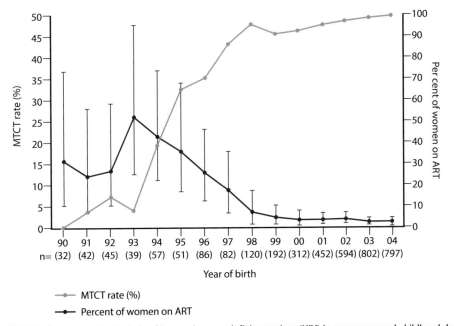

Figure 9.6 UK data from the national study of human immunodeficiency virus (HIV) in pregnancy and childhood demonstrating efficacy of maternal antiretroviral therapy (ART) in preventing mother-to-child transmission (MTCT) of HIV. (Adapted from CROI data, 2007.)

skin (such as fetal scalp electrodes) or increase maternal blood in the birth canal; however, these risks are reduced by effective control of maternal HIV.

Even in the presence of well-controlled HIV, transmission rates to the infant during breastfeeding are up to 3%, so in circumstances where formula feeding is safe, this is preferable. Where breastfeeding is safer than formula, exclusive breastfeeding for the first 6 months with rapid weaning so that no mixed feeding occurs is the safest option, as mixed feeding results in the highest rates of MTCT.

Conclusion

Knowledge of the modern tests and management of STIs and related conditions have been summarized in this chapter. This is important in gynaecological practice as these conditions are common in women and have serious implications, but can be effectively managed to minimize the risk of complications and transmission. HIV in particular has been transformed from a life-limiting condition to a chronic manageable condition, although offering testing and appropriate management of the condition and associated comorbidities and of reproductive health in HIV-positive women is crucial.

Further reading

The British Association for Sexual Health & HIV: http://www.bashh.org/BASHH/Guidelines/Guidelines/BASHH/Guidelines/Guidelines.aspx.
The British HIV Association: http://www.bhiva.org/guidelines.aspx.
The Centres for Disease Control and Prevention CDC: http://www.cdc.gov/std/tg2015/.
The International Union against STIs: http://iusti.org/sti-information/guidelines/default.htm.
United States HIV treatment guidelines: https://aidsinfo.nih.gov/guidelines
Spotting the signs of child sexual exploitation: http://www.bashh.org/documents/Spotting-the-signs-A%20national%20proforma%20Apr2014.pdf.
The University of Liverpool HIV Drug interactions website: http://www.hiv-druginteractions.org/.

Self assessment

CASE HISTORY

A 29-year-old woman presents to the emergency gynaecology unit with a 5-day history of lower abdominal and pelvic pain that has got progressively worse over the last 24 hours. She also feels generally unwell with chills and rigors. She has had several partners in recent months and was found to have chlamydia a few weeks ago. She is not sure whether she completed the whole course of treatment and did not go back to get tested. She does not use any form of contraception and has had unprotected intercourse recently.

On examination, she looks unwell. She has a raised temperature at 38°C and is tachycardic.

She is very tender on abdominal examination with guarding. On speculum examination, the cervix appears inflamed with a profuse mucopurulent discharge. A high vaginal swab, endocervical swab and a urethral swab are taken. On pelvic examination there is marked cervical tenderness. She is also generally tender to palpate throughout the pelvis and is unable to tolerate the examination. A pregnancy test is negative.

A What is the diagnosis?
B What tests are required?
C What is the management?

ANSWERS

A The clinical diagnosis is suggestive of acute PID with pelvic peritonitis.

B Vulvovaginal, high vaginal and cervical swabs (as available depending on your local microbiology service) are taken, as well as a midstream urine sample, full blood count and C-reactive protein (CRP). A pelvic ultrasound shows the possibility of an adnexal mass with some free fluid in the pelvis.

C She is admitted and started with intravenous antibiotics (ceftriaxone + metronidazole) and oral doxycycline. She is also supported with intravenous fluids, analgesics and regular paracetamol.

She continues to be unwell with a raised temperature even after 48 hours of antibiotics. Thus, a decision is taken to perform a laparoscopy. Usually conservative management is preferred, but when it is unsuccessful after 24–48 hours laparoscopy is indicated. At the operation, she is found to have a 7-cm enlarged tubo-ovarian abscess and marked inflammation of the uterus and other tube. The abscess is drained and the patient markedly improves after the surgery. She is found to have chlamydia on the endocervical swab with anaerobes on the high vaginal swab.

She improves over the course of a few days and is treated with oral antibiotics for 2 weeks. She is counselled regarding the implications of the infection and is encouraged to contact her present and previous partners for testing, of whom one tested positive for chlamydia and was subsequently treated. In the future she would require referral to fertility services early if she failed to conceive. An early scan in pregnancy is indicated to confirm intrauterine pregnancy, as the risk of an ectopic pregnancy is increased.

SBA QUESTIONS

1 A 32-year-old woman presents at the community reproductive clinic with altered vaginal discharge and mild abdominal pain. On examination there is a profuse mucopurulent discharge from an inflamed cervix.

What is the appropriate management? Choose the single best answer.

A Treat with cephalosporin for a presumed gonorrhoeal infection.

B Perform NAAT testing, treat presumptively with wide-spectrum antibiotic.

C Treat with penicillin and test for other STIs.

D Treat with cephalosporin and azithromycin and perform NAAT testing if unresponsive.

E Perform NAAT testing and culture and sensitivity, test for other STIs and treat with cephalosporin and azithromycin.

ANSWER

E The likely diagnosis is GC and accepted management is to test for other STIs as dual infection is common. NAAT testing for chlamydia, gonorrhoea or dual infection is performed but culture and sensitivities are also performed, as increasingly there is resistant infection. Meanwhile treatment is commenced with cephalosporins and azithromycin, and, of course, contact tracing as for all such visits. If bimanual examination demonstrates cervical motion and adnexal tenderness, then 2 weeks of doxycycline and metronidazole should also be given.

2 Which of the following infections can be diagnosed on wet mount microscopy? Choose the single best answer.

A Candidiasis.

B Gonorrhoea.

C Trichomoniasis.

D Syphilis.

E BV.

ANSWER

B Each of these pathogens/infections have specific features on microscopy, but some only on Gram stain. *Candida* has pseudo-hyphae, *Neisseria gonorrhoeae* is a gram-negative intracellular diplococcus, syphilis is caused by a spirochaete bacterium that is visible on dark light microscopy and BV is associated with Clue cells. Trichomoniasis is caused by a flagellate protozoan, *Trichomonas vaginalis* visible on a simple wet mounted swab.

Urogynaecology and pelvic floor problems

DOUGLAS TINCELLO

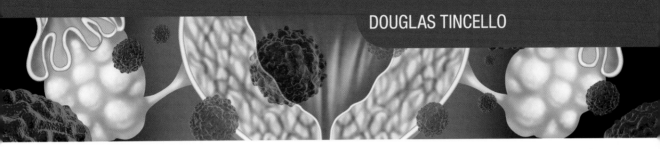

LEARNING OBJECTIVES

- Understand the anatomy of supporting ligaments and fascia of the female pelvic organs.
- Understand the mechanism of continence in women, and how disorders of this lead to symptoms.
- Appreciate the relationships between anatomical prolapse and functional symptoms, including urinary, bowel and sexual dysfunction.

- Learn how to assess the patient with incontinence or prolapse by means of history, examination and relevant investigations.
- Understand the principles of urodynamic testing.
- Understand the principles of treatment of prolapse and incontinence and be able to describe the effectiveness of each treatment, together with an understanding of potential side-effects and complications.

Urinary symptom terminology

Urinary symptoms can be divided into those relating to urine storage and those relating to voiding. The symptom of stress incontinence (leaking with cough, straining, exercise, etc) may be isolated, but most patients present with mixed incontinence, which is where stress incontinence occurs with frequency, urgency and urge incontinence. The combination of frequency, urgency and/or urge incontinence is given the term overactive bladder (OAB). Voiding symptoms are uncommon in women who have not had previous continence surgery.

Urine storage symptoms

- Frequency: patient considers he/she voids too often by day.
- Nocturia: waking at night one or more times to void.
- Urgency: a sudden compelling desire to pass urine, which is difficult to defer.
- Urge incontinence: involuntary leakage accompanied by or immediately preceded by urgency.
- Stress incontinence: involuntary leakage on effort, exertion, sneezing or coughing.
- Nocturnal enuresis: the loss of urine occurring during sleep.

Urine voiding symptoms

- Slow stream: perception of reduced urine flow.
- Splitting or spraying: where the stream or urine is not a single flow.
- Intermittent stream: urine flow that stops and starts.
- Hesitancy: difficulty in initiating micturition resulting in a delay in the onset of voiding.
- Terminal dribble: a prolonged final part of micturition, when the flow has slowed to a trickle or dribble.

Relevant functional anatomy

In health the bladder stores, and then voids, urine. This is known as the micturition cycle. Most of the time, the detrusor muscle of the bladder is relaxed allowing storage of increasing urine volumes with no increase in pressure. As bladder capacity is reached, sensory signals from stretch receptors in the bladder wall send the sensation of bladder filling. The sphincter mechanism is closed. As an adult, voluntary delay of micturition until socially convenient is achieved by cortical inhibition of the spinal voiding reflex arc. Before voiding begins, this inhibition is removed and the pelvic floor and urethral sphincters relax in a coordinated fashion, to allow detrusor contraction and bladder emptying. The detrusor muscle is innervated by muscarinic cholinergic nerves of the parasympathetic nervous system (causing detrusor muscle contraction), and the urethral sphincter by noradrenergic neurons of the sympathetic nervous system (sphincter contraction) and somatic fibres (voluntary contraction and relaxation) from the pudendal nerves.

In women the urethral sphincter mechanism is a functional system that includes the internal (smooth muscle) and external (striated muscle) sphincters, the muscles of the pelvic floor and the pubourethral ligament supporting the urethra within the abdominal cavity. Increases in abdominal pressure are transmitted equally to the bladder and bladder neck (**Figure 10.1A**). In the premenopausal woman the urethral epithelium has a rich blood supply and contributes to continence by acting as a seal.

Stress incontinence

In isolation, the symptom of stress incontinence is a reasonably good predictor of the presence of an incompetent urethral sphincter. Urethral sphincter weakness in most cases is due to hypermobility, where the pelvic floor and ligaments cannot retain the urethra in position and it falls through the urogenital hiatus during increases in abdominal pressure, leading to loss of pressure transmission to the urethra and hence leakage of urine (**Figure 10.1B**).

Intrinsic sphincter deficiency (ISD) is less common and occurs where urethral closure pressure is low without any urethral mobility. ISD is due to weakness of the sphincter muscles and loss of the cushioning seal effect in the urethra.

Urethral sphincter weakness is associated strongly with a history of vaginal childbirth and various related risk factors, and with some non-obstetric factors. Obstetric risk factors act by a combination effect of stretching/damage to the pudendal nerves and overstretching, or even avulsion, of the pelvic floor muscles from their insertions on the pelvic side wall. Direct muscle damage results in loss of pelvic floor support and hence urethral hypermobility. Pudendal nerve damage causes both weakening of the pelvic floor muscles and urethral sphincter. It is now possible to identify levator muscle defects in symptomatic women by means of magnetic resonance imaging or transperineal/transvaginal ultrasound. Most risk factors may not be modifiable (with exceptions noted by asterisks below).

- Multiparity (particularly vaginal births).
- Forceps delivery*.
- Perineal trauma.
- Long labour*.
- Epidural analgesia.
- Birthweight >4 kg.
- Increasing age.
- Postmenopause.
- Obesity studies have shown that significant weight loss among obese women is associated with major improvements in urinary leakage symptoms.
- Connective tissue disease.
- Chronic cough (e.g. bronchiectasis or chronic obstructive pulmonary disease).
- Doxazocin (alpha-adrenergic antagonist) for hypertension causes relaxation of the urethral sphincter*.

Detrusor overactivity

Detrusor overactivity (DO) is characterized by involuntary detrusor contractions during the filling phase of micturition (which can be seen during a urodynamic investigation as described later). Women with DO will often complain of symptoms of OAB, but may not be incontinent unless the urethral sphincter function is compromised or the detrusor contractions are of very high pressure amplitude and overcome urethral resistance (**Figure 10.1C**).

The aetiology of DO is poorly understood but laboratory studies have identified differences in sensory and interstitial nerves in the bladder wall of patients compared to controls, and alterations in the expression of several different neurotransmitters and their receptors.

Fewer risk factors for DO have been identified, of which the most modifiable are obesity and smoking. All continence surgery carries a risk of 5–10% of new DO.

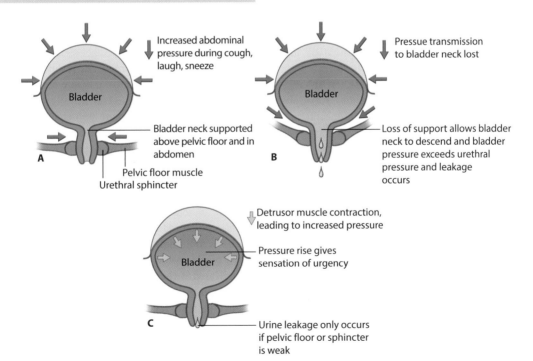

Figure 10.1 Mechanism of continence. In normal women, the bladder neck is supported above the pelvic floor and so abdominal pressure increases are transmitted to the bladder neck (**A**). Loss of bladder neck support results in descent of the bladder neck and loss of pressure transmission, resulting in leaking when coughing, straining, etc (stress incontinence) (**B**). Detrusor overactivity causes increased sensation; leakage only occurs if the contraction pressure exceeds the pelvic floor and sphincter pressure (**C**).

Risk factors for detrusor overactivity

- Childhood bedwetting.
- Obesity.
- Smoking.
- Previous hysterectomy.
- Previous continence surgery.

Clinical assessment of incontinence

A detailed history should be taken to elicit the patient's presenting symptoms, to identify whether the patient has only stress incontinence symptoms, only OAB symptoms or mixed symptoms. If there are mixed symptoms, an assessment should be made as to which predominate. It is useful to record measures of severity, including: the number of episodes per day of frequency, urgency and leakage; whether continence pads are needed, and if so how many and what size; whether the patient needs to change her underclothes or outer clothes because of leakage; and what behaviour changes have been employed. Commonly, women will have reduced their fluid intake and may limit their social activities to places where they already know about the position and cleanliness of toilet facilities. Associated symptoms of prolapse (see later), faecal incontinence symptoms (which patients rarely offer spontaneously) and any sexual difficulties should be sought, as well as a detailed medical history to identify potential predisposing factors and to identify any ongoing medical or surgical conditions that may impact on treatment (including comorbidities that may increase the risk of anaesthesia, or present cautions or contraindications to drug therapy). Remember to be alert for 'red flag' signs suggesting malignancy such as haematuria, rectal bleeding or significant pain.

Physical examination should include general examination and an abdominal and pelvic examination. Abdominal examination will identify any surgical scars, evidence of obesity and the presence or absence of any pelvic mass that may be a factor in urinary frequency. The presence of a large fibroid uterus or ovarian cyst filling the pelvis is an uncommon finding, but will cause urinary frequency by occupying the space in the pelvis where the full bladder would normally lie. In such cases, surgical removal of the mass will be indicated and should improve the urinary symptoms. Pelvic examination of the incontinent woman ideally should be done in the lithotomy position using a right-angled Sims speculum (see **Figure 2.4**) to assess each vaginal wall adequately for associated prolapse (see later). Visible leakage during coughing or Valsalva manoeuvre should be sought, and an assessment of the patient's ability to contract and hold the contraction of her pelvic floor muscles is essential.

All patients should be asked to provide a fresh midstream specimen of urine to exclude overt infection or asymptomatic bacteriuria. Additional simple investigations include a patient bladder diary (for 3 days is usually adequate) to record the amount, type and frequency of drinks taken and to record the timing, frequency and volume of voids (**Figure 10.2**). This can be a useful exercise for the patient herself to take note of exactly what she is drinking and her voiding habits. The bladder diary will also allow the patient to record leakage episodes and urgency. Many clinicians will also ask patients to complete one of a range of disease-specific quality of life instruments to assess the impact of the patient's problem and this can be repeated after treatment to allow collection of outcomes, which is extremely useful for the purpose of service audit and for individual clinician appraisal and revalidation. It is possible to obtain an objective measure of urine leak by conducting a pad test. This is an investigation where the patient wears one or more preweighed sanitary pads for a variable length of time (between 1 hour in clinic and 24 hours at home) while performing specific provocation tests (e.g. hand washing, climbing stairs, coughing) or activities of daily living. The change in weight (g) is a measure of the amount of urine lost (ml). Only the 24-hour home pad test has been shown to be reliable and reproducible, and pad tests have become much less commonly done in the last 5–10 years.

A pelvic and/or renal tract ultrasound may be indicated if there are symptoms of pelvic pain, clinical suspicion of a pelvic mass, haematuria, bladder pain or recurrent urinary tract infection. For patients with mixed symptoms, or those with recurrent problems after previous treatment, it is good practice to discuss management plans within a multidisciplinary team (MDT) meeting, including a gynaecologist, urologist, continence nurse, physiotherapist and possibly a medicine for the elderly consultant. Within the UK, current guidance to

Date: Sunday 27th November 2016

I got up at...7 am   I went to bed at...10.30 pm

Time	Record drinks taken (type and amount)	Volume of urine passed (ml)	Each time you leak, circle whether you were:	Each time you pass water, circle how severe the urgency was:
6 am			Almost Dry Damp Wet Soaked	None Mild Moderate Severe
7 am		400 ml	Almost Dry Damp Wet Soaked	None Mild Moderate Severe
8 am	1 cup of tea 200 ml		Almost Dry Damp Wet Soaked	None Mild Moderate Severe
9 am		200 ml	Almost Dry Damp Wet Soaked	None Mild Moderate Severe
10 am	1 cup of tea 200 ml		Almost Dry Damp Wet Soaked	None Mild Moderate Severe
11 am		200 ml	Almost Dry Damp Wet Soaked	None Mild Moderate Severe
Mid-day	1 glass of wine 150 ml 1 cup of coffee 200 ml	100 ml 150 ml	Almost Dry Damp Wet Soaked	None Mild Moderate Severe
1 pm			Almost Dry Damp Wet Soaked	None Mild Moderate Severe
2 pm	1 glass of orange 200 ml		Almost Dry Damp Wet Soaked	None Mild Moderate Severe
3 pm		250 ml	Almost Dry Damp Wet Soaked	None Mild Moderate Severe
4 pm		100 ml	Almost Dry Damp Wet Soaked	None Mild Moderate Severe
5 pm	1 cup of tea 200 ml		Almost Dry Damp Wet Soaked	None Mild Moderate Severe
6 pm		200 ml	Almost Dry Damp Wet Soaked	None Mild Moderate Severe
7 pm			Almost Dry Damp Wet Soaked	None Mild Moderate Severe
8 pm	1 can of coke 240 ml	100 ml	Almost Dry Damp Wet Soaked	None Mild Moderate Severe
9 pm		100 ml	Almost Dry Damp Wet Soaked	None Mild Moderate Severe
10 pm	1 cup of hot chocolate 150 ml	100 ml	Almost Dry Damp Wet Soaked	None Mild Moderate Severe
11 pm			Almost Dry Damp Wet Soaked	None Mild Moderate Severe
Mid-night			Almost Dry Damp Wet Soaked	None Mild Moderate Severe
1 am			Almost Dry Damp Wet Soaked	None Mild Moderate Severe
2 am			Almost Dry Damp Wet Soaked	None Mild Moderate Severe
3 am			Almost Dry Damp Wet Soaked	None Mild Moderate Severe
4 am			Almost Dry Damp Wet Soaked	None Mild Moderate Severe
5 am			Almost Dry Damp Wet Soaked	None Mild Moderate Severe

Reminders

1. Don't forget to record the time you woke up in the morning and the time you went to sleep
2. Don't forget to record what happened overnight
3. Try and make a record of things just after they happen
4. Record things to the nearest hour
5. Record type and amount of drinks taken (e.g. 2 cups of tea, 1 can of coke)

Urgency severity scale

NONE: no urgency

MILD: awareness of ugency but easily tolerated

MODERATE: enough urgency discomfort that it interferes with usual activities/tasks

SEVERE: extreme urgency discomfort that abruptly stops all activities/tasks

Figure 10.2 An example of a bladder diary, including columns for recording fluid intake (volume and amount), voided volume, the amount of leakage and the severity of urgency.

best practice is that all women (even primary cases) should be discussed in such a meeting before initiating surgical treatment of any type.

KEY LEARNING POINTS

- Stress incontinence is typically a result of a weak urethral sphincter, often as a consequence of childbirth.
- DO causes urgency, frequency and nocturia, but not all patients will have leakage.
- History should include direct questions about faecal leakage or leakage during sexual intercourse.
- Clinical examination should exclude pelvic masses (e.g. fibroid uterus) and assess the patient's ability to contract her pelvic floor muscles and the strength of that contraction.
- Women with pain, haematuria or recurrent infections should have the renal tract investigated radiologically and by cystoscopy.

Treatment for incontinence

Conservative treatment and the role of urodynamic assessment

For many years, most gynaecologists and urologists would perform urodynamic investigation on all women before initiating treatment. However, it has become clear that urodynamic testing has an appreciable false-negative rate, carries a small risk of urinary tract infection and does not reliably identify women at risk of complications after surgery or those who are likely to benefit from drug treatment. It has also become apparent that a package of conservative treatment will deliver significant symptom benefit for women with stress incontinence, OAB and mixed incontinence, irrespective of the underlying urodynamic findings (**Figure 10.3**).

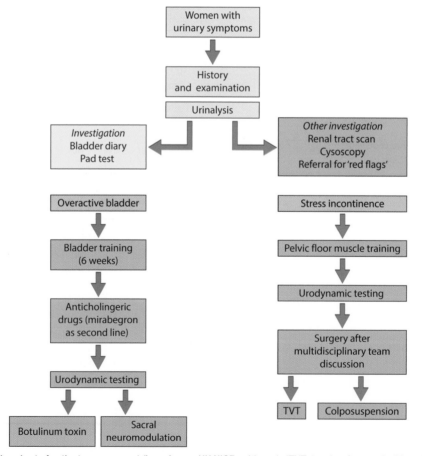

Figure 10.3 Flowchart of patient management (based upon UK NICE guidance). (TVT, tension-free vaginal tape.)

For these reasons, the first-line treatment of choice for women with any form of incontinence, once the basic investigations have ruled out serious pathology, is for a package of conservative treatment measures that can be delivered and supervised by a continence nurse, clinical nurse specialist or physiotherapist. Fluid balance is important; obviously excessive intake (over 2.5 litres) will result in frequency, but paradoxically, reducing fluid intake (which many patients do) can result in an increase in the sensation of urgency, due to the more concentrated urine. Women should be encouraged to drink between 1.5 and 2.5 litres of water a day, reducing or avoiding caffeinated beverages and also artificially sweetened or carbonated (fizzy) drinks, since experimental evidence suggests some artificial sweeteners can increase detrusor contractility *in vitro*.

> **Elements of conservative treatment for urinary incontinence**
>
> - Advice about fluid balance.
> - Reduction of caffeine intake.
> - Bladder retraining.
> - Pelvic floor muscle exercise.

Pelvic floor muscle exercise

In parallel with fluid management, most women are taught 'pelvic floor exercises' where they contract their pelvic floor muscles by direct coaching while being examined vaginally to ensure correct identification of the levator muscle complex. Without confirmation by direct examination, only 40% of women will be able to correctly initiate a contraction of the pelvic floor. Individualized exercise programmes are devised for each patient, to increase both the number of contractions that can be performed consecutively and also to increase the duration of 'hold' of each contraction. This two-pronged approach is important to build both strength and endurance of the muscle, both of which are essential to improve continence function. Successful adherence to a programme of pelvic floor exercises can lead to cure in over 50% of women and improvement in 75% or more. The major barrier to success is the woman's willingness to persevere with the exercises over a period of several weeks, in order to achieve maximum benefit, but the most obvious advantage

is that a course of exercise carries no risk of complications! Pelvic floor exercises work for both stress incontinence and OAB. In the latter case, it is likely that the benefit is from improving muscle strength to give women the confidence to resist the urge without fear of leakage, and also by pelvic floor contraction having a reflex inhibition action on detrusor muscle contraction.

Bladder retraining

For women with OAB or mixed incontinence, pelvic floor muscle training is combined with a form of bladder drill or bladder retraining. Bladder drill involves re-educating the patient (and her bladder) to increase the interval between voids, to re-establish normal frequency. For many women with OAB, the urgency and associated leakage (or fear of leakage) leads them to establish a pattern of voiding whenever they are aware of bladder filling sensations. An awareness of bladder filling is a normal physiological signal that occurs once or more than once as the bladder fills, but before full bladder capacity is reached. Bladder retraining (in conjunction with pelvic floor muscle training) includes teaching the woman about normal bladder sensation, the rate of urine production (usually 1–2 ml/min) and normal bladder capacity (350–500 ml), and then encouraging her to practice delaying voiding for several minutes beyond when she would normally void. It is usual do to this in a stepwise fashion, to push back voiding in 5 or 10 minute steps, rather than trying to hold for a whole hour. Bladder retraining can be very successful in reducing frequency and urgency, but like pelvic floor exercises, it requires perseverance and determination on the part of the patient.

It is important to counsel women about the benefits of weight loss, for those who are overweight or obese. Obesity is associated with increased risk and severity of stress incontinence, due to the increase in abdominal pressure, but it is also associated with increased severity of OAB. Several studies have demonstrated that weight loss leads to improvement in both stress incontinence and OAB, and can result in cure.

Urodynamic testing

The purpose of urodynamic testing is to reproduce a micturition cycle (bladder filling and voiding) while recording abdominal and bladder pressure and attempting to reproduce the patient's symptoms, to provide a diagnosis.

Common urodynamic diagnoses

- DO: the presence of a detrusor contraction, with or without sensation, during the filling phase of urodynamics.
- DO incontinence: leakage from the urethra in association with a detrusor contraction and increase in bladder pressure.
- Urodynamic stress incontinence: leakage from the urethra in association with a rise in abdominal pressure (e.g. coughing) without a detrusor contraction (a sign of urethral sphincter weakness).
- Mixed incontinence: the presence of both urodynamic stress incontinence and DO.

A fine pressure catheter is placed in the bladder through the urethra and a second catheter in the rectum, and the bladder is filled with warm saline while pressure recordings are made with the patient sitting on a commode that records leakage (**Figure 10.4A**). The pressure generated by any contraction of the detrusor can be inferred by subtraction (bladder pressure − abdominal pressure = detrusor pressure). During filling the patient is asked to declare the onset of bladder filling sensation (usually around 150 ml volume), a strong desire to void (around 350 ml and the onset of urgency (up to 500 ml, depending on bladder capacity) (**Figure 10.4B**). When urgency is reported (and functional bladder capacity is reached) filling is stopped and the patient performs various actions to provoke leakage and/or detrusor contractions (e.g. coughing, star jumps, listening to running water), before voiding while the pressure catheters remain in place. A urodynamic test will provide evidence of urethral sphincter weakness (**Figure 10.4B**) or DO (**Figure 10.4C**), as well as identifying normal or abnormal voiding function.

Urodynamic testing is reserved for patients who fail to improve with conservative measures, and also for patients with recurrent symptoms or those with complex histories or who have undergone previous surgery for incontinence or prolapse (**Figure 10.4**).

For women with OAB, many clinicians will initiate drug treatment before urodynamic testing (see below) and only perform the investigation when considering second-line interventions.

However, the relationship between urinary symptoms and urodynamic diagnoses is not strong. Although the symptom of stress incontinence in isolation is a good predictor of identifying urethral sphincter weakness on urodynamic testing, OAB symptoms are much less reliably associated with evidence of DO on testing (**Figure 10.5**). Evidence is lacking to show that urodynamic testing improves the outcome of surgery, reliably predicts postoperative voiding dysfunction or is of benefit in women with the symptom of stress incontinence alone. For women with mixed incontinence or OAB, it remains good practice to perform urodynamic testing before considering second-line treatments, after oral medication and conservative measures have failed.

 KEY LEARNING POINTS

- Conservative treatment with fluid advice, pelvic floor exercises and bladder retraining is the first line for all patients with incontinence or OAB and ideally should be delivered in primary care.
- Patient motivation is important for success of conservative treatment.
- Urodynamic investigation is not always necessary before commencing drug treatment or before surgery in women complaining only of stress incontinence.
- A urodynamic assessment should be done for women who fail to respond to anticholinergic medication or in women with mixed symptoms for whom surgery is being considered.

Medical treatment

Medical treatments for urinary incontinence are primarily aimed at treatment of OAB symptoms and DO. Because the parasympathetic nerves stimulate the detrusor muscle to contract, anticholinergic medications have been the mainstay of medical treatment for many years. There is a wide range of different compounds and preparations available. The main site of action of anticholinergic drugs is the motor end-plate of the neuromuscular

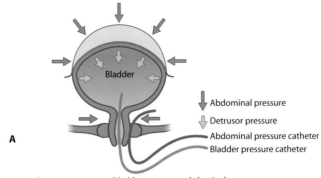

Detrusor pressure = bladder pressure − abdominal pressure

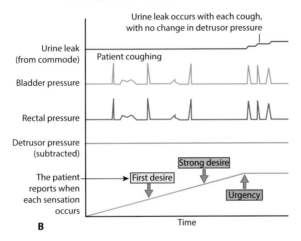

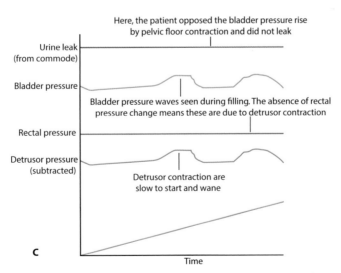

Figure 10.4 A urodynamic investigation (cystometry) records bladder pressure and abdominal pressure (usually via a rectal pressure catheter), and calculates detrusor pressure by subtraction (**A**). During filling, the patient is asked to report the occurrence of first desire to void (usually about 150 ml), strong desire and urgency (at functional bladder capacity) (**B**). With urodynamic stress incontinence, leakage is seen with increases in abdominal pressure (e.g. coughing) with no change in detrusor pressure (**B**). With detrusor overactivity, detrusor contractions are seen during the filling phase (**C**). These may or may not result in leakage, but normally will be associated with increased sensation.

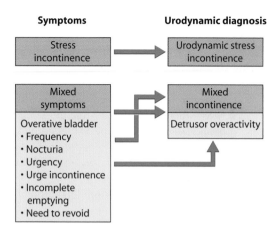

Figure 10.5 The relationship between symptoms and urodynamic diagnosis.

junction, where they antagonize the action of acetylcholine at the muscarinic receptors and inhibit detrusor contraction. In the last 5 years, it has become apparent that acetylcholine is also an important neurotransmitter in the afferent, sensory pathways in the bladder and thus the drugs also have a direct effect in reducing the perceived sensations of bladder filling by inhibiting receptor-mediated afferent signals.

Anticholinergic medications

- Oxybutynin: 2.5–5 mg up to three times daily; first-choice medication recommended by the UK National Institute for Health and Care Excellence (NICE); modified release preparation 5 mg once daily; increase weekly by 5 mg up to 20 mg daily.
- Propiverine: 15 mg one to three times daily.
- Trospium: 20 mg twice daily.
- Tolterodine: 2 mg twice daily; reduced to 1 mg in hepatic impairment; modified release preparation 4 mg once daily.
- Fesoterodine: 4 mg once daily, maximum 8 mg once daily (fesoterodine is related to tolterodine).
- Solifenacin: 5 mg once daily; can be increased to 10 mg once daily.
- Darifenacin: 7.5 mg once daily.

All anticholinergic drugs have similar efficacy, with published randomized studies demonstrating a decrease in urgency and incontinence episodes in the range of 1–2 per day, compared with placebo. The side-effect profile is similar across all drugs, with dry mouth, constipation and blurred vision being the most common.

Mirabegron is a more recently developed medication for OAB, which is a beta 3-adrenergic agonist. Mirabegron acts upon the sympathetic neurones innervating the bladder, to enhance relaxation of the detrusor. Therefore it is acting more on the storage function of the bladder than do anticholinergic medications, which act by suppressing voiding. Mirabegron can be used simultaneously with an anticholinergic drug.

In postmenopausal women topical vaginal oestrogen for 3 months can provide dramatic improvement in bladder sensation and associated urgency.

Duloxetine is used very occasionally for incontinence. It is a combined serotonin and noradrenaline reuptake inhibitor, and has a dual licence for the treatment of depression in higher doses. Duloxetine acts at the micturition centre in the sacral spinal cord to increase the sympathetic nerve output to the urethral sphincter and increase sphincter tone. Randomized trials have shown a 50% improvement or more in leakage symptoms in over one-half of the patients treated. However, the side-effects, including nausea, cause many women to stop treatment.

Surgical treatment

Stress incontinence

For women with stress incontinence (based on a history of only stress leakage or on urodynamic assessment) surgery is a highly effective option for treatment. The most effective and thus the first-choice procedures are either a synthetic midurethral tape procedure (**Figure 10.6**) or a Burch colposuspension (**Figure 10.7**). In much of the UK, Europe and the USA, midurethral tape procedures almost entirely replaced colposuspension as primary treatment during the 1990s and later, although our developing understanding of potential complications may lead to a return to colposuspension. Certainly, in settings where synthetic tapes are not available, colposuspension remains a safe and effective operation.

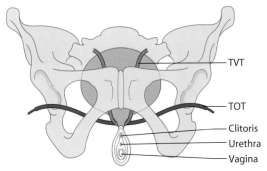

Figure 10.6 The position of tension-free vaginal (TVT) and transobturator (TOT) midurethral tapes. The TVT lies under the midurethra and in the retropubic space between the pelvis and bladder. The introducing trocars pass through the urogenital diaphragm and the rectus sheath. The TOT lies in a more horizontal position under the midurethra and exits through the obturator foramen, piercing the obturator muscle and the adductor longus tendon in the thigh.

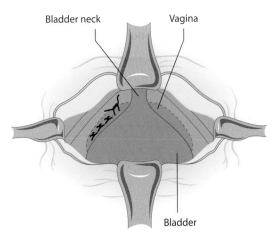

Figure 10.7 A sketch of a colposuspension through a Pfannenstiel incision. The patient's head is at the bottom of the picture, and interrupted sutures are being placed in the paravaginal fascia at the level of the bladder neck through the pectineal ligament on the posterior surface of the superior pubic ramus.

There are now several variations of midurethral tapes available, but the underlying principle is the same. A permanent, non-absorbable mesh of polypropylene woven into a tape approximately 1 cm wide is placed through a small vaginal incision under the midurethra and into a U shape behind the pubic symphysis, via two small suprapubic incisions (a retropubic placement), or into a hammock shape behind the inferior pubic rami and through the obturator foramen, via a small incision in each

groin (a transobturator placement) (**Figure 10.6**). The midurethral tapes have a cure rate for stress incontinence of 80–85%, and this high success rate persists in the long term (10 years or more). Complications specific to midurethral tapes relate to the non-absorbable polypropylene they are manufactured from. There is a low rate of the tape interfering with vaginal wound healing, leading to exposure of the central portion of tape, or of later erosion of the tape through the vaginal skin at other places along its length.

Common operative complications include:

- Voiding difficulty (usually short term) in 2–5%.
- Bladder perforation during the procedure (2–5%).
- Onset of new OAB symptoms after surgery (5%).

Burch colposuspension was the primary procedure for stress incontinence for many years before the midurethral tapes were developed. At colposuspension, the retropubic space is opened via a Pfannenstiel incision in the abdomen, and the bladder reflected medially on each side to allow the placement of two or three sutures (either absorbable or permanent) into the paravaginal fascia on each side at the level of the bladder neck (**Figure 10.7**). These sutures are placed through the pectineal ligament on the pubic ramus on the same side, and then tied to provide support to the bladder neck and prevent descent during coughing or straining. The cure rate for incontinence is the same as for midurethral tapes (80–85%), and complications are similar.

Colposuspension carries a long-term risk of developing posterior vaginal prolapse (5–10%) due to lifting of the anterior vaginal wall.

A third option for surgery is periurethral injections of material that bulk up the bladder neck and coat the urethral mucosa to prevent leakage. Three products are widely available (Macroplastique, Durasphere and Bulkamid). These are all synthetic polymer materials, either as microscopic beads or viscous liquid. The procedure is performed under local anaesthetic and is available for women deemed too medically unfit or frail for a formal anaesthetic, or for women with residual leakage after a tape or colposuspension (**Figure 10.8**). Cure rates after these procedures are of the order of 60–80% but longer-term cure is less effective, so some patients require two or more treatments. High-quality data

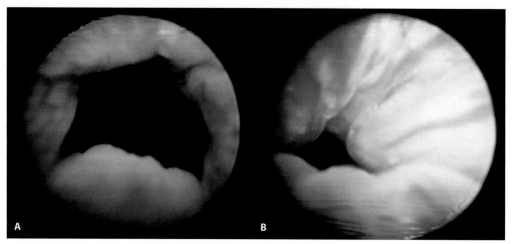

Figure 10.8 Cystoscope images showing an open bladder neck (**A**) before injection and a closed bladder neck after injection (**B**).

from randomized trials of these products are lacking, so most clinicians will use these as third-line or 'rescue' therapy, although in some settings women are choosing injectables as first-line treatment in view of the possibility of being treated in an 'office' setting.

Detrusor overactivity

For DO, a surgical option may be considered as second-line treatment (**Figure 10.3**). The neurotoxin botulinum toxin A (marketed as Botox or Dysport) has been shown in recent randomized trials to be a highly effective treatment. Botulinum toxin is a long-acting molecule that prevents the release of neurotransmitter vesicles from the motor end-plate and causes a flaccid paralysis in the treated muscle. A single intramuscular injection can last for 3–6 months. Botulinum toxin is administered via a flexible or rigid cystoscope and injected in multiple sites across the dome of the bladder, to abolish the involuntary detrusor contractions that cause symptoms. Reduction of urgency and leakage episodes of over 50–80% have been reported, and continence rates in excess of 40%. The major drawback of this treatment is a voiding difficulty rate of 8–15% which, if it occurs, can persist for the duration of treatment effect and be troublesome for the patient to manage. However, many patients are able to self-catheterize with little difficulty and still find that this gives them a high degree of social independence, compared to before treatment.

Sacral neuromodulation is also an effective surgical management option.

 KEY LEARNING POINTS

- Surgery for stress incontinence is highly effective with cure rates of 85% or higher.
- Midurethral tapes and colposuspension are equally effective, but tape surgery is more cost-effective due to the short hospital stay and rapid return to normal activities.
- Patients should be warned of the risk of voiding dysfunction, bladder injury and new OAB symptoms after surgery.
- Mesh-related complications are uncommon after midurethral tape surgery but can be difficult to treat; patients should be fully informed of the risks, and of the potential for further surgery to deal with these complications.
- Botulinum toxin and sacral neuromodulation are highly effective second-line treatments for detrusor overactivity.

Prolapse

Symptoms from pelvic organ prolapse

Pelvic organ prolapse can cause symptoms directly due to the prolapsed organ or indirectly due to organ dysfunction secondary to displacement from the anatomical position. Proplase symptoms include a sensation of vaginal bulge, heaviness or a visible protrusion at or beyond the introitus. Patients may also describe lower abdominal or back pain, or a dragging discomfort relieved by lying or sitting.

Indirect symptoms will depend on which other organs are involved in the prolapse but may include difficulty in voiding urine or emptying the bowel (termed obstructive defaecation), and sensations of incomplete emptying of bladder or rectum. Patients may have to support or reduce the prolapse with their fingers to be able to void or evacuate stool completely (termed digitation, distinct from manual evacuation of the rectum). Urinary or faecal incontinence may also be present. It is important to ask about sexual activity, even in the older patient, and to enquire about difficulty achieving penetration, pain or discomfort during intercourse and loss of sensation and difficulty achieving orgasm due to vaginal or introital laxity.

Patients may experience vaginal bleeding from a prolapse that is external and becomes ulcerated or abraded, but in women with a uterus, one must remember to exclude endometrial carcinoma by biopsy and ultrasound.

Risk factors predisposing to prolapse are very much similar to those predisposing to stress incontinence. Research has shown the pudendal nerves to be damaged after childbirth, with increased nerve conduction times, and ultrasound studies of the pelvic anatomy of women with prolapse have demonstrated thinning or avulsion of the puborectalis muscle from its insertion on the pubic ramus, on either one or both sides in a high proportion of cases.

Relevant anatomy

Uterovaginal prolapse is caused by failure of the interaction between the levator ani muscles and the ligaments and fascia that support the pelvic organs. For a detailed description of the relationships and function of these structures, see the review by Wei & De Lancey in Further reading. The levator ani muscles are puborectalis, pubococcygeus and iliococcygeus. They are attached on each side of the pelvic side wall from the pubic ramus anteriorly (pubococcygeus), over the obturator internus fascia to the ischial spine to form a bowl-shaped muscle filling the pelvic outlet

and supporting the pelvic organs (see Chapter 1, The development and anatomy of the female sexual organs and pelvis). There is a gap between the fibres of the puborectalis on each side to allow passage of the urethra, vagina and rectum, called the urogenital hiatus. The levator muscles support the pelvic organs and prevent excessive loading of the ligaments and fascia.

There are three levels of supporting ligaments and fascia, which work together to provide a global and dynamic system to support the uterus, vagina and associated organs (**Figure 10.9**). Level 1 (apical) support is provided by the uterosacral ligaments, which attach the cervix to the sacrum. Obviously, support at this level is crucial in contributing to support of the vaginal walls that are attached to the cervix (**Figure 10.10A**). Defects in level 1 support can be seen on examination by the descent of the uterus within the vagina. Level 1 support remains critical even after hysterectomy, so it is important during that procedure to reattach the uterosacral ligaments to the vaginal vault. In women who have previously undergone hysterectomy, level 1 support defects will manifest as vaginal vault prolapse (**Figure 10.10B**).

Level 2 support is provided by the fascia that surrounds the vagina, both anteriorly and posteriorly, lying between the vagina and the bladder (pubocervical fascia) or rectum (rectovaginal fascia). These fascial sheets fuse together at the vaginal edge and then are attached to the pelvic side wall, fusing to the fascia overlying obturator internus. These fascial attachments result in the vagina lying as a flattened tube (laterally) at rest. Defects in the fascia providing level 2 support will lead to prolapse of the vaginal wall into the vaginal lumen (causing anterior or posterior vaginal prolapse) (**Figure 10.10C, D**). The bladder or rectum will prolapse behind the vaginal wall due to the fascial attachment to it. On examination, the affected vaginal wall will be seen bulging into the vagina.

Level 3 support is provided by the fascia of the posterior vagina, which is attached at its caudal end to the perineal body. The perineal body is a dense connective tissue mass underneath the lower third of the posterior vaginal wall and is the insertion of the posterior vaginal fascia, fibres of levator ani and the transverse perineal muscles. It is the perineal body that is torn or cut (by episiotomy) during childbirth. Defects of the perineal body

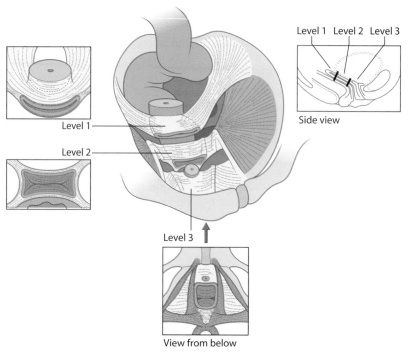

Level 1

Level 2

Level 3

Side view

View from below

Figure 10.9 Fascial supports of the pelvic organs. Level 1 support is provided by the uterosacral ligaments, suspending the uterus and attached vaginal vault. Level 2 (midvagina) support is provided by the fascia lying between the vagina and the bladder or rectum that fuses laterally and runs to attach on the pelvic side wall. Level 3 support is provided by the perineal body, which has the posterior vaginal fascia fused to its upper surface.

usually cause the development of lower posterior vaginal wall prolapse, but the loss of the perineal body increases the size of vaginal opening and therefore predisposes to anterior vaginal prolapse as well (**Figure 10.10C, D**).

KEY LEARNING POINTS

- The levator ani muscles (puborectalis, pubococcygeus and iliococcygeus) support the pelvic organs and relieve excessive pressure from the ligaments and fascia.
- The uterosacral ligaments provide essential apical support (level 1 support).
- Vaginal fascia supports the vagina (level 2 support).
- The perineal body is very important in supporting the lower vagina (level 3 support).
- All the structures provide a dynamic and integrated support to the pelvic organs.

Clinical assessment of prolapse

The history should elicit the presenting symptom(s) and severity, and include questions to ascertain if the patient has any coexisting urinary, faecal or sexual symptoms as discussed above for the incontinent patient. One should be sensitive to the emotional aspect of the problem, but specific questions should be asked about sexual discomfort and difficulty achieving orgasm. For women who are not sexually active, it should be discussed whether this is due to the prolapse symptoms or other personal or social issues (e.g. health of the partner). For some women, intercourse is avoided because of anxieties or embarrassment over the appearance of the genitalia and a loss of perceived attractiveness.

Clinical examination should ideally be done in the lithotomy position with a Sims speculum (see Chapter 2, Gynaecological history, examination and investigations, **Figure 2.4**). This allows retraction of the anterior

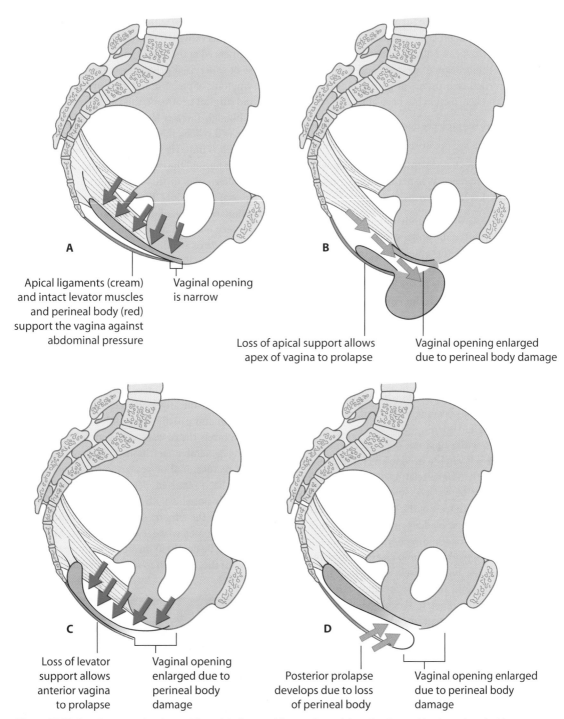

A Apical ligaments (cream) and intact levator muscles and perineal body (red) support the vagina against abdominal pressure

Vaginal opening is narrow

B Loss of apical support allows apex of vagina to prolapse

Vaginal opening enlarged due to perineal body damage

C Loss of levator support allows anterior vagina to prolapse

Vaginal opening enlarged due to perineal body damage

D Posterior prolapse develops due to loss of perineal body

Vaginal opening enlarged due to perineal body damage

Figure 10.10 Development of prolapse. The pelvic floor and ligaments work together to provide support against increases in abdominal pressure (**A**). Prolapse is almost invariably associated with perineal body damage causing an enlarged vaginal opening. Prolapse can then occur if the apical (level 1) support is lost (**B**), or if the pelvic floor muscles are ineffective (**C**) or directly as a result of perineal body deficiency (**D**). Often, a combination of factors is at work.

and posterior vaginal wall in turn, to allow full assessment of the degree of prolapse and to assess how much descent of the cervix and uterus is present. Prolapse is described in three stages of descent, and note should be made of whether it occurs at patient straining or at rest and whether traction has been applied:

- Stage I where the prolapse does not reach the hymen.
- Stage II where the prolapse reaches the hymen.
- Stage III when the prolapse is mostly or wholly outside the hymen. When the uterus prolapses wholly outside this is termed procidentia.

In women who have undergone hysterectomy, the vaginal vault can prolapse (**Figure 10.10B**). Vaginal prolapse of the anterior vagina (the anterior compartment) is also known as cystocele in the upper half or urethrocele in the lower half. Posterior vaginal prolapse (the posterior compartment) is also known as enterocele in the upper third, or rectocele below this (**Figure 10.10D**). Vaginal prolapse is formally staged using the methods mentioned above, but the most important assessment is whether the vaginal prolapse reaches to, or beyond, the hymen. Finally, it is important to assess whether the perineal body is intact or has become attenuated, resulting in an enlarged vaginal opening.

For women with symptoms of pressure or vaginal bulge only, there is rarely a need to arrange any investigations, other than those relating to anaesthetic pre-assessment (see Chapter 17, Gynaecological surgery and therapeutics). In view of the complex relationship between prolapse and bladder or bowel functions, if women have additional indirect symptoms, then it is prudent to arrange urodynamic assessment or functional tests of the lower bowel, which may include endoanal ultrasound to check for anal a sphincter defects, rectal manometry, flexible sigmoidoscopy and a defaecating proctogram. Ideally, such patients should be reviewed with the completed investigations in a MDT meeting including a gynaecologist, colorectal surgeon, continence nurse and physiotherapist.

Treatment for prolapse

Conservative treatment

Conservative treatment for prolapse includes pelvic floor muscle exercises and the use of supportive vaginal pessaries. For women with urinary or bowel symptoms as well, conservative treatment for these symptoms can be commenced at the same time as for the prolapse. A course of supervised pelvic floor exercises will reduce the symptoms of prolapse and for women who are keen to avoid surgical treatment, this can be an effective first step, although there is less evidence that pelvic floor exercise will reduce the anatomical extent of the prolapse and it is unlikely to be helpful for women whose prolapse is beyond the vaginal introitus.

An alternative to this is to insert a vaginal support pessary to reduce the prolapse, which leads to resolution of many of the symptoms. Pessary use can be very effective at relieving symptoms and has the advantage of avoiding surgery and the associated risks, which can be extremely useful in the medically unfit and elderly. A range of shapes of pessary is available (**Figure 10.11**). Ring pessaries are usually tried first, but an intact perineal body is necessary for these to be retained. Shelf pessaries, Gelhorn pessaries and others are useful for women with deficient perineal bodies. It is usual practice to replace a pessary every 6 months and to examine the patient for signs of vaginal ulceration, although this frequency is traditional and not based on any evidence. Complications are uncommon and usually minor (bleeding, discharge), although rarely the pessary can become incarcerated, requiring general anaesthesia to remove, and rare cases of rectovaginal or vesicovaginal fistula formation have been reported. Sexual intercourse remains theoretically possible with a well-placed ring pessary, but not with the others, so would not generally be suitable for women who are sexually active. Motivated patients can be taught to insert and remove their own pessaries if they do wish to remain sexually active.

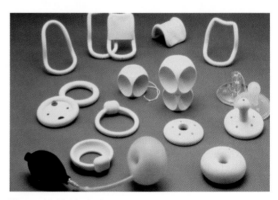

Figure 10.11 Vaginal support pessaries.

Surgery for pelvic organ prolapse

Surgical treatment for prolapse is common, and can be offered if conservative treatments have failed or if the patient chooses surgery from the outset. There are a wide range of specific procedures that are described further in Chapter 17, Gynaecological surgery and therapeutics. The procedure chosen depends on which compartment is affected, whether the woman wishes to retain her uterus and whether the vaginal or abdominal route of surgery is chosen. The essential principles of prolapse surgery apply for all procedures. Prolapse surgery is performed through the vagina to restore the ligamentous tissue supports to the apex, anterior and posterior vagina (anterior repair, posterior repair) and repair of the perineal body. The vaginal route can also be used for posthysterectomy vault prolapse, attaching the vaginal vault to the right sacrospinous ligament with non-absorbable or slowly absorbable sutures, but here an abdominal approach to perform a sacrocolpopexy is an option that will provide excellent, durable long-term cure. The relative merits of abdominal compared to vaginal surgery and the usual recovery times are discussed in Chapter 17, Gynaecological surgery and therapeutics. In the last 3–5 years, there has been an increasing number of women wishing to avoid hysterectomy during prolapse surgery, so both sacrospinous fixation and sacrocolpopexy can be performed by attaching a mesh or sutures to the cervix rather than the vaginal vault.

Vaginal repair using mesh improves the anatomical outcome and reduces the risk of recurrent prolapse. However, the available long-term data do not demonstrate a difference in symptom relief between standard repair and mesh repair. Mesh repair carries the risk of later erosion and need for removal, which is challenging surgery. Therefore, many surgeons will only consider mesh repair for women with recurrent vaginal prolapse, and only proceed after careful and full counselling of the woman about the relative benefits and potential risks of surgery.

KEY LEARNING POINTS

- Uterovaginal prolapse causes troublesome symptoms but is not life threatening.
- A course of pelvic floor exercises can reduce symptoms and may reduce prolapse progression in women with mild/moderate prolapse.
- Vaginal pessaries are a useful conservative treatment but do not suit all women.
- Surgery for prolapse is effective, but has a recurrence rate of about 5%.
- It is not essential to perform hysterectomy for prolapse.
- Mesh repairs for prolapse give a better anatomical cure, but there is no convincing evidence that symptom relief is different from standard surgery.
- Mesh complications are common and can be extremely difficult to manage.

Principles of prolapse surgery

- Remove/reduce the vaginal bulge.
- Restore the ligament/tissue supports to the apex, anterior and posterior vagina.
- Replace associated organs in their correct positions.
- Retain sufficient vaginal length and width to allow intercourse.
- Restore the perineal body.
- Correct or prevent urinary incontinence.
- Correct or prevent faecal incontinence.
- Correct obstructed defaecation.

Further reading

Dmochowski RR, Blaivas JM, Gormley EA, *et al.* (2010). Update of AUA guideline on the surgical management of female stress urinary incontinence. *J Urol* **183**:1906–14.

Smith A, Bevan D, Douglas HR, James D (2013). Management of urinary incontinence in women: summary of updated NICE guidance. *BMJ* **347**:f5170. doi: 10.1136/bmj.f5170.:f5170.

Wei JT, De Lancey JO (2004). Functional anatomy of the pelvic floor and lower urinary tract. *Clin Obstet Gynecol* **47**:3–17.

Self assessment

CASE HISTORY

A 47-year-old patient, who is a lawyer, presents to clinic with symptoms of leaking urine on coughing, sneezing and exercise, and when she has the urge to pass urine.

A   *Describe the important parts of the history to be taken.*
B   *Describe the investigations required.*
C   *Describe the best treatment.*

ANSWERS

A   Take a standard gynaecological history first, noting any severe menstrual symptoms (in case a hysterectomy should be considered), AUB or menopause. Note number and mode of deliveries. Note any abdominal surgery. When taking the history have a mind to both the effect on the patient's life and indications for, or against, medical or surgical treatment.

Next a detailed urogynecological history is required as discussed in this chapter.

The patient reveals on direct questions that she has no menstrual problems, has had three vaginal deliveries and no abdominal surgery. She is fit and not overweight and exercises regularly. She drinks a normal volume of fluids, has a few caffeinated drinks per day. She avoids red wine as it makes her bladder worse.

She notes leakage on exercise, coughing and sneezing and on intercourse. She is getting some burning on passing urine in the last few weeks. She has an urge to pass urine when her bladder is not very full, and the urge is very strong. She leaks urine when this happens. She passes urine about eight times a day and once at night.

On examination she has a deficient perineum, a moderate cystocele and minimal rectocele. She has poor pelvic tone.

B   A midstream urine sample (MSU) should be taken as the symptoms are quite new. Urodynamics are not the first line of treatment because their relation to detruser instability is not good.

C   The first-line of management is supervised pelvic floor exercises. If the MSU shows infection antibiotics should be prescribed.

EMQ

A   Urodynamic assessment.
B   Urgent flexible cystoscopy.
C   Renal tract ultrasound.
D   Insertion of midurethral tape.
E   Immediate release oyxbutynin.
F   Topical oestrogen.
G   Oral antibiotics.
H   Botulinum toxin injection.
I   Duloxetine.

For each description below, choose the SINGLE most appropriate answer from the above list of options. Each option may be used once, more than once or not at all.

1   Immediate management of a 73-year-old woman with frequency, urgency and haematuria.

2   Management of a 38-year-old woman with symptoms of only stress incontinence who has completed a course of pelvic floor exercises without improvement.

3   Should be performed after failed conservative and/or medical management before second-line treatments for incontinence.

4   First-line drug treatment for OAB.

ANSWERS

1B Because of the haematuria, cystoscopy is required to exclude a malignancy.

2D It is reasonable to insert a midurethral tape without further investigations in this situation, because there are no symptoms of mixed incontinence.

3A Urodynamic assessment will exclude a picture of mixed incontinence, which is necessary before more invasive treatment.

4E Immediate release oxybutynin will effectively treat overactive bladder symptoms and no further investigations are required before treatment.

SBA QUESTIONS

1 A 45 year old woman attends outpatients complaining of a 3-year history of stress incontinence, urgency and urge incontinence. She leaks urine about four times a day, has to wear sanitary pads all the time and rarely travels due to the urgency and need to pass urine 8 or 9 times during the day. Examination reveals her to be of normal BMI, with a weak pelvic floor muscle strength.

What would be the recommended first line of management? Choose the single best answer.

A Commence the patient on an oral anticholinergic medication for 8 weeks.

B Arrange urodynamic assessment to define the underlying cause of her problems.

C Arrange a 6–8 week course of supervised pelvic floor exercises and bladder retraining.

D Admit the patient for a cystoscopy.

E Test the urine for infection and treat with antibiotics.

ANSWER

C Pelvic floor strengthening exercises will improve up to 50% of stress incontinence problems and may avoid the need to treat urge incontinence with anticholinergics. Urodynamics are not necessary before first-line treatment. Although a urinary tract infection must be excluded before investigations or treatment, it is not a first-line investigation and does not fit with the symptoms or signs. No bladder abnormality is expected here to necessitate a cystoscopy.

2 A 73-year-old woman attends clinic with a large prolapse. She underwent abdominal hysterectomy at the age of 42 for heavy periods, and later required a second laparotomy for a large left-sided ovarian cyst, which was complicated by dense abdominal adhesions. She has no other significant history. On examination she has a vaginal vault prolapse that extends beyond the introitus and also has a very deficient perineum with a large vaginal opening. She is married and wishes to be able to resume intercourse.

What is the best option for treatment for this patient? Choose the single best answer.

A Insertion of a vaginal pessary.

B Colpocleisis.

C Abdominal sacrocolpopexy.

D Vaginal repair with sacrospinous fixation.

E Antero-posterior repair.

ANSWER

D Abdominal surgery must be avoided in this woman because of the adhesions. A vaginal pessary will not help her to resume intercourse. Repair of the vaginal walls will not help her deficient perineum or vault prolapse. Colpocleisis is the closure of the vagina, performed in older women who do not wish to have intercourse, to effectively treat prolapse.

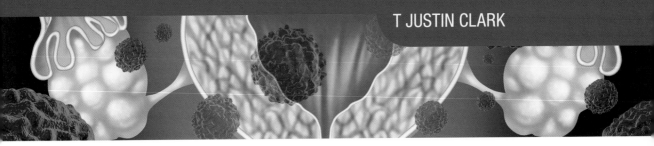

Benign conditions of the ovary and pelvis

CHAPTER

11

T JUSTIN CLARK

LEARNING OBJECTIVES

- Describe the types of benign ovarian cysts, their symptoms, diagnosis and treatment.
- Describe the presentation and management of acute pelvic pain.
- Understand the pathology of endometriosis and recognize its involvement in chronic pelvic pain and subfertility.

- Understand how to diagnose and treat endometriosis.
- List potential causes for chronic pelvic pain (CPP).
- Appreciate the multifactorial nature of CPP and potential management options.

Benign diseases of the ovary

Benign ovarian tumours are listed in *Table 11.1*. Most benign ovarian tumours will be diagnosed following investigation of women complaining of acute pelvic pain or chronic pelvic pain (CPP), or noticing the presence of an abdominal mass. They may also be found incidentally during a gynaecological examination or pelvic ultrasound scan (USS). The differential diagnosis of a pelvic mass includes tumours of adjacent structures (uterus, bladder and bowel) and pregnancy.

The presentation with the different types of benign ovarian tumours varies with age. Functional cysts are common in young girls, adolescents and women in their reproductive years. Germ cell

The differential diagnosis of a pelvic mass

- Gynaecological: benign or malignant ovarian cyst; torsion; para-ovarian cyst; ectopic pregnancy; hydrosalpinx; pyosalpinx; tubo-ovarian abscess; tubal malignancy; pregnancy; fibroids; uterine malignancy.
- Gastrointestinal: small or large bowel obstruction; diverticular/appendicular abscess; intussusception; malignancy.
- Urological: hydronephrosis; pelvic kidney; renal/bladder malignancy.
- Other: pelvic lymphocele; peritoneal cyst; psoas muscle abscess; lymphoma; neuroblastoma; aortic aneurism.

155

Table 11.1 Types of benign ovarian cyst

Functional	Follicular cyst
	Corpus luteal cyst
	Theca luteal cyst
Inflammatory	Tubo-ovarian abscess
	Endometrioma
Germ cell	Benign teratoma (dermoid cyst)
Epithelial	Serous cystadenoma
	Mucinous cystadenoma
	Brenner tumour
Sex cord stromal	Fibroma
	Thecoma

tumours occur more commonly in young women, whereas benign epithelial tumours are more prevalent in older and postmenopausal women.

Diagnosis may be made by symptoms of pelvic discomfort or pressure on the bowel or bladder.

Ovarian torsion

- Torsion of an ovary refers to a situation where there is rotation of the vascular pedicle supplying the ovary, which compresses and cuts its blood supply. Torsion is more likely with enlargement of the ovary as is seen in the presence of an ovarian cyst. Up to 15% of dermoid cysts present acutely with torsion.

- Presenting symptoms are usually acute onset of lower abdominal pain associated with nausea and vomiting. Pelvic USS with Doppler measurement of blood flow may be useful in the diagnosis, to confirm the presence of a cyst and comment on blood flow to the ovary. Torsion of a normal ovary is very unlikely.

- Emergency surgical treatment to untwist the ovary and its attached pedicle is required to restore blood flow, and the ovarian cyst should then be removed. However, if this complication is not recognized within a few hours of presentation, infarction and gangrene may result, necessitating removal of the necrotic ovary. Decision making to operate should be based on clinical findings, with transvaginal ultrasound scan (TVUSS) support.

Acute pain may represent torsion of a cyst, rupture or haemorrhage into it. Abdominal and bimanual pelvic examination may elicit a pelvic/abdominal mass that may be tender and will be separate from the uterus.

The first-line investigation for women with a suspected pelvic mass or pelvic pain is an USS. A TVUSS has better resolution for pelvic masses. A transabdominal ultrasound scan (TAUSS) is indicated in women who have never been sexually active, or in combinations with a TVUSS where large ovarian masses extending beyond the pelvis and into the abdomen are present. Additional imaging with computed tomography (CT) scanning or magnetic resonance imaging (MRI) can further characterize the nature of ovarian cysts, especially where they are thought to be potentially malignant. Serological tumour markers should also be taken to help determine the type of ovarian cyst and differentiate between a benign and malignant neoplasm (Table 11.2 and Chapter 14, Malignant disease of the ovary). A pregnancy test should be performed to exclude pregnancy. Inflammatory markers, such as C-reactive protein (CRP) and white cell count (WCC), are important if the differential diagnosis includes appendicitis or a tubo-ovarian abscess.

Table 11.2 Tumour markers used in the investigation and follow-up of ovarian cysts

Tumour marker	Ovarian tumour type	Uses
Ca 125	Epithelial ovarian cancer (serous), borderline ovarian tumours	Preoperative, follow-up
Ca 19-9	Epithelial ovarian cancer (mucinous), borderline ovarian tumours	Preoperative, follow-up
Inhibin	Granulosa cell tumours (type of sex cord stromal tumour)	Follow-up
β-hCG	Dysgerminoma, choriocarcinoma (germ cell tumours)	Preoperative, follow-up
AFP	Endodermal yolk sack, immature teratoma (germ cell tumours)	Preoperative, follow-up

AFP, α-fetoprotein; hCG, human chorionic gonadotrophin.

Functional ovarian cysts

This group of ovarian cysts includes follicular, corpus luteal and theca luteal cysts. The risk of developing functional cysts is reduced by the use of the combined oral contraceptive pill (COCP). Little is known about their aetiology, but diagnosis is made when the cyst measures more than 3 cm (normal ovulatory follicles measure up to 2.5 cm). They rarely grow larger than 10 cm and appear as simple unilocular cysts on ultrasound (**Figure 11.1A**). Management depends on symptoms: if asymptomatic, the patient can be reassured and a repeat USS performed to check resolution or non-enlargement and thereafter the patient can be discharged; if symptomatic, she can be booked for laparoscopic cystectomy if necessary.

Corpus luteal cysts occur following ovulation and may present with pain due to rupture or haemorrhage, typically late in the menstrual cycle (**Figure 11.1B**). Treatment is expectant, with analgesia. Occasionally, surgery may be necessary if there has been significant bleeding to wash out the pelvis and perform an ovarian cystectomy.

Theca luteal cysts are associated with pregnancy, particularly multiple pregnancy, and are often diagnosed incidentally at routine ultrasound. They are often bilateral. Most resolve spontaneously during pregnancy.

> ▶ **eResource 11.1**
>
> Ovarian cysts
> http://www.routledgetextbooks.com/textbooks/tenteachers/gynaecologyv11.1.php

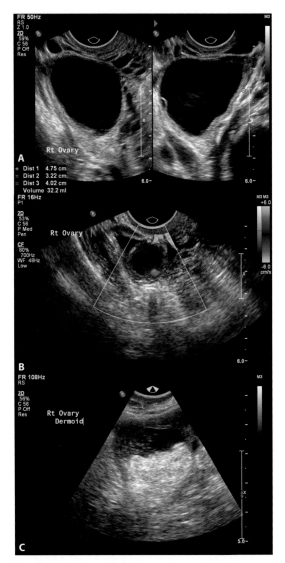

Figure 11.1 Transvaginal ultrasound scan. **A**: Simple ovarian cyst; **B**: corpus luteum cyst; **C**: dermoid cyst.

Inflammatory ovarian cysts

Inflammatory ovarian cysts are usually associated with pelvic inflammatory disease (PID) (see Chapter 9, Genitourinary problems), and are most common in young women. The inflammatory mass may involve the tube, ovary and bowel and can be described on imaging as a mass or an abscess. Occasionally, the tubo-ovarian mass can develop from other infective causes, for example appendicitis or diverticular disease.

Diagnosis is similar to that for PID: inflammatory markers are helpful and treatment may include antibiotics, surgical drainage or excision. Definitive surgery is usually deferred until after the acute infection has resolved, due to the risks of perioperative systemic infection and bleeding from handling acutely inflamed and infected tissue.

Patients may present with endometriomas, often known as 'chocolate cysts' due to the presence of altered blood within the ovary. They have a characteristic 'ground glass' appearance on USS. Further management of endometriosis is discussed in the next section.

Germ cell tumours

These are the most common ovarian tumours in young women aged 20–40 years, accounting for more than 50% of ovarian tumours in this age group with a peak incidence in the early 20s. The most common form of benign germ cell tumour is the mature dermoid cyst (cystic teratoma), which contains fully differentiated tissue types derived from all three embryonic germ cell layers (mesenchymal, epithelial and stroma). Hair, teeth, fat, skin, muscle, cartilage, bone and endocrine tissue are frequently present. Up to 10% of dermoid cysts are bilateral. The risk of malignant transformation is rare (<2%), usually occurring in women over 40 years. Diagnosis is usually confirmed with a pelvic USS (**Figure 11.1C**) and because of the high fat content present in dermoid cysts, MRI may also be useful where there is uncertainty. In general, ovarian cystectomy is indicated because spontaneous resolution is unlikely. Surgery is especially indicated if the dermoid cyst is symptomatic (**Figure 11.2**), is more than 5 cm in diameter or is enlarging. Cystectomy will prevent ovarian torsion and provide tissue for histological analysis.

Epithelial tumours

Benign epithelial tumours increase in frequency with age and are most common in perimenopausal women. The most common epithelial tumours are serous cystadenomas, accounting for 20–30% of benign tumours in women under 40. Serous cystadenomas are typically unilocular and unilateral, whereas mucinous cystadenomas are large multiloculated cysts that are bilateral in 10% of cases.

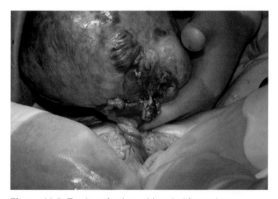

Figure 11.2 Torsion of a dermoid cyst at laparotomy.

Brenner tumours are small tumours often found incidentally within the ovary. They contain urothelial-like epithelium and may rarely secrete oestrogen.

Sex cord stromal tumours

Ovarian fibromas are the most common sex cord stromal tumours. They are solid ovarian tumours composed of stromal cells. They present in older women, often with torsion due to the heaviness of the ovary. Occasionally, patients may present with Meig syndrome (pleural effusion, ascites and ovarian fibroma). Following removal of the ovarian fibroma, the pleural effusion will usually resolve.

Thecomas are benign oestrogen-secreting tumours. They often present after the menopause with manifestations of excess oestrogen production, usually postmenopausal bleeding. Although benign, they may induce an endometrial carcinoma.

Other ovarian cysts

Other non-ovarian cysts can occasionally present as ovarian tumours. Fimbrial cysts and paratubal cysts originate from the adjacent Fallopian tube and broad ligament. The uncommon embryologically derived paraovarian cysts of Morgani are large collections of grape-like cysts derived from the paraoopheron.

Endometriosis

Endometriosis is a common condition that is defined as endometrial tissue lying outside the uterine cavity. It is usually found within the pelvis, being commonly located on the peritoneum lining the pelvic side walls, pouch of Douglas, uterosacral ligaments and bladder. This 'ectopic' endometrial-like tissue can induce fibrosis and be found infiltrating into deeper tissue such as the rectovaginal septum and bladder. When endometrial tissue is implanted into the ovary an endometrioma forms. This cyst may be large and contains old, altered blood that has a thick brown appearance, and for this reason is frequently referred to as a 'chocolate cyst'. Less commonly, endometriotic deposits can be found in other sites such as umbilicus, abdominal scars and the pleural cavity.

Endometriotic tissue responds to cyclical hormonal changes and therefore undergoes cyclical bleeding and local inflammatory reactions. These regularly repeated episodes of bleeding and healing lead to fibrosis and adhesion formation between pelvic organs, causing pain and infertility. In extreme cases a 'frozen pelvis' results, where extensive adhesions tether the pelvic organs and obliterate normal pelvic anatomy.

Adenomyosis is a uterine condition often seen with endometriosis, where islands of endometrial tissue are found deep within the underlying myometrium (see Chapter 12, Benign conditions of the uterus, cervix and endometrium).

Incidence

Endometriosis occurs in approximately 5–10% of women of reproductive age. It is found in at least one-third of women undergoing a diagnostic laparoscopy for pelvic pain or infertility. It is a condition that is oestrogen dependent and therefore it resolves after the menopause or when treatment is directed towards inducing a pseudomenopause.

Aetiology

The aetiology of endometriosis is unknown although there are several theories. There is unlikely to be a single theory that explains its aetiology, but the two most commonly accepted theories are:

- Sampson's implantation theory: menstrual blood can be seen within the pelvis during laparoscopy at the time of menses. Sampson's implantation theory postulates that it is this retrograde menstrual regurgitation of viable endometrial glands and tissue along patent Fallopian tubes, and that subsequent implantation on the pelvic peritoneal surface causes endometriosis. Using animal/primate models endometriosis has been induced with menstrual blood. Implantation of endometrium within human surgical scars after caesarean section or perineal repair following delivery lends support to this theory.
- Meyer's 'coelomic metaplasia' theory: coelomic epithelium transformation describes the dedifferentiation of peritoneal cells lining the Müllerian duct back to their primitive origin, which then transform into endometrial cells. This transformation into endometrial cells may be due to hormonal stimuli or inflammatory irritation.

Genetic and immunological factors

It has been suggested that genetic and immunological factors may alter the susceptibility of a woman and allow her to develop endometriosis. There appears to be an increased incidence in first-degree relatives of patients with the disorder and racial differences, with increased incidence among oriental women and a low prevalence in women of Afro-Caribbean origin.

Vascular and lymphatic spread

Vascular and lymphatic embolization to distant sites has been demonstrated and explains the rare findings of endometriosis in sites outside the peritoneal cavity, such as the lung.

Clinical features

Classical clinical features are severe cyclical non-colicky pelvic pain restricted to around the time of menstruation, sometimes associated with heavy menstrual loss. Symptoms may begin a few days before menses starts until the end of menses. However, women often also complain of chronic non-cyclical pelvic pain and severe fatigue. It is well recognized that there is a lack of correlation between the extent of the disease and the intensity of symptoms.

Pelvic pain presenting with colicky pain throughout the menstrual cycle may be associated with irritable bowel syndrome symptoms. Deep pain with intercourse (deep dyspareunia) and on defaecation (dyschezia) are key indicators of the presence of endometriosis deep within the pouch of Douglas.

Endometriosis in distant sites can cause local symptoms, for example cyclical epistaxis with nasal passage deposits and cyclical rectal bleeding with bowel deposits (*Table 11.3*).

Diagnosis

Physical examination

The accuracy of clinical examination in diagnosing endometriosis is limited and so the condition should be suspected even if the vaginal examination is normal. Positive examination findings indicative of endometriosis include thickening or nodularity of the uterosacral ligaments, tenderness in the pouch of Douglas, an adnexal mass or a fixed retroverted uterus. However, pelvic tenderness alone is non-specific, and differential diagnoses for restricted mobility of the uterus include chronic PID and uterine,

Table 11.3 Symptoms of endometriosis in relation to site of lesion

Site	Symptoms
Female reproductive tract	Dysmenorrhoea
	Lower abdominal and pelvic pain
	Dyspareunia
	Rupture/torsion endometrioma
	Low back pain
	Infertility
Urinary tract	Cyclical haematuria/dysuria
	Loin/flank pain (ureteric obstruction)
Gastrointestinal tract	Dyschezia (pain on defaecation)
	Cyclical rectal bleeding
	Obstruction
Surgical scars/ umbilicus	Cyclical pain, swelling and bleeding
Lung	Cyclical haemoptysis
	Haemopneumothorax

ovarian or cervical malignancy. In these conditions, other suggestive features are usually present, and imaging would rule out features of malignancy.

Ultrasound

TVUSS can detect endometriosis involving the ovaries (endometriomas or chocolate cysts) but its use in diagnosing smaller lesions is limited, although findings such as ovaries fixed together or to the back of the uterus (kissing ovaries) add strength to the diagnosis. In women with symptoms and signs of rectal endometriosis, TVUSS may be useful for identifying rectal disease, although again a negative scan does not exclude the disease.

 eResource 11.2

TVUSS of the pelvis with endometriosis
http://www.routledgetextbooks.com/textbooks/tenteachers/gynaecologyv11.2.php

Magnetic resonance imaging

MRI can detect lesions >5 mm in size, particularly in deep tissues, for example the rectovaginal septum. This can allow careful presurgical planning in difficult cases.

Laparoscopy

Although laparoscopy remains the traditional method for diagnosis, it is based on the accuracy of the visual diagnosis of endometriotic lesions, which is dependent on the experience of the surgeon. The endometriotic lesions can be red, puckered, black 'matchstick' or appear white and fibrous (**Figure 11.3**). The advantage of laparoscopy is that it allows lesions to be biopsied for histological

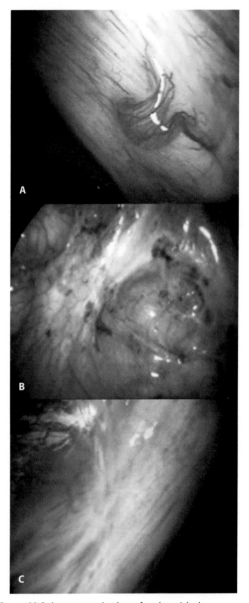

Figure 11.3 Laparoscopic view of endometriosis. **A**: Red lesions on peritoneum; **B**: black 'matchstick' lesions; **C**: white fibrous lesion.

confirmation of diagnosis and it affords concurrent surgical diathermy and/or excision of the endometriotic lesions and also staging of the disease. The patency of the Fallopian tubes can also be checked.

Biomarkers

There has been recent interest in the diagnosis of endometriosis using immunological biomarkers, such as CA125, in plasma, urine or serum. However, to date these non-invasive diagnostic approaches are too inaccurate for use in clinical practice.

Endometriosis and infertility

It is estimated that between 30% and 40% of patients with endometriosis complain of difficulty in conceiving. In many patients, there is a multifactorial pathogenesis to this subfertility (see Chapter 7, Subfertility). It is uncertain if and why minimal endometriotic deposits might render a patient subfertile. However, in the more severe stages of endometriosis, there is commonly anatomical distortion, with periadnexal adhesions and destruction of ovarian tissue when endometriomas develop. A number of possible and variable mechanisms have been postulated to connect mild endometriosis with infertility (*Table 11.4*).

From the balance of available evidence, medical treatment of endometriosis does not improve fertility and should not be given to patients wishing to conceive. However, surgical ablation/excision of minimal and mild endometriosis does improve fertility chances. It is uncertain whether surgical treatment of endometriomas increase spontaneous or in-vitro fertilization (IVF) pregnancy rates, as the removal of the endometriomas must be balanced against damage to ovarian tissue. The consensus from fertility specialists at present is to leave endometriomas alone prior to IVF unless they are symptomatic or reduce access for egg collection.

Management

Analgesics and hormonal ovarian suppression can be effective for treating cyclical and non-cyclical pelvic pain associated with endometriosis. Medical treatment of presumed endometriosis can be started if the clinical examination and TVUSS are normal, without the need for more invasive laparoscopy. However, if no symptom relief is obtained after 3–6 months of treatment, a laparoscopy should be considered. Patients

Table 11.4 Infertility and endometriosis – possible mechanisms

Ovarian function	Luteolysis caused by prostaglandin F2
	Oocyte maturation defects
	Endocrinopathies
	Luteinized unruptured follicle syndrome
	Altered prolactin release
	Anovulation
Tubal function	Impaired fimbrial oocyte pick-up
	Altered tubal mobility
Coital function	Deep dyspareunia – reduced coital frequency
Sperm function	Antibodies causing inactivation
	Macrophage phagocytosis of spermatozoa
Early pregnancy failure	Prostaglandin induced Immune reaction Luteal phase deficiency

with endometriosis are often difficult to treat, not only from a physical point of view, but also often because of associated psychological issues associated with their pain. Long-term therapeutic strategies should be formulated where possible. Coexisting additional diseases such as irritable bowel syndrome and constipation (present in up to 80% of cases) should also be treated to improve overall success rates. Endometriosis is known to recur throughout reproductive life and it is impossible to guarantee complete cure. Treatment should therefore be tailored for the individual according to her age, symptoms, extent of the disease and her desire to have children. In a significant proportion of patients there is little progression of the disease over time, and this may be reassuring. Due to the variation in presentation it has been shown that there is a significant delay to diagnosis, with research indicating around 6 years on average, and some patients will be relieved by a positive laparoscopy that validates their symptoms.

Medical therapy
Analgesics

Non-steroidal anti-inflammatory drugs (NSAIDs) are potent analgesics and are helpful in reducing the severity of dysmenorrhoea and pelvic pain. However, they have no specific impact on the disease and hence their use is for symptom control only. The additional use of codeine/opiates should be avoided as the coexisting irritable bowel symptoms can be worsened, exacerbating pelvic pain symptoms.

Combined oral contraceptives

In the absence of contraindications (see Chapter 6, Contraception and abortion) or desire for pregnancy, the COCP should be considered because it has been shown to reduce endometriosis-associated dyspareunia, dysmenorrhoea and non-menstrual pain as well as providing cycle control and contraception. The COCP can be taken sequentially with the usual 7-day pill-free break but may be more effective in alleviating pain symptoms, especially cyclical dysmenorrhoea, if it is tricycled (where three packets are taken back to back) or taken continuously without a break, inducing amenorrhoea. If the COCP achieves symptomatic relief, then this therapy can be continued for several years until pregnancy is intended. If symptoms persist, the diagnosis should be reviewed and common coexisting conditions such as irritable bowel disease and constipation treated (e.g. encouraging a high-fibre diet and adequate fluid intake). Alternative medical or surgical treatments should be discussed (see below).

Progestogens

In those where there are risk factors for the use of a COCP, progestogens should be used to induce amenorrhoea. The long-acting reversible contraceptives (LARCs), depot-medroxyprogesterone acetate and the levonorgestrel intrauterine system (LNG-IUS) (Mirena®) are particularly useful in providing a long-term therapeutic effect particularly after surgical treatment. The effect is probably related to 100% compliance with treatment.

Gonadotrophin-releasing hormone agonists

Gonadotrophin-releasing hormone agonists (GnRH-a) are effective in relieving the severity and symptoms of endometriosis. GnRH has been discussed in Chapter 4, Disorders of menstrual bleeding. Despite their side-effects, the drugs are well tolerated by some and they have become established agents in the diagnosis (if CPP is of a gynaecological origin [e.g. endometriosis], then symptoms will be eradicated) and treatment of endometriosis. They are

available as multiple, daily-administered intranasal sprays but are usually administered as slow-release depot formulations, each lasting for 1 month or more. Long-term use over 6 months is precluded because drug-induced osteoporosis results The recurrence of symptoms on cessation of therapy is usually rapid.

Other hormonal agents

In the past, the ovarian suppressive agents danazol and gestrinone were used to good effect, but are no longer appropriate as newer treatment have become available, notably LNG-IUS. They had a number of androgenic side-effects, such as weight gain, greasy skin and acne as well as causing alterations in lipid profiles and liver function and potential deepening of the voice.

There has been some interest in a newer class of drug called aromatase inhibitors that inhibit the action of the enzyme aromatase, which converts androgens into oestrogens and is over expressed in endometriotic tissue. Further research is ongoing for their use in refractory cases.

Surgical treatment
Fertility-sparing surgery

Most surgery for endometriosis can be achieved laparoscopically. Symptomatic endometriotic chocolate cysts should not just be drained but the inner cyst lining should be excised to reduce the risk of recurrence; however, this will be associated with damage to functional ovarian tissue. Therefore, when drainage is performed as an adjunct to fertility treatment, drainage only may be considered. Deposits of superficial peritoneal endometriosis can be easily ablated or excised during laparoscopy using diathermy or laser energy.

Specialist surgery is needed to treat endometriosis where the disease has caused extensive adhesions distorting normal pelvic anatomy or involved other organs such as the rectum, large bowel or bladder, or when there are rectovaginal nodules of disease. Recurrent risks following conservative surgery are as high as 30% and therefore concurrent long-term medical therapy is often necessary and started straight after surgery.

Hysterectomy and oophorectomy

Hysterectomy with removal of the ovaries and all visible endometriosis lesions should be considered only in women who have completed their family and failed to respond to more conservative treatments. Women should be informed that hysterectomy will not necessarily cure the symptoms or the disease. Oestrogen-only hormone replacement therapy (HRT) can be started immediately following surgery once the patient is mobile, but some surgeons prefer to defer commencing HRT for up to 6 months to prevent activation of any residual disease. Combined (oestrogen and progestogen) HRT can also be considered as a suppressive treatment, where reactivation of new or residual disease is suspected.

Chronic pelvic pain

CPP is a debilitating symptom among women, which has a major impact on health-related quality of life, work productivity and health care utilization. The Royal College of Obstetricians and Gynaecologists (RCOG) has defined CPP as 'intermittent or constant pain in the lower abdomen or pelvis of a woman of at least 6 months in duration, not occurring exclusively with menstruation (dysmenorrhoea) or intercourse and not associated with pregnancy'.

Incidence

CPP presents in primary care as frequently as migraine, asthma or low back pain and accounts for 20% of all outpatient appointments in gynaecological secondary care. Estimates of prevalence vary widely but are thought to be between 10% and 20%.

Aetiology

The potential causes of CPP in women are listed in *Table 11.5*. In contrast to acute pelvic pain, there is often more than one underlying cause contributing to CPP. The experience of pain is affected by physical, psychological and social factors.

Table 11.5 Causes of chronic pelvic pain in women

Gynaecological	Endometriosis and adenomyosis* Adhesions including chronic PID* Uterine fibroids Ovarian cysts
Central and peripheral nervous system	Changes in both afferent and efferent nerve pathways in the central and peripheral nervous systems modifying pain perception (e.g. 'visceral hyperalgesia' and 'neuropathic pain')
Gastrointestinal	Irritable bowel syndrome* (a functional bowel disorder characterized by the presence of a cluster of symptoms and signs that include cramping, abdominal pain, increased gas, altered bowel habits, food intolerance, and bloating) Constipation Inflammatory bowel disease Coeliac disease (gluten sensitivity)
Urological	Bladder pain syndrome (previously known as interstitial cystitis, consisting of pain, pressure or discomfort related to the bladder along with at least one other urinary symptom [e.g. urgency or frequency], in the absence of any other pathology) Recurrent urinary tract infections Urinary tract calculi
Musculoskeletal	Pain arising from the joints in the pelvis or from damage to the muscles in the abdominal wall or pelvic floor (e.g. degenerative joint disease, spondylolisthesis)
Nerve entrapment	Nerve entrapment within scar tissue, fascia or a narrow foramen may result in pain and dysfunction in the distribution of that nerve, which is highly localized and exacerbated by particular movements
Psychological and social issues	Depression, anxiety and sleep disorders are common in women with chronic pain and may be a consequence rather than a cause of pain Physical and sexual abuse

* Most commonly encountered. PID, pelvic inflammatory disease.

Diagnosis

A thorough history should include questions about the pattern of the pain and its association with other problems, such as psychological, bladder and bowel symptoms, and the effect of movement and posture on the pain. An abdominal and pelvic examination should look for areas of tenderness and pelvic masses as well as distortion or tethering or prolapse of pelvic organs.

Investigations

Investigations to consider when evaluating women with CPP are shown in *Table 11.6*. Findings from the history and examination will dictate the need for further testing; CPP refractory to medical treatment or associated with abnormal examination findings, such as enlargement, tenderness, irregularity or fixity of pelvic structures, would indicate the need for further investigation. TVUSS is the least invasive and first-line method of imaging the pelvis. Diagnostic laparoscopy is the most invasive test for evaluating the female pelvis and has been regarded as the 'gold standard' investigation for CPP. However, depending on the preceding work-up, 40% of diagnostic laparoscopies fail to show any cause for the CPP symptoms. Structural pathologies identified at laparoscopy can often be surgically treated at the same time.

Management

The multifactorial nature of CPP should be discussed and explored with the patient from the start. General health advice including the importance of diet, hydration, exercise and sexual health should be given. Analgesia such as NSAIDs, opiates and paracetamol to control pain should be discussed. Where clinical examination and USS are normal, women with cyclical CPP should be offered a therapeutic trial using hormonal treatment to suppress ovarian function for a period of 3–6 months before having a diagnostic laparoscopy. Hormonal treatments include the COCP, systemic and local (LNG-IUS) progestogens and GnRH-analogues. Structural pathologies can be treated surgically, usually via laparoscopy, including removal of adnexal masses, treatment of endometriosis and adhesiolysis.

If the nature of the CPP is thought to be primarily non-gynaecological then referral to the relevant health care professional such as gastroenterologist, urologist, genitourinary medicine physician, physiotherapist, psychologist or psychosexual counsellor should be made. If, despite the above interventions, pain is not adequately controlled, consideration should be given to referral to a pain management team or a specialist pelvic pain clinic.

Table 11.6 Common investigations for chronic pelvic pain (CPP)

Investigation	Indication	Potential diagnoses
Genital tract swabs	All sexually active women should be offered screening for STIs such as *Chlamydia trachomatis* or gonococcus	Pelvic infection/PID
Pelvic USS	Suspected pelvic masses	Adnexal masses – ovarian cysts including endometriomas, hydrosalpinges, tubo-ovarian abscesses Uterine pathology – adenomyosis, fibroids
MRI	Further assessment of pelvic masses or suspected deep infiltrating endometriosis	Further characterize masses seen on USS Rectovaginal endometriosis
Laparoscopy	Where pelvic masses, endometriosis or adhesions are suspected	Superficial and deep infiltrating endometriosis Abdominopelvic adhesions Pelvic masses

MRI, magneic resonance imaging; PID, pelvic inflammatory disease; STI, sexually-transmitted infection; USS, ultrasound scan.

KEY LEARNING POINTS

- Commonly encountered benign ovarian tumours include functional cysts, teratomas (dermoid cysts) and endometriomas.

- Ovarian cysts can be asymptomatic or present with pain or as an abdominal mass. Acute pain may arise because of an ovarian cyst 'accident' such as haemorrhage, rupture or torsion.

- TVUSS is the primary test used to diagnose different types of ovarian cyst. Along with the CA125 serological tumour marker, ultrasound can be used to help differentiate between benign and malignant ovarian tumours.

- Treatment is based on the symptoms, size and type of cyst. Ovarian cystectomy or even oophorectomy may be required and this is usually undertaken using a laparoscopic approach.

- Endometriosis refers to the finding of endometrial glands and stroma outside of the uterus and is one of the commonest conditions seen in gynaecology, affecting 5–10% of women of reproductive age.

- Endometriosis usually presents with cyclical non-colicky pelvic pain around the time of menstruation, and is sometimes associated with heavy menstrual loss. However, affected women may also complain of chronic non-cyclical pelvic pain, dyspareunia, dyschezia and severe fatigue.

- Endometriosis is associated with tubal and ovarian damage and the formation of adhesions and can compromise fertility.

- Medical treatment of endometriosis involves suppressing oestrogen levels to induce amenorrhoea using the COCP, progestogens or GnRH agonists.

- Conservative laparoscopic surgical treatment of endometriosis involves excising or ablating visible lesions. More radical excisional laparoscopic surgery may be required for deeply infiltrating endometriosis involving the bowel and rectovaginal septum. Total hysterectomy and bilateral salpingo-oophorectomy is often undertaken for refractory symptoms.

- CPP is usually multifactorial involving physical, psychological and social factors. Management should be directed at the underlying causes and include general health advice, analgesics, hormonal therapies and surgery. Multidisciplinary pelvic pain clinics are necessary to manage severe, refractory cases.

Further reading

Dunselman GA, Vermeulen N, Becker C, *et al.* (2014). ESHRE guideline: management of women with endometriosis. *Hum Reprod* **29**(3):400–12. doi: 10.1093/humrep/det457.

NHS Clinical Knowledge Summaries on Endometriosis. Available from: www.cks.nhs.uk/endometriosis. April 2015.

RCOG Green-top Guideline No. 34: Ovarian cysts in postmenopausal women. RCOG 2010 [on line source: https://www.rcog.org.uk/globalassets/documents/guidelines/gtg34ovariancysts.pdf].

RCOG Green-top Guideline No. 41: The initial management of chronic pelvic pain. RCOG 2012 [on line source https://www.rcog.org.uk/globalassets/documents/guidelines/gtg_41.pdf].

RCOG Green-top Guideline No. 62: Management of suspected ovarian masses in premenopausal women. RCOG 2011 [on line source: https://www.rcog.org.uk/globalassets/documents/guidelines/gtg_62.pdf].

Self assessment

CASE HISTORY

A 26-year-old law student presents with a 2-year history of CPP. She admits to a poor diet but is otherwise fit and healthy. She contracted genital chlamydial infection from a previous relationship 3 years ago, but is currently in a new and stable relationship. A urinary pregnancy test has been performed and the result is negative.

A *What questions would you ask about the presenting complaint?*

B *What features of the history would suggest a gynaecological cause for the pain?*

C What features from a bimanual pelvic examination would suggest a gynaecological cause for the pain?

D List likely gynaecological causes of CPP.

E List likely non-gynaecological causes of CPP.

F Suggest diagnostic tests you would perform.

G How might you manage this patient?

ANSWERS

A Establish the nature of the pain, such as using 'SOCRATES' – Site, Onset (e.g. relationship to chlamydial infection), Character, Radiation (gynaecological pain may be bilateral and into the back, groins and vagina), Associations, Time course (especially relationship to the menstrual cycle), Exacerbating/relieving factors (e.g. sexual intercourse, voiding and defaecation), Severity (e.g. effect on activities of daily living, use of analgesics, etc).

B Onset or exacerbation in relation to the menstrual cycle along with deep dyspareunia is suggestive of a gynaecological origin for the pain, although CPP is often multifactorial.

C Presence of a pelvic mass may suggest the presence of an adnexal mass (e.g. ovarian cyst, hydrosalpinx) or enlarged uterus (e.g. fibroids, adenomyosis). Tenderness, fixed, immobile pelvic organs (suggestive of adhesions secondary to endometriosis or infection) and nodularity of the uterosacral ligaments (indicative of deep infiltrating endometriosis) are other features to assess.

D Chronic PID causing adhesions and/or a chronic tubo-ovarian abscess should be considered given the history of a sexually transmitted infection. Endometriosis is common in women of reproductive age and usually presents in the second or third decade.

An ovarian cyst should form part of the differential diagnosis.

E Gastrointestinal causes such as irritable bowel syndrome or constipation in light of her poor diet. A negative pregnancy test excludes an ectopic pregnancy. Genitourinary problems such as bladder pain syndrome, musculoskeletal causes, neuropathic pain and psychological contributors should be evaluated depending on the history and examination.

F Genital tract swabs and a midstream urine specimen (if there are symptoms). First-line imaging should be a pelvic USS in order to identify uterine and adnexal masses. Laparoscopy to detect adhesions and endometriosis if the pain is resistant to medical treatment or the gynaecological examination is abnormal.

G This depends on the cause. General health advice, analgesics and hormonal treatments (e.g. the COCP, systemic and local [LNG-IUS]) to suppress ovulation for at least 3–6 months assuming a likely gynaecological origin for the chronic pain and the absence of an adnexal mass requiring surgical removal. Laparoscopic surgery should be considered in the presence of adhesions (adhesiolysis), endometriosis (excision or ablation of endometriotic deposits) or adnexal pathology (removal of adnexal masses [e.g. ovarian cystectomy]).

EMQ

A Endometriosis.
B Adenomyosis.
C Bladder pain syndrome.
D Irritable bowel syndrome.
E Constipation.
F Depression.
G Nerve entrapment.
H Torted ovarian cyst.
I Endometrioma.
J Dermoid cyst (benign teratoma).
K Functional ovarian cyst.
L Tube–ovarian abscess.

For each description below, choose the SINGLE most appropriate answer from the above list of options. Each option may be used once, more than once or not at all.

1 A recently divorced 36-year-old woman presents with 6 months of generalized pelvic pain, insomnia, fatigue, constipation and headaches. On further questioning she admits to being anxious and tearful.

2 A parous, 30-year-old woman complains of increasingly heavy menstrual periods that are painful throughout their 5 day duration. She is pain free for the rest of the month. On examination she has an enlarged 'bulky' uterus.

3 A 22-year-old woman presents with a history of CPP and dyspareunia. She has a history of chlamydial infection when she was 19 years old. On vaginal examination a tender mass is palpable and pelvic USS confirms the presence of bilateral complex adnexal masses.

4 A 24-year-old woman presents with long-standing pelvic pain. Her periods are painful for the first day but are regular and light.

She has occasional pain with sexual intercourse. She admits to being an anxious person and weight conscious, exercising daily. She opens her bowels on alternate days and sometimes has loose stools as well as feeling bloated, especially prior to her period.

5 A 38-year-old woman complains of pelvic pain for the last 5 years. The pain can be worse cyclically but she has not noted a definite pattern to it. She has been treated for recurrent urinary tract infections by her general practitioner (GP) because of pain and pressure on voiding urine along with urgency and frequency. However, many of these infections have not been confirmed on microbiological examination of midstream urine specimens (MSUs). A laparoscopy 3 years ago was normal.

ANSWERS

1F The generalized somatic symptoms of depression are clear here, and abdominal pain is common in this scenario. If the pain persisted after the emotional problems had passed then further investigations would be indicated. Investigations at this point may increase anxiety, unless of course there were clear clinical findings.

2B The key symptom here is pain with the bleed that persists throughout the period. This makes endometriosis unlikely, as this is associated with premenstrual pain as a rule. Tubo-ovarian pathology would not cause cyclical menstrual pain.

3L Pelvic inflammaory disease can cause the tubes to be obstructed and swell to cause hydrosalpinges. Subsequently, infection can turn the tubes into abscesses that can envelop the ovary, a tubo-ovarian abscess. This may be bilateral. The inflammation surrounding this can cause a 'frozen pelvis', where the pelvic organs become stuck together and immobile, causing pain. The differential diagnosis would be endometriosis, but the history and the TVUSS findings make this unlikely. TVUSS with severe endometriosis would show the presence of ovarian endometriomas, but usually the tubes would not be involved.

4D The normal periods (pain on day 1 being a common and non-pathological complaint), and lack of symptoms in the pelvis specifically, makes a gynaecological cause for pain unlikely. Patients are frequently seen to exclude a gynaecological cause of pain, because it can be difficult to pinpoint the site of pain. The alteration in the bowel habit and the bloating is the key to diagnosing irritable bowel. Irritable bowel is often worse premenstrually because the progesterone of the luteal phase causes a relaxation of the smooth muscle in bowel.

5C The symptoms point to the bladder as the site of pain. It is useful that the GP has performed MSUs to exclude recurrent urinary tract infections. Occasionally there is a spot of endometriosis causing bladder pain, but the laparoscopy 3 years previously excludes this.

SBA QUESTIONS

1 A 25-year-old parous woman is admitted to hospital with acute left-sided, colicky pain. She has no abnormal vaginal discharge nor urinary or bowel symptoms. She is apyrexial and tachycardic. On examination her abdomen is soft, not distended and non-tender. She has not missed a menstrual period and her urinary pregnancy test is negative. She requires morphine for pain relief.

Which diagnostic test would you consider first-line in this situation? Choose the single best answer.

A   Serum βhCG.

B   MRI.

C   CT scan.

D   Transabdominal + transvaginal pelvic USS.

E   Laparoscopy.

ANSWER

D   The clinical assessment of this woman suggests that she has considerable pain necessitating narcotic analgesia but does not have an acute surgical abdomen. Thus immediate surgery in the form of laparoscopy or laparotomy is not indicated. In the absence of genitourinary or gastrointestinal symptoms or a temperature or significant abdominal tenderness on examination, infection and/or peritonitis is unlikely. An ovarian cystic accident is the most likely gynaecological diagnosis. Of the radiological imaging tests listed, pelvic USS is the safest and most readily available and provides excellent images of adnexal cystic masses. An early pregnancy complication such as an ectopic pregnancy is improbable given that she has not missed a period and the urinary pregnancy test (UPT) is negative; a UPT has high sensitivity and so serum quantification of βhCG levels is unnecessary.

2 A 32-year-old woman has a pelvic TVUSS as part of investigations for primary subfertility. The scan shows bilateral 5 cm 'kissing' ovarian cysts in the pouch of Douglas, both of which contain diffuse, low-level echoes giving a solid 'ground-glass' appearance. She reports severe dysmenorrhoea and dyspareunia.

What type of ovarian cysts are these most likely to be? Choose the single best answer.

A   Haemorrhagic functional ovarian cysts.

B   Dermoid cysts.

C   Endometriomas.

D   Tubo-ovarian abscesses.

E   Serous cystadenomas.

ANSWER

C   The age of this woman and her history of subfertility and cyclical pain are consistent with the presence of endometriosis ('chocolate cysts'). Furthermore, the close proximity of both ovaries, known as 'kissing ovaries', is caused by adhesions, which is considered a sign of pelvic endometriosis and would cause pain with sexual intercourse. The description on ultrasound of homogenous, low-level 'echoes' represents old altered blood are also characteristic of endometriomas. However, the solid appearance could also reflect a haemorrhagic cyst, dermoid cyst or chronic tubo-ovarian abscess. A tubo-ovarian abscess can also be associated with subfertility and dyspareunia although not typically cyclical pain. The other cysts listed are usually asymptomatic or present with non-cyclical pelvic pain. Serous cystadenomas are rarely bilateral, usually asymptomatic unless large (>10 cm) and clear without solid components.

Benign conditions of the uterus, cervix and endometrium

T JUSTIN CLARK

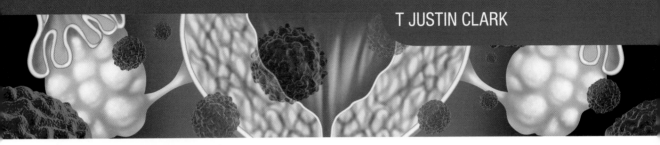

LEARNING OBJECTIVES

- Describe the common benign conditions that affect the uterus according to their tissue of origin: the cervix, the endometrium and the myometrium.

- Understand the presenting symptoms and examination findings associated with benign uterine pathology.

- Describe the common tests used to evaluate the uterus and endometrial cavity.

- Explain the available treatment options for uterine fibroids and adenomyosis and the rationale for selection.

Uterine cervix

The cervix is the cylindrical lower extremity of the uterus and consists mainly of collagen fibres. The vaginal part of the cervix, called the ectocervix, is lined by thick non-keratinized stratified squamous epithelium and has a pink appearance. The external os is visible in the centre of the ectocervix as a dark circular or slit-like area and is the opening to the endocervical canal, which is lined by simple columnar epithelium. There is a clear demarcation of this transformation between the two types of epithelium, called the 'squamocolumnar junction'. This anatomical junction fluctuates under hormonal influence as described further in Chapters 1, The development and anatomy of the female sexual organs and pelvis, and Chapter 16, Premalignant and malignant disease of the lower genital tract. Benign lesions can occur on the surface or structure of the cervix.

Benign cervical surface lesions

Cervical ectropion

In women of reproductive age the columnar epithelium is visible on the ectocervix as a circular, red area surrounding the external cervical os (**Figure 12.1A**). This is a normal finding and should not be called 'cervical erosion' because this erroneously implies it is an ulcer. An ectropion commonly develops under the influence of the 'three Ps': puberty, pill and pregnancy. The fragile, glandular columnar epithelium of a large cervical ectropion may predispose to intermenstrual and postcoital bleeding (IMB, PCB). Some women may present with an excessive, clear, odourless mucus-type discharge. To reduce the ectropion and associated symptoms women should be changed from oestrogen-based hormonal contraceptives. The other option is cervical ablation where the visible glandular producing columnar cells are ablated, usually with cryocautery, as an outpatient. Prior to treatment end, cervical and lower genital tract swabs are taken to exclude chlamydia and other sexually-transmitted infections and normal cervical cytology should be confirmed to exclude cervical premalignancy and malignancy (see Chapter 16, Premalignant and malignant disease of the lower genital tract).

Nabothian follicles

Sometimes the columnar glands within the transformation zone become sealed over, forming small, mucus-filled cysts visible on the ectocervix. These are termed 'nabothian follicles' and are of no pathological significance. No treatment is usually required although extremely large ones can be drained using a large-bore needle (**Figure 12.1B**).

Cervical polyps

Cervical polyps are benign tumours arising from the endocervical epithelium and may be seen as smooth, reddish protrusions. They are usually asymptomatic, being identified incidentally during a routine cervical smear, but as with a cervical ectropion they can cause vaginal discharge, IMB and PCB. They are easily removed by avulsion with polyp forceps as an outpatient.

Cervical stenosis

Cervical stenosis refers to pathological narrowing of the endocervical canal and is usually an iatrogenic phenomenon caused by a surgical event. Treatment of premalignant disease of the cervix using a cone biopsy or loop diathermy can cause cervical stenosis, as can endometrial ablation affecting the os. The ensuing trapped blood in the uterus (haematometra) causes cyclical dysmenorrhoea with no associated menstrual bleeding. Treatment is by surgical dilatation of the cervix under ultrasound or hysteroscopic guidance.

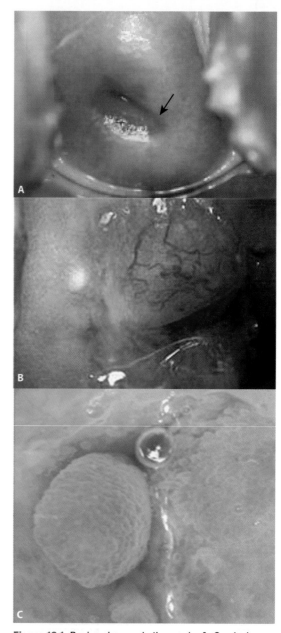

Figure 12.1 Benign changes in the cervix. **A**: Cervical ectropion; **B**: nabothian follicle; **C**: cervical polyp.

Benign endometrial lesions

Endometrial polyps

Endometrial polyps are focal endometrial outgrowths containing a variable amount of glands, stroma and blood vessels, which influence their

▶ eResource 12.1

Endometrial polyps
http://www.routledgetextbooks.com/textbooks/tenteachers/gynaecologyv12.1.php

macroscopic appearance. Endometrial polyps may be asymptomatic but can cause abnormal uterine bleeding (AUB) (heavy menstrual bleeding [HMB], IMB and postmenopausal bleeding [PMB]) and adversely impact on fertility. They are common and estimated to be present in around 10–20% of women with AUB and 10% of women with subfertility. Risk factors for endometrial polyp development include obesity, late menopause, the use of the partial oestrogen agonist tamoxifen and possibly the use of hormone replacement therapy (HRT). Most polyps do not appear to be subject to the normal cellular mechanisms that regulate the endometrium. Consequently, they are relatively insensitive to cyclical hormonal changes, leading them to persist and cause unscheduled vaginal bleeding. Endometrial polyps contain hyperplastic foci in 10–25% of symptomatic cases and 1% is frankly malignant. The risk of polyps harbouring serious endometrial disease is increased after the menopause and with the use of tamoxifen. Endometrial polyps may be pedunculated or sessile, single or multiple and vary in size (0.5–4 cm).

Endometrial polyps can be diagnosed by transvaginal ultrasound scan (TVUSS) but because they are focal, intracavity pathologies the most accurate tests are outpatient hysteroscopy (OPH) and saline infusion sonography (SIS), because these investigations involve distending the uterine cavity with fluid, thereby aiding detection (**Figure 12.2**). Smaller endometrial polyps can spontaneously resolve but most persist such that once diagnosed,

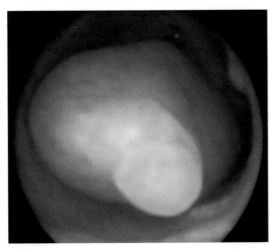

Figure 12.2 A hysteroscopic view of an endometrial polyp.

removal is indicated (polypectomy) in order to alleviate AUB symptoms, optimize fertility and exclude hyperplasia or cancer. Polypectomy is a simple procedure that can be performed as a day-case under general anaesthesia, but is now increasingly performed as an outpatient with or without local anaesthesia. A hysteroscope is used to visualize the polyp(s) and to allow miniature instruments to be passed down its operating channel in order to remove the polyp with scissors, electrodes or morcellators.

Asherman syndrome

Irreversible damage of the single layer thick basal endometrium does not allow normal regeneration of the endometrium. The endometrial cavity undergoes fibrosis and adhesion formation, termed 'Asherman syndrome'. The result is reduced, or absent, menstrual shedding and subfertility. This usually occurs after pregnancy where there has been uterine infection (endometritis) or following overzealous curettage of the uterine cavity during surgical management of miscarriage or following secondary postpartum haemorrhage. In this 'soft' uterine state, the myometrium (including the basal layer) can be inadvertently excavated while attempting to evacuate these retained products of conception (RPOC) using metal instruments or suction cannulae. Prevention of uterine scarring by adopting conservative or less traumatic surgical approaches to managing RPOC and preventing endometritis is important given its adverse impact on fertility. To treat Asherman syndrome hysteroscopic surgical techniques are needed to manually break down the intrauterine adhesions (adhesiolysis). However, treatment can be difficult and risks further uterine trauma.

Surgical treatments to deliberately destroy the basal layer have been developed for treatment of HMB, called endometrial ablation (see Chapter 4, Disorders of menstrual bleeding).

Benign lesions of the myometrium

Uterine fibroids and adenomyosis are the two most prevalent conditions affecting the myometrium.

Fibroids

Classification

A fibroid is a benign tumour of uterine smooth muscle termed a 'leiomyoma'. The gross appearance is of a well-demarcated, firm, whorled tumour. They are highly prevalent, being found in approximately 40% of women overall, and are more common in nulliparous and obese women and in those with a family history or of African descent. They are usually multiple and can substantially increase the size of the uterus. Fibroids are classified according to their location in relation to the uterine wall (**Figure 12.3**). Uncommonly, fibroids can arise separately from the uterus, especially in the adjacent broad ligament, presumably from embryonal remnants.

Symptoms caused by fibroids

Most fibroids are small and asymptomatic, but they can be associated with the following conditions:

- AUB (usually HMB and IMB).
- Reproductive failure.
- Subfertility.
- Recurrent pregnancy loss.
- Bulk effects on adjacent structures in the pelvis.
- Pressure and pain.
- Bladder and bowel dysfunction.
- Abdominal distension.

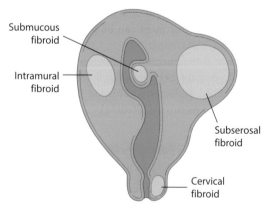

Figure 12.3 Diagram showing the typical sites of uterine fibroids.

Submucous fibroid

Intramural fibroid

Subserosal fibroid

Cervical fibroid

Natural history

Fibroids are benign, oestrogen-dependent tumours that can enlarge during pregnancy in response to the hyperoestrogenic state, become common with advancing reproductive age and shrink after the menopause when ovarian oestrogen production ceases. They can undergo degenerative change usually in response to outgrowing their blood supply. Three forms of degeneration are recognized:

- Red – haemorrhage and necrosis occurs within the fibroid typically presenting in the midsecond trimester pregnancy with acute pain.
- Hyaline – asymptomatic softening and liquefaction of the fibroid.
- Cystic – asymptomatic central necrosis leaving cystic spaces at the centre. Degenerative changes can initiate calcium deposition leading to calcification. Rarely, malignant or sarcomatous degeneration can occur but the incidence of this is 1:350 cases or less. The suspicion is greatest in the postmenopausal period when there is a rapidly increasing size of the fibroid.

Clinical features

Fibroids can cause several gynaecological complaints and are one of the commonest indications for hysterectomy. However, the vast majority of fibroids are asymptomatic. Abdominal examination might indicate the presence of a firm mass arising from the pelvis. Unless fibroids cause symptoms they do not require any treatment. Common presenting symptoms include menstrual disturbance and pressure or 'bulk' symptoms, especially urinary frequency, and infertility. Pain is unusual, except in the special circumstance of acute red degeneration or torsion of a pedunculated fibroid (**Figure 12.4**).

Subfertility may result from mechanical distortion or occlusion of the Fallopian tubes, and an endometrial cavity grossly distorted by submucous fibroids may prevent implantation of a fertilized ovum. Removal of submucosal fibroids can enhance fertility and also outcomes with assisted reproductive techniques such as in-vitro fertilization (IVF). However, the effectiveness of surgically removing the other types of fibroids is less clear and risks hysterectomy in 1% of cases because of significant intraoperative bleeding. Thus, these fibroids should only be

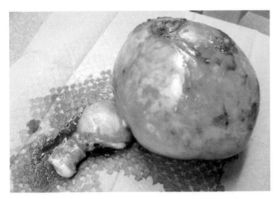

Figure 12.4 Pedunculated, subserosal fibroid on a hysterectomy specimen.

removed if symptomatic and where there is proven, otherwise unexplained, infertility. Once a pregnancy is established, however, the risk of miscarriage is not increased. In late pregnancy, fibroids located in the cervix or lower uterine segment may cause an abnormal lie. After delivery, postpartum haemorrhage may occur due to inefficient uterine contraction.

Examination findings suggestive of uterine fibroids

- General: signs of anaemia.
- Abdominal examination: visible and/or palpable abdominal mass arising from the pelvis*.
- Bimanual examination: enlarged, firm, smooth or irregular, non-tender# uterus palpable.

---

* See Chapter 2, Gynaecological history, examination and investigations, and imaging for determining the pelvic origin of a mass; # tenderness may suggest red degeneration.

Diagnosis

Often the clinical features obtained from the history and examination alone will be sufficient to establish the diagnosis. A full blood count should be taken in women with HMB; severe anaemia associated with HMB invariably indicates the presence of significant fibroids.

Abdominopelvic ultrasound (TAUSS and TVUSS) is the mainstay of diagnosis and helps delineate the origin of a clinically-detected pelvic mass (i.e. distinguishing between a uterine fibroid and an ovarian tumour, and locating the position and size of fibroids). In the presence of large fibroids, ultrasonography is

Useful tests where uterine fibroids are suspected

- TVUSS: good for detecting and locating submucous fibroids and small intramural fibroids.
- Transabdominal ultrasound scan (TAUSS): good for detecting larger intramural and subserosal fibroids and excluding hydronephrosis secondary to pressure from fibroids obstructing the ureters.
- SIS: good for detecting and locating submucosal fibroids and endometrial polyps.
- Hysteroscopy:
  - good for detecting submucosal fibroids and endometrial polyps;
  - good for planning subsequent hysteroscopic surgical treatment;
  - surgical hysteroscopy can remove polyps, adhesions and submucosal fibroids.
- Magnetic resonance imaging (MRI):
  - good for describing the morphology and location of fibroids;
  - indicated prior to uterine artery embolization and to monitor treatment response.

also helpful to exclude hydronephrosis from pressure on the ureters. MRI is occasionally used to demarcate the morphology, size and location of uterine fibroids prior to radiological or surgical intervention (**Figure 12.5**).

Treatment of fibroids

Medical treatment

Conservative management is appropriate where asymptomatic fibroids are detected incidentally. The main types of medical treatment for HMB (see Chapter 4, Disorders of menstrual bleeding) namely the levonorgestrel intrauterine system (LNG-IUS), tranexamic acid, mefenamic acid and the combined oral contraceptive pill (COCP) tend to be ineffective in the presence of a submucous fibroid or an enlarged uterus that is palpable abdominally (>12 weeks size). The only effective medical treatment is to use injectable gonadotrophin-releasing hormone (GnRH) agonists, which induce a menopausal state by shutting down ovarian oestradiol production. However, GnRH treatment is not tolerated by all women because of severe menopausal symptoms.

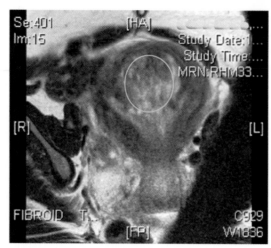

Figure 12.5 Magnetic resonance imaging of an enlarged fibroid uterus.

More recently, the selective progesterone receptor modulator (SPRM) ulipristal acetate has been shown to be as effective as GnRH agonists in reducing fibroid volume and alleviating HMB symptoms, although it is not yet widely accepted into clinical practice. In addition to being an oral tablet, this SPRM does not induce a menopausal state and associated symptoms. However, neither GnRH nor SPRM represent a viable long-term treatment option. Moreover, when ovarian function returns, the fibroids regrow to their previous dimensions.

Surgical treatment

The choice of surgical treatment is determined by the presenting complaint and the patient's aspirations for menstrual function and fertility. Minimally invasive hysteroscopic surgery can be used to cut away a submucous fibroid or fibroid polyp, helping to resolve HMB symptoms even in the presence of other types of fibroid (see Chapter 4, Disorders of menstrual bleeding and Chapter 17, Gynaecological surgery and therapeutics).

Where a bulky fibroid uterus causes pressure symptoms or where HMB is refractory to medical interventions, the options are myomectomy to surgically remove fibroids with uterine conservation, or hysterectomy. Myomectomy will be the preferred option where preservation of fertility is required, and this procedure can be performed through a laparotomy incision or, increasingly, laparoscopically where 'power morcellation' of the removed fibroids is

▶ **eResource 12.2**

Surgical treatment of fibroids
http://www.routledgetextbooks.com/textbooks/tenteachers/gynaecologyv12.2.php

required to debulk the tumour to facilitate removal through a small 15 mm laparoscopic port site. An important point for the preoperative discussion during the consent process for myomectomy is that there is a small but significant risk of uncontrolled life-threatening bleeding during myomectomy, which could lead to hysterectomy.

Hysterectomy and myomectomy may be facilitated by GnRH agonist pretreatment over a 3-month period to reduce the bulk and vascularity of the fibroids. Useful benefits of this approach are to enable a suprapubic (low transverse) rather than a midline abdominal incision, or to facilitate vaginal rather than abdominal hysterectomy, both of which are conducive to more rapid recovery and fewer postoperative complications. GnRH agonist pretreatment can obscure tissue planes around the fibroid making surgery more difficult but, on the positive side, blood loss and the likely need for transfusion are reduced.

Radiological

Uterine artery embolization (UAE) is a technique performed by interventional radiologists. It involves embolization of both uterine arteries under radiological guidance. A small incision is made in the groin under local anaesthesia and a cannula placed into the femoral artery and guided into the uterine arteries. Embolization particles are then injected, reducing the blood supply to the uterus, which induces infarction and degeneration of fibroids such that the overall reduction in fibroid volume is around 50%. Following UAE, patients usually require admission overnight because of pain following arterial occlusion, requiring opiate analgesia. Complications include fever, infection, fibroid expulsion and potential ovarian failure.

Women wishing to retain their fertility should be counselled carefully before undergoing UAE as the effects on subsequent reproductive function are uncertain. Pregnancies have been reported in the literature, but concerns remain over premature ovarian failure and effects on the endometrium that may lead to abnormal placentation. The procedure is equivalent to myomectomy for alleviating fibroid-related HMB and pressure symptoms. However, one-third of women subsequently require further medical, radiological or surgical intervention within 5 years of UAE. Thus, when counselling women about treatment options for symptomatic fibroids it is important to balance the less invasive nature of UAE compared with surgical myomectomy against the much higher likelihood of needing further treatments.

Adenomyosis

The endometrium is usually well demarcated from the underlying myometrium. Adenomyosis is a disorder in which endometrial glands and stroma are found deep within the myometrium. Adenomyosis can only be definitively diagnosed following histopathological examination of a hysterectomy specimen, where it is identified in 40% of uteri from a general female population of reproductive age.

Relative advantages and disadvantages of treatments for symptomatic uterine fibroids

Medical

- Tranexamic acid /non-steroidal anti-inflammatory drugs [NSAIDs]/COCP/LNG-IUS (Mirena®): all are simple and fertility sparing (although COCP/LNG-IUS are contraceptive) and avoid more invasive interventions, but they are generally less effective in the presence of submucosal fibroids or a uterus >12 weeks size where an enlarged uterine cavity can be expected.
- COCP: contains oestrogen, which may increase the growth of oestrogen-dependent fibroids.
- LNG-IUS: increased likelihood of expulsion if cavity is enlarged or distorted by submucosal fibroids.
- GnRH-agonists: reduce fibroid volume prior to surgery but induce a temporary oestrogen deficient 'menopausal' state precluding long-term use.
- Ulipristal acetate (SPRM): oral medication and, as with GnRH-agonists, it reduces fibroid volume prior to surgery, but more data about safety with long-term use are needed.

Surgical

- Hysteroscopic myomectomy: minimally invasive, day-case procedure for submucous fibroids that avoids surgical incisions and is effective in resolving HMB and improving fertility. Will not treat other types of fibroid.
- Myomectomy: fertility sparing and will treat HMB and bulk symptoms. Usually requires a laparotomy, but a less invasive laparoscopic approach is possible with smaller and fewer fibroids. Associated with intraoperative bleeding from vascular fibroids, a 1% risk of unplanned hysterectomy and postoperative intra-abdominal adhesions.
- Hysterectomy: indicated for women with no future fertility desires. May be achieved vaginally, laparoscopically or via open surgery depending on the size of the uterus. Definitive, guaranteeing amenorrhoea but as invasive as myomectomy.

Radiological

- Uterine artery embolization: minimally invasive, avoids general anaesthesia and surgery. Although fertility sparing there are concerns over effect on subsequent reproductive function. Equivalent patient satisfaction compared with myomectomy but the need for further treatments much higher.
- Novel radiological treatments are currently being explored to destroy fibroids through thermal ablation. These include MRI-guided transcutaneous focussed ultrasound and transcervical intrauterine ultrasound-guided radiofrequency ablation. However, the effectiveness and safety of these interventions need further study before they can be considered for use in routine clinical practice.

This ectopic endometrium is responsive to cyclical hormonal changes that result in bleeding within the myometrium, leading to increasingly severe secondary dysmenorrhoea (pain throughout menses), uterine enlargement and HMB.

Women with adenomyosis are usually multiparous and diagnosed in their late 30s or early 40s. Examination may reveal a bulky and sometimes tender 'boggy' uterus, particularly if examined perimenstrually. Ultrasound examination of the uterus may be helpful for diagnosis when adenomyosis is particularly localized, showing haemorrhage-filled, distended endometrial glands. Sometimes this may give an irregular nodular

development within the uterus, very similar to that of uterine fibroids. MRI is the investigation of choice although expensive, as it provides excellent images of the myometrium, endometrium and areas of adenomyosis (**Figure 12.6**).

Given the practical difficulty in making the diagnosis of adenomyosis preoperatively, conservative surgery and medical treatments are so far poorly developed. In general, any treatment that induces amenorrhoea will be helpful as it will render the ectopic endometrium quiescent, relieving pain and excessive bleeding. Thus, the use of the progestin-containing long-acting reversible contraceptives (LARCs, see Chapter 6, Contraception and abortion) such as the LNG-IUS and depot Provero and short-term GnRH agonists should be considered. On ceasing treatment, however, the symptoms rapidly return in the majority of patients, and hysterectomy remains the only definitive treatment.

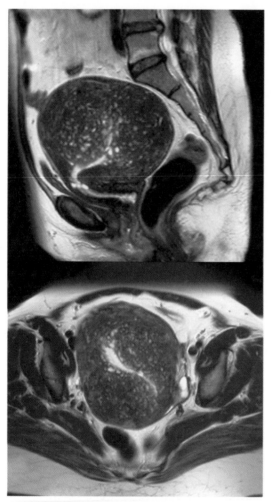

Figure 12.6 MRI showing adenomyosis – note the bright reflections of the central endometrium and flecks of ectopic endometrium in the underlying myometrium.

 KEY LEARNING POINTS

- A cervical ectropion is a normal finding in women of reproductive age and is usually due to hormonal influence – the three Ps: puberty, pill and pregnancy.
- Tests to evaluate the uterus include TVUSS, SIS, MRI, hysteroscopy and endometrial biopsy.
- Endometrial polyps are common, usually benign focal lesions arising from the endometrium. They can cause abnormal patterns of uterine bleeding including HMB, IMB and PMB.
- Surgical removal of endometrial polyps, known as polypectomy, is a simple procedure usually performed under direct vision with the aid of a hysteroscope as an outpatient or day-case.
- Fibroids (leiomyomas) are common, oestrogen-dependent, benign tumours of the myometrium and are estimated to be present in about 40% of women over 30 years of age. Fibroids undergo shrinkage after the menopause. Malignant change to leiomyosarcomas occurs in 1:350 fibroids and is usually associated with rapid fibroid growth and AUB in a postmenopausal women.
- Fibroids are classified according to their relationship to the uterine wall, being described as submucosal or intramural and subserosal. Fibroids can be detected on abdominal and/or bimanual pelvic examination as an enlarged pelvic mass of uterine origin.

- Fibroids can cause HMB and pressure 'bulk'-related abdominal symptoms and in some cases subfertility. However, the vast majority of fibroids are asymptomatic. Treatment is indicated for symptomatic fibroids. Surgical or radiological intervention is often required because medical treatments are generally less effective.

- Surgical removal of fibroids is termed myomectomy. Submucous fibroids protrude into the uterine cavity and so can be removed using hysteroscopic techniques. Intramural and subserosal fibroids are removed via a laparotomy incision or laparoscopically depending on their size, location and number.

- Adenomyosis is a disorder in which endometrial glands and stroma are found deep within the myometrium, which can cause dysmenorrhoea, HMB and uterine enlargement. The mechanism whereby fibroids affect fertility is unclear.

- Medical treatments such as the LNG-IUS (Mirena®) that can induce amenorrhoea will alleviate symptoms associated with adenomyosis. Hysterectomy remains the only definitive treatment.

Further reading

American Association of Gynecologic Laparoscopists (2012). AAGL practice report: practice guidelines for the diagnosis and management of endometrial polyps. *J Minim Invasive Gynecol* **19**:3–10.

Garcia L, Isaacson K (2011). Adenomyosis: review of the literature. *J Minim Invasive Gynecol* **18**:428–37.

Gupta JK, Sinha A, Lumsden MA, Hickey M (2014). Uterine artery embolization for symptomatic uterine fibroids. *Cochrane Database Syst Rev* **12**:CD005073.

Munro MG, Critchley HOD, Fraser IS (2012). The FIGO systems for nomenclature and classification of causes of abnormal uterine bleeding in the reproductive years: who needs them? *Am J Obstet Gynecol* **207**:259–65.

Owen C, Armstrong AY (2015). Clinical management of leiomyoma. *Obstet Gynecol Clin North Am* **42**:67–85.

Self assessment

CASE HISTORY

A 34-year-old woman presents with increasingly heavy menstrual periods and an abdominal mass. She is known to have uterine fibroids. She is due to get married next month and plans to start a family soon. Several hormonal and non-hormonal medical treatments prescribed by her GP have failed in the past 5 years.

A What questions would you ask in order to further explore the presenting complaint?

B What examination would you perform and what diagnostic tests would you perform or request?

C What medical treatments would you consider and explain why?

D What surgical or radiological treatments would you consider and explain why?

E Do you think she may be worried about anything in relation to her presenting complaint?

ANSWERS

A Assess the nature and severity of the menstrual bleeding (e.g. the chronicity of the symptoms, the duration, regularity and amount [e.g. 'flooding' through sanitary protection] of menstrual loss and the adverse impact on health-related quality of life [e.g. impact on work, social and emotional relationships, physical and sexual functioning]). Establish whether there is any IMB or PCB that may indicate cervical pathology.

Enquire about dysmenorrhoea and whether this is primary, spasmodic and short lived at the onset of menses or secondary lasting throughout the period, which may suggest other gynaecological pathology especially if there is associated chronic pelvic pain. Information relating to the pelvic mass should be obtained (e.g. when was it first noticed and how, is it enlarging and/or causing bulk, pressure symptoms and how were uterine fibroids diagnosed?). Fertility plans/desires should be established from the outset in addition to past 'failed' treatments as this information will influence suitable management options.

Gastrointestinal causes such as irritable bowel syndrome or constipation should be considered in light of her poor diet. A negative pregnancy test excludes an ectopic pregnancy. Genitourinary problems such as bladder pain syndrome, musculoskeletal causes, neuropathic pain and psychological contributors should be evaluated depending on the history and examination.

B A gynaecological examination should be undertaken to better characterize the nature and origin of the mass; the size, regularity, mobility and tenderness of the mass should be determined. Investigations to consider include a pelvic USS and possibly a MRI scan if the fibroids are large, rapidly enlarging or morphologically abnormal on ultrasound. An endometrial biopsy is generally unnecessary in women under 45 years of age unless they have risk factors for endometrial hyperplasia (e.g. erratic cycles, obesity, polycystic ovaries). An outpatient hysteroscopy may be indicated if submucosal fibroids are suspected or seen on radiological imaging.

C As she plans to start a family soon, contraceptive hormonal treatments should be avoided although may be used in the short term. Tranexamic acid and NSAIDs are good options although it is likely these have already been tried, given the long-standing history. HMB in the presence of substantial uterine fibroids are more resistant to medical treatments and so surgery should be considered.

D In this instance it should be fertility conserving so hysterectomy and endometrial ablation are contraindicated. Myomectomy can be performed but as there is a small risk of emergency hysterectomy because of severe intraoperative bleeding, this should probably be avoided unless she is unable to conceive within a year of trying. In contrast, hysteroscopic myomectomy is indicated if submucosal fibroids are detected as the operation is minimally invasive, can treat HMB and can optimize subsequent fertility. UAE is another option, although the impact on subsequent reproductive function remains unclear.

E She may be worried about the effect of fibroids on her fertility and subsequent pregnancy in view of her forthcoming marriage. She may also be worried about the possibility of cancerous change if she feels the uterine mass has increased in size.

EMQ

A Endometrial biopsy (EB).
B SIS.
C Outpatient hysteroscopy (OPH).
D TVUSS.
E TAUSS.
F MRI.
G Genital tract swabs.
H Laparoscopy.
I Computed tomography (CT) scan.
J Cervical smear.
K Colposcopy +/– cervical biopsy.
L Hysterosalpingogram (HSG).

For each description below, choose the SINGLE most appropriate answer from the above list of options. Each option may be used once, more than once or not at all.

1 An obese, diabetic 49-year-old woman presenting with erratic, heavy and prolonged menstrual bleeding.

2 A 32-year-old woman with IMB, subfertility and a suspected 2 cm endometrial polyp seen on pelvic USS.

3 A 22-year-old virgin with HMB and a pelvic mass palpated on abdominal examination.

4 An obese 44-year-old woman with regular, heavy and painful menstrual bleeding and some PCB. Examination of the genital tract appears normal and she has a normal and up-to-date cervical smear history.

5 A 32-year-old woman with a history of amenorrhoea and secondary subfertility since a postpartum dilatation and curettage (D&C) for RPOC 2 years ago.

6 A 44-year-old woman considering a UAE for a 34 weeks sized fibroid uterus.

ANSWERS

1A This woman is at high risk for endometrial carcinoma. As per HMB guidelines and in view of risk, EB is indicated. Other tests such as cervical smear, swabs and TVUSS may also be necessary later, depending on the history.

2C The IMB is likely to be due to the polyp, which may also be affecting implantation. OPH will afford direct vision and resection. SIS is not necessary as the polyp has been visualized already, HSG is also unnecessary at this point.

3E Visualization of the uterus is necessary but TVUSS is not suitable as she is a virgin, and anyway the mass is large. No further imaging such as CT or MRI is indicated yet, and would be unnecessarily expensive and invasive. Operative procedures are not indicated here, nor are smears, swabs or colposcopy.

4D Further examination of the cervix is unnecessary given her normal smear history. TVUSS is required to image the uterus and the cervical structure. Swabs may prove necessary later, depending on history. More expensive and invasive imaging such as MRI and CT are unnecessary.

5C The history indicates an endometrial cause for the amenorrhoea. Although a TVUSS may show scarring as a bright line in the endometrium and SIS may show an occluded endometrium, OPH will afford the opportunity to treat any scarring by resection. It is therefore the most efficient next step.

6F Prior to UAE a MRI is essential to identify the size and exact location of the fibroids, and to ensure that the UAE is possible. TVUSS will also show very good identification of the fibroids, but MRI is a better imaging modality to review specific fibroids at a later date.

SBA QUESTIONS

1 A parous 35-year-old woman complains of cyclical heavy and painful menstrual bleeding. On examination she is found to have an enlarged, 'boggy' uterus and a TVUSS suggests the possibility of adenomyosis. She has completed her family and currently relies on condoms for contraception. She smokes 10 cigarettes per day but is otherwise fit and well.

Which treatment would you consider most appropriate? Choose the single best answer.

A LNG-IUS (Mirena®).
B COCP.
C Hysterectomy
D GnRH analogues.
E Endometrial ablation.

ANSWER

A Although adenomyosis can only be definitively diagnosed following histological examination of the uterus after hysterectomy, the history, examination and scan findings are suggestive of this benign condition of the uterus. As she has completed her family a hysterectomy could be considered, but this should not be considered a first-line treatment given its greater potential morbidity. Any treatment that induces amenorrhoea will be helpful as it will render the ectopic endometrium quiescent, relieving symptoms of pain and excessive bleeding. Local progestogen treatment using the LNG-IUS can induce amenorrhoea and also provide more effective contraception so seems the best option. GnRH analogues are not a long-term treatment and endometrial ablation is primarily a treatment for HMB of endometrial origin in the absence of other pathology.

2 Submucous fibroids are not associated
with which of the following presentations?
Choose the single best answer.

A IMB.

B Subfertility.

C Pregnancy loss.

D HMB.

E Pressure and pain.

ANSWER

E Submucous fibroids are most commonly diagnosed when investigating abnormal uterine bleeding
or subfertility. Pressure and pain is not a feature of uterine fibroids confined to the uterine cavity
unless submucous fibroids coexist with other intramural and/or subserosal fibroids, leading to a
substantially enlarged uterus.

Benign conditions of the vulva and vagina, psychosexual disorders and female genital mutilation

LEILA CG FRODSHAM

LEARNING OBJECTIVES

- Describe the presentation and management of common benign conditions of the vulva and vagina.
- Describe the causes of superficial and deep dyspareunia.
- Understand the impact of vulval and vaginal conditions on sexual function.
- Understand the definition of psychosexual disorders.
- Describe the diagnosis, impact and management of psychosexual disorders.

Anatomy and histology

The vulva is the term used to describe the external female genitalia – the sexual organs. It includes the labia majora and minor, clitoris and fourchette. The vulval vestibule is defined anatomically as the area between the lower end of the vaginal canal at the hymenal ring and the labia minora. The different anatomical areas of the external genitalia have different histological characteristics and embryological origins. Both the labia minora and majora are covered with keratinized, pigmented, squamous epithelium. The labia majora are two large folds of adipose tissue covered by skin containing hair follicles and sebaceous and sweat glands. In contrast, the labia minora are devoid of adipose tissue and hair follicles, but contain sebaceous follicles. The normal vulval vestibule is covered with non-keratinized, non-pigmented squamous epithelium and is devoid of skin adnexa. Within the vulval vestibule are the ducts of the minor vestibular glands, the periurethral glands of Skene, the urethral meatus and the ducts of the Bartholin's glands. The Bartholin's glands (major vestibular glands) are the major glands of the vestibule and lie deep within the perineum. Both the major and the minor vestibular glands contain mucus-secreting acini with ducts lined by transitional epithelium. The ducts of the Bartholin's glands exit at the introitus just above the fourchette at approximately five and seven o'clock on the perineum, and those of the minor vestibular glands are distributed throughout the vulval vestibule. The vagina and vulva are commonly known as the lower genital tract with the vagina leading to the upper genital tract (uterus, cervix, tubes and ovaries).

The vagina has is a tubular structure but has anterior and posterior walls that lie in opposition.

Vulval skin has different physiological properties when compared to other regions of the body such as the forearm. Transepidermal water loss is twice the amount in vulval skin compared to forearm skin. This suggests that the stratum corneum, the protective layer of vulval skin, functions poorly as a skin barrier when compared to other skin areas and may explain why vulval skin is more prone to irritancy.

Vulval overview

Benign vulval conditions have a far ranging impact on women's health and lifestyles and yet there are a dearth of clinicians able to provide a holistic approach to care. Approximately 20% of women will have vulval symptoms such as itching, skin changes or pain at any time. Effective management of vulval diseases incorporates skills in dermatology, oncology, infectious diseases and psychosexual medicine. Current training in these areas for gynaecologists are scanty and so women are at best seen in vulval clinics with a multidisciplinary team (MDT) approach. At worst, they may be passed between primary, secondary and tertiary care feeling increasingly frustrated and disgruntled that no one seems to understand or be able to help them. In turn, this can make the speciality less appealing to clinicians. The recent survey, Tomorrow's Specialist, by the Royal College of Obstetricians and Gynaecologists (RCOG) suggests that women expect psychosexual, dermatological and surgical skills from their gynaecologist and, while this chapter does not aim to cover all these areas in detail, it is hoped to give an overview in the management of these cases in order

that a sole clinician can manage the majority of cases themselves. Of course, there will always be cases where tertiary care is required, but the bulk should remain in primary and secondary care.

Assessment

A full history and clinical examination (with optional vaginal swabs and biopsies) are essential to make the diagnosis. Vulval skin is an extension of general skin surfaces and it is important in the history to ask about general skin problems as this might point towards the diagnosis; for example, psoriasis or eczema can synchronously affect the vulva and the limbs. The history should focus on the presenting complaint. It is important to discuss current methods of skin care (e.g. use of scented products that can aggravate symptoms), which topical treatments are being used (e.g. some creams such as antifungals can aggravate the problem) and the impact of the symptoms on sexual functioning. The clinical examination should include all skin surfaces and the vulval area should be examined systematically with a good light source.

Vulval pruritus, pain and superficial dyspareunia are common symptoms and *Table 13.1* illustrates the differential diagnoses of different symptoms, although this is not an exhaustive list. Confusingly for the clinician, most patients have more than one symptom.

Vulval itching (pruritis) and discomfort

The most common presenting symptoms of benign vulval conditions are itching, discomfort, pain,

Table 13.1 Differential diagnosis of vulval complaints

Vulval pruritus	Vulval pain	Superficial dyspareunia
Infections (e.g. candidiasis, *Trichomonas vaginalis*)	Infections (e.g. candidiasis)	Skin conditions (e.g. lichen sclerosus [causes vulval splitting])
Skin conditions (e.g. lichen sclerosis, eczema, VIN)	Skin conditions (e.g. lichen sclerosis, eczema, VIN)	Vulvodynia
Contact dermatitis	Vulvodynia	Vulval fissures
	Bartholin gland infection	Skin bridges of the vulva

VIN, vulval intraepithelial neoplasia.

discharge and dyspareunia (painful sex). Women with vulval disease present at all ages but there is a preponderance of postmenopausal women with benign dermatological conditions. This group particularly lend themselves to a polypharmacy, as pathology may have multiple aetiologies (e.g. atrophic vaginitis and vulvitis or lichen sclerosus), and a more holistic approach. Women in this age group may be disinclined to seek advice early and sexual dysfunction is already more common in both women and their partners. Additionally, this patient group can feel very 'alone' with their disease and can really benefit from joining support groups that run regular educational workshops such as the Vulval Pain Society.

Older women can be particularly distressed by pruritis and can be mortified to find their partners woken by their nocturnal involuntary itching. As a result of nocturnal itching some women can present with dysuria as urine burns their excoriated vulval skin and the gross pathology can look alarming. It is also important to consider the effects of both urinary and faecal incontinence as this can damage the skin barrier function and form a vulval dermatitis in itself.

Reduction in allergens

The appearance of vulval dermatitis is often not specific and is strongly associated with a history of atopy and other dermatoses. It is therefore prudent to reduce allergens in all patients presenting with symptoms of vulval pruritis.

It is advisable to discourage women from washing with any soaps or detergents (including feminine washes), which disrupt the bacterial balance of the vagina and can cause a vulval dermatitis. Water is preferable but some women find olive (or other natural unperfumed) oils offer moisturization and a better clean. Women who wish to have a scented, moisturizing bath can use either similar oils with a few drops of tea tree oil.

Women should be encouraged to wear cotton underwear (with minimal dyes) and wash clothing with an unperfumed non-biological washing powder/fabric conditioner. It is also worth considering the effect of sanitary protection/pads for urinary incontinence. It is not uncommon to see women who have marked vulval dermatitis from popular sanitary brands (particularly the super-thin gel-filled variety of sanitary towel) and they may benefit from sourcing unbleached, organic protection, washable pads or the 'Moon Cup'.

Recurrent use of antifungals

Women will frequently both self-source and be prescribed multiple courses of antifungals such as clotrimazole cream and pessaries, often without examination. While this can soothe in the initial stages, it can precipitate a hypersensitivity reaction that increases symptoms, and yet women feel obliged to use what is offered as the 'doctor is the expert' and their symptoms, are so distressing.

The vulval and vaginal condition of candidal infection or 'thrush' is common and particularly affects women of reproductive age (or using hormone replacement therapy, HRT) where oestrogen levels are high (and there is an increased prevalence in pregnancy). It is uncommon in prepubescent girls and postmenopausal women and other causes for irritation should be sought rather than relying on readily available antifungals. Hypo-oestrogenic women, therefore, should be checked for other causes of itching and examined before prescription of antifungals. It is very important to consider diabetes as a cause of recurrent thrush. Once excluded, a genuine case of candidal infection should be treated with a course of 150 mg clotrimazole nightly over 3 consecutive nights. In menstruating women this is most useful postmenstrually when candida is more common due to alteration of the vaginal pH. Oral fluconazole is a second-line treatment after clotrimazole. A combination of reduction of allergens and the above is sufficient in most cases. It is unnecessary to treat partners unless they have symptoms themselves and there is no proven benefit in doing so. A referral to genitourinary medicine (sexual health) can be of great benefit in recurrent cases of treatment-resistant candida.

Low ferritin

About 5% of women with vulval pruritis may have low ferritin and correction of this will improve symptoms, so it should always be checked in the early stages.

Biopsy in vulval disease

Biopsy should only be performed in first-line treatment if there is a concern regarding malignancy.

If there is a diffuse leukoplakia or erythema, treatment with steroids and emollients is recommended and, if symptoms do not resolve, biopsy should be considered. The Keyes punch biopsy is a 4-mm sample of skin that can be taken under local anaesthetic in the clinic (**Figure 13.1**). A pathology sample allows an accurate diagnosis to be made and the correct treatment to be instigated. Biopsies should be carried out when there is a pigmented lesion, a raised or indurated area and a persistent ulcer.

Lichen planus

Lichen planus is an autoimmune disorder affecting 1–2% of the population (particularly in people over 40) and affects the skin, genitalia and oral and gastrointestinal mucosa. There is no known precipitating factor although pressure can increase symptoms (for example restrictive underwear), but symptoms are often pruritis and/or superficial dyspareunia. Lesions in the mouth may be reticular-like cobwebs, and oral inspection should be performed if the diagnosis is suspected. Lesions can occur on the shins and there can be characteristic appearances to the nail bed such as longitudinal ridging and sandpaper effect.

Genital lesions can be longitudinal, annular, ulcerative, hyperpigmented or bullous and may cause vaginal stenosis and resulting sexual dysfunction. Treatment is by high-dose topical steroids. Sexual dysfunction is common due to pain and stenosis. If there is a vaginal stenosis, it is preferable to try dilatation with manual (fingers or dilators) rather than surgical means in the first instance.

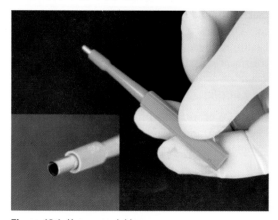

Figure 13.1 Keyes punch biopsy.

Lichen sclerosus

Lichen sclerosus is a destructive inflammatory skin condition that affects mainly the anogenital area of women. It is believed to affect 1 in 300 women and the cause is believed to be autoimmune. Many patients have other autoimmune conditions, such as thyroid disease and pernicious anaemia. The destructive nature of the condition is due to underlying inflammation in the subdermal layers of the skin, which results in hyalinization of the skin. This leads to a fragility and white 'parchment paper' appearance of the skin and loss of vulval anatomy. The condition can involve the foreskin of men to produce a phimosis. Lichen sclerosus is evident elsewhere on the body in 15% of patients. The main symptoms on the vulva are itching and subsequent soreness of the vulva, usually due to scratching. A biopsy can confirm the diagnosis and treatment is a combination of good skin care and strong steroid ointments such as those containing clobetasol. Lichen sclerosus is associated with vulval cancer, but is not a cause. Many women with vulval cancer have lichen sclerosis at the time of diagnosis and it is estimated that there is a low risk of cancer developing in a women with lichen sclerosus (around 3–5%).

Lichen sclerosus characteristically presents in a 'figure of 8' pattern around the vulva and anus. There is frequently hypopigmentation, loss of anatomy, vaginal stenosis and cracking (particularly in the posterior fourchette) but appearances can be subtle in early-stage disease (**Figure 13.2**). Treatment of both lichen planus and sclerosus is by high-dose topical steroids (clobetasol proprinate), applying a pea-sized amount daily for 1 month, alternate days for the second month and twice a week for the third month. If there is not complete resolution of symptoms, biopsy is indicated. Women should be advised to seek advice if the lesions become raised or resistant to treatment. Once the course of treatment is completed, the steroid cream can be used by women as and when required.

Vulval cysts

Bartholin's cysts, Skene gland cysts and mucous inclusion cysts can affect the vulval area and cause a lump with or without vulval discomfort. If they do not cause the patient any problem, they can be either

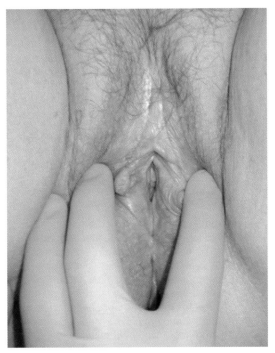

Figure 13.2 Lichen sclerosus.

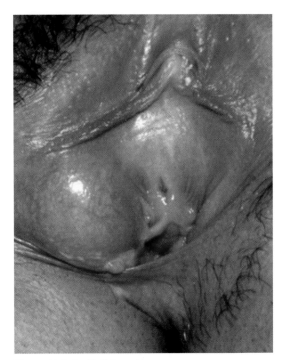

Figure 13.3 Bartholin's cyst.

monitored or excised. A Bartholin's cyst is the most common type of cyst and develops in the region of the Bartholin's gland (**Figure 13.3**). The Bartholin's gland has a long duct which, when blocked, causes fluid to build up and eventually forms a cyst. It is not uncommon for these cysts to get infected and cause a Bartholin's abscess that usually presents acutely and may require incision and drainage. Marsupialization of the cyst is the term used when the internal aspect of the cyst is sutured to the outside of the cyst to create a window so that the cyst does not reform. Marsupialization of Bartholin's cysts is usually an elective procedure under general or spinal anaesthesia. Outpatient drainage is also possible, sometimes followed by the insertion of a tiny catheter into the incision, which remains in place for several weeks to maintain its patency.

Vulvodynia

Vulvodynia is the condition of pain on the vulva most often described as a burning pain, occurring in the absence of skin disease or infection. It is akin to a neuropathic pain syndrome. The pain can be further classified by the anatomical site (e.g. generalized, localized or clitoral) and also by whether pain is provoked or unprovoked. Vulvodynia can occur at any age, and causes huge distress to sufferers. It is essential to exclude physical causes such as dermatitis. The Vulval Pain Society can be an invaluable source of information and support for sufferers. There is recent evidence that neuromodulators are of limited benefit in vulvodynia but some women find them useful (particularly if pain inhibits sleep, when a sedative neuromodulator such as amitrytiline can be used).

It is important to take a detailed history about the onset of symptoms and the timing and relation to the sexual history. Women with vulvodynia may have primary or secondary psychosexual dysfunction as described below. Some women can benefit from perineal massage, which may aid vulval desensitization, reduce muscular spasm and reassociate women with their own genitalia. Oils (such as coconut) may act as a barrier to precipitating factors (allergens, chafing from sports or clothing) and enable better lubrication for sexual function. While this can be initiated on guidance from a gynaecologist, the women's health physiotherapists are doing invaluable work and research in this area and there should be a low threshold for referral in this patient group.

Many women with vulvodynia will see multiple clinicians and have tried conventional and alternative therapies with no resolution of symptoms until they have worked on a combination of perineal massage and consideration of their feelings surrounding the diagnosis and their relationships. Women need support to regain their sex lives. Ideally this should be by someone who appreciates the physical and psychosexual aspects of their pain, not a 'specialist' but a health care professional with an empathetic ear who is able to work with the patient. A management of symptoms rather than complete resolution of pain is most realistic.

Patient insight

'For 8 years I have felt that I am not living my life but managing my pain on a daily basis. I have seen numerous specialists, used every possible cream and tablet and felt like a disappointment to doctors who want to help me to get better but can't. In recent months my pain patch has reduced, my sex life improved and I can see that one day, like a butterfly, it will just fly away'. Vulvodynia sufferer.

Dyspareunia

Dyspareunia is defined as pain during sexual intercourse. Dyspareunia may be associated with many gynaecological problems and is described as superficial or deep, the latter sometimes associated with pathology such as endometriosis or pelvic inflammatory disease (PID). On many occasions, despite appropriate investigations, no cause can be found and psychological support should be offered.

Dyspareunia

- Definition: pain during or after sexual intercourse, which can be classified as superficial affecting the vagina, clitoris or labia, or deep with pain experienced within the pelvis.
- Epidemiology: the estimated prevalence is between 10% and 20%, although this may be an underestimate as many women may

not present. Risk factors include female genital mutilation (FGM), suspected PID and endometriosis, peri/postmenopausal status, depression or anxiety states and history of sexual assault.

- Clinical evaluation:
  - the clinical history should explore the nature and onset of pain, the relationship to intercourse, associated chronic pelvic pain symptoms, reproductive and past medical history. A psychosexual history should be considered especially for superficial dyspareunia;
  - abdominal and pelvic examination should look for lower genital tract lesions (e.g. skin disorder, scarring, anatomical abnormality), vaginismus (involuntary contraction of vaginal muscles during vaginal examination), areas of tenderness within the lower and upper genital tract and evidence of pelvic disease (masses, tenderness, fixity of organs).
- Investigations:
  - superficial dyspareunia: consider a biopsy of lower genital tract lesions and swabs;
  - deep dyspareunia: consider transvaginal ultrasound scan (TVUSS), swabs and laparoscopy.
- Treatment:
  - superficial dyspareunia: treat any identifiable cause;
  - deep dyspareunia: treat as for chronic pelvic pain.

Psychosexual medicine

Psychosexual problems may be primary or secondary.

Psychosexual dysfunction

- Primary psychosexual dysfunction describes sexual difficulties where there may be psychosomatic pain.
- Secondary psychosexual dysfunction describes sexual difficulties resulting from pain or emotional issues.

How to approach consultations

Vulval disorders are invariably linked with female (and occasionally secondary male) sexual dysfunction. Whether primary or secondary, and regardless of the aetiology, it is important to explore this in the consultation.

The Institute of Psychosexual Medicine uses the LOFTI model to aid with consultation.

The LOFTI model

Listening

- Open questions and periods of silence allow the patient to divulge and elaborate on essential information.
- What is their tone/style of language?
- What is/is not said? How and when?

Observing

- Patterns of behaviour (e.g. frequent cancellations/avoidance of appointments).
- Urgency, demeanour, style of dress and mannerisms.
- Referral letters from the general practitioner (GP) may be detailed and pressurized, emphasizing the urgency of the referral (an example of transference, the unconscious redirection of feelings from the patient to the GP).

Feelings

- Be aware of feelings in the room.
- How does the patient make you feel?
- Feelings aroused in any doctor by the patient's language, behaviour and the attitude of the doctor to the patient are seen as possible evidence of the patient's own less than conscious feelings.

Thinking

- Note what sort of doctor you are being in the consultation – a parent? Teacher?
- Why is the patient presenting now? How did the patient come to have the consultation/what is their motivation?
- Note how you feel before and after the consultation.

Interpreting

- Assess the overall picture – is the patient displaying certain types of behaviour or attitude as a defence mechanism or a means of hiding anxiety or fear such as tears or anger?
- Defence mechanisms include regression, dissociation, introjection, sublimation or denial.
- What do you notice from genital examination? Is there avoidance (i.e. patients menstruating at every appointment or always having difficulties with smears)?

Vaginismus and non-consummation

Vaginismus cases are often some of the most challenging for both gynaecologists and psychosexual therapists. Vaginismus can lead to non-consummation and all gynaecologists should appreciate the huge impact of such sexual dysfunction on their patients' relationships and lives.

There is often a pressure of time (fertility or relationship issues), in addition to the patients concerns about a physical anomaly, that may lead the gynaecologist to a physical intervention such as a Fenton's procedure. While this may satisfy a short-term desire for a patient to widen what appears to be an impossibly small hole, it very rarely succeeds in providing an answer to non-consummation and the underlying vaginismus that will defeat the partner from penetration.

Patient insight

'Please will you just drive something through the blockage whilst I'm asleep so my husband can get in there?' Patient with non-consummation.

Traditionally, both doctors and sex therapists have used vaginal dilators to enable the woman to 'overcome her blockage' but they often become very adept at satisfying the doctor in going up the sizes but, anecdotally, rarely translate this into sexual activity. Although frequently prescribed, the use of dilators has no proven benefit and the evidence in favour of their use remains anecdotal, without evidence of efficacy if there is no physical pathology. More research is needed in this area.

Patient insight

'He gave me vaginal dilators, but when I used them it felt like an extension on the doctors fingers and got me no closer to having sex with my husband'. Vaginismus patient.

Practitioners undertaking psychosexual training will begin to recognize the transference of the partner's feelings onto themselves and a drive to open the vagina and achieve penetration that may exhibit itself subconsciously as a frustration and irritation with the patient. Additionally, they may feel inhibited from examining women with vaginismus and willingly accept the 'everlasting period' as a means of avoiding examination as a result of the patient's fear of the vagina and thus examination. In addition, this may further lead to a temptation to provide an examination under anaesthesia and manual dilation, which may positively reinforce the patient's perception of a physical issue that might eventually lead to further unnecessary surgery.

Women with vaginismus may make the most progress with a professional who is able to address the physical concerns by psychological 'flooding' (for example paying close attention to wording and action). Instead of responding to 'too small' by using the small speculum and thereby positively reinforcing the phantasy, examination might be performed with the patient involved, for example using a mirror, allowing them control during the examination and encouraging self-exploration at home with perineal massage and stretching of the vagina with their or their partner's fingers. The practitioner will always question the patient's reluctance to engage with their own genitalia because ultimately this might precipitate disclosure of a phantasy (physical fantasy). Genital examination may lead to the 'moment of truth' in consultation where the patient recognizes the influence of the mind over the body in their sexual problem. It is often tempting to reassure patients that their anatomy is normal, but more powerful to encourage them to see and feel that themselves.

Additionally, women with vaginismus are covertly in control of their sex lives (although this is largely subconscious in both partners). Empowering them to to recognize this and take overt control, by encouraging them to tell their partners that penetrative sex is 'off the menu' for a specified period of time, can be therapeutic. This is called modified sensate focus, and might help them to enable penetration when in combination with perineal massage and exploration of their subconscious defences (for example always wearing fleece pyjamas to bed, or avoiding the same bed time).

In summary, it is advisable to use the consultation to recognize and reflect the patient's anxieties and consider carefully whether surgery is the best option. The Institute of Psychosexual Medicine does not aim to turn doctors and allied health professionals into experts on sexual dysfunction, but to refine their skills to enable them to see that the patient is the expert, who has the answers but requires a 'professional mirror' to see them. All health professionals act as chameleons in consultation (for example, they adapt their tone of voice, body language or demeanour), but those trained in psychosexual medicine also recognize what is coming from the patient, and reflect it back.

Female genital mutilation

There are four degrees of FGM practiced in different geographical areas as shown in **Figures 13.4, 13.5**. Widely regarded in Western countries as a barbaric and unacceptable procedure, the prevalence remains extremely high with physical, psychological and social ramifications. The World Health Organization (WHO)'s position on FGM is shown below. FGM is frequently performed in girls from the age of 8 onwards without analgesia or adequate sterility.

FGM is defined as: 'Any procedure involving partial or total removal of the external genitalia and/or injury to the female genital organs whether for cultural, religious or other non-therapeutic reasons' (WHO 2006).

FGM is a practice that has far reaching implications to women's health in the acute and chronic timeframe. The implications are physical, psychological and psychosexual and may, in the worst case scenario, lead to renal failure from urinary obstruction and infection. There is now a legal obligation in the UK to document all cases in the medical notes and report all cases through the safeguarding team in NHS Trusts to reduce the incidence of this practice in young girls and women in the UK. In cases where FGM is suspected in minors, this is classified as child sexual abuse and social services and the police should be involved.

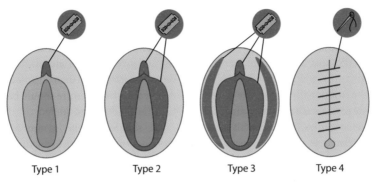

Type 1   Type 2   Type 3   Type 4

Figure 13.4 Types of female genital mutilation.

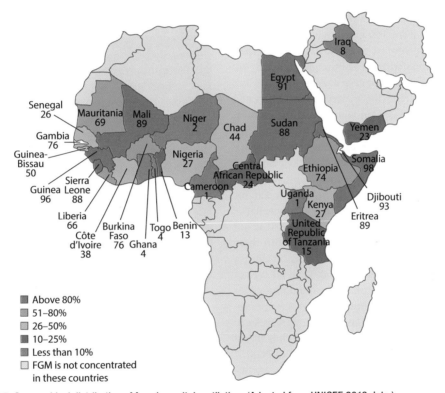

Figure 13.5 Geographical distribution of female genital mutilation. (Adapted from UNICEF 2013 data.)

The four main types of FGM are shown in **Figure 13.4**:

- Type 1 Clitoroidectomy: excision of prepuce (clitoral hood) with or without the removal of the clitoris.

- Type 2 Excision of clitoris and partial or total removal of the labia minora.

- Type 3 Excision of part or all of the external genitalia and stitching/narrowing of the vagina – infundibulation.

- Type 4 Piercing the clitoris, cauterization, cutting the vagina, inserting corrosive substances. This also includes any plastic surgery procedures done as an adult.

There is often an extremely fine line between cosmetic surgery on the vulva and FGM and the gynaecologist must seek advice before considering such procedures. Prevalence of requests for labioplasty procedures have risen dramatically in recent years (possibly as a result of accessibility of pornography and 'photoshopping' on the web) and many health care providers have withdrawn funding for such procedures on the NHS. This has, in turn, increased private practice in this area, which may offer less vigorous support for the emotionally vulnerable patient. Pre- and postsurgery patients are now attending NHS psychosexual medicine clinics for help with sexual dysfunction either related to body dysmorphia or side-effects of surgery. A useful tool for women to use is 'The Great Wall of Vagina', by Jamie McCartney, a British artist who has taken hundreds of plaster casts of vulvas. Women are often pleasantly surprised to see how 'normal' their vulva is after looking at this.

It is difficult for UK gynaecologists to appreciate the cultural context of FGM, particularly when working in areas where it is infrequently seen. The novel 'Possessing the Secret of Joy' by Alice Walker is an essential read for gynaecologists interested in the impact of FGM on women and the cultural influences behind the practice. The main character chooses FGM after puberty to feel more 'in tune with her culture' and eloquently describes the emotional and physical impact of her decision.

The obstetrician must be alert to form a plan for such patients in labour and delivery in hospital is advised with a clear plan of care detailed. It is not fully known whether labour is obstructed in these women from the evidence to date, but is certainly a possibility in Type 3 FGM. Depending on the type of FGM, it may be necessary to perform midline episiotomy for safe delivery. However, what is far preferable is to enquire early in the pregnancy and refer to a specialist centre for deinfundibulation. It is illegal to resuture (which many women request) an FGM.

Reversal of infundibulation (deinfundibulation)

Ideally women should be identified preconceptually and sent to a specialist centre but can be managed antenatally. It should be rare that women are managed on the labour ward, as all women felt to be at risk should be identified by their booking midwives and, if this is the case, a senior obstetrician should be present.

Deinfundibulation should be performed with adequate analgesia to avoid flashbacks to the FGM procedure (local anaesthetic can be used but may distort anatomy). The incision should be made along the vulval incision scar and the urethra identified before surgery commences to reduce damage. All women should have prior urinary infection screening and given appropriate antibiotic therapy, as bladder obstruction and urinary infection rates are high. A fine absorbable suture should be used and prophylactic antibiotics considered.

It should not be assumed that both sexual dysfunction and emotional distress is resolved by deinfundibulation and specialist centres will be able more adequately to access specialist services and support groups for affected women.

KEY LEARNING POINTS

- Women with vulval disease often present late with extensive and debilitating disease that affects their daily lives and intimate relationships.
- Vulval disease may cause pruritis and good skin care and steroid treatment may help.
- Biopsy may aid diagnosis and exclude malignancy.
- Dyspareunia is described as deep or superficial.
- Patients with psychosexual disorders are often frustrated and angry and so may feel 'difficult' to manage, but provide an opportunity to use the skills that all gynaecologists possess in a holistic manner to help them improve symptoms, live with their disease and achieve a satisfactory sexual life.
- FGM is frequently performed on girls worldwide, and it is essential to recognize and offer deinfundibulation.

Further reading

British Association for Sexual Health and HIV UK National Guideline on the Management of Vulval Conditions 2014.

McEwan I (2007). *On Chesil Beach*. Jonathan Cape.

Royal College of Gynaecologists and Obstetricians. Female Genital Mutilation and its Management (Green-top Guideline No. 53) 2015.

Skrine R, Montford H. *Psychosexual Medicine: An Introduction*, 2nd Edition. Hodder Arnold, 2001.

Walker A (1992). *Possessing the Secret of Joy*. Harcourt Brace Jovanovich.

Useful websites:
The Institute of Psychosexual Medicine
www.ipm.org.uk
College of Sexual and Relationship Therapies
www.cosrt.co.uk
www.csp.org.uk

Self assessment

CASE HISTORY

A 25-year-old woman has been seen by her community midwife and disclosed previous 'cutting'. The midwife has urgently referred her to your antenatal clinic. She is now 28 weeks pregnant.

What are the next steps that you should take?

ANSWERS

Initial examination is helpful to determine the degree of FGM (1–4) as this will affect the management initially and of labour. The safe guarding team must be aware, and it essential that documentation, dated and timed, is present in the notes. These are legal requirements. Ensure that a translator is available if necessary for all visits. Depending on the type of FGM, midline episiotomy in labour may be necessary. Early deinfundibulation is preferable. Suturing postdelivery should be performed by a senior obstetrician. In the UK it is illegal to perform restoration of the FGM, even on request.

SBA QUESTIONS

1 A 36-year-old obese woman presents with recurrent thrush, increased thirst and frequency of urination. What test is essential in this case? Choose the single best answer.

A   Serum ferritin.
B   High vaginal swab.
C   Vulval biopsy.
D   Fasting blood glucose.
E   Skin prick allergy testing.

ANSWER

D   There is a association of diabetes and recurrent candida, due to the increased serum glucose. This patient has symptoms of diabetes as well as risk factor.

2 A 30-year-old woman presents with her partner unable to consummate her marriage. She asks you to assist her in achieving penetrative penile sex.

What should be your first step? Choose the single best answer.

A   Prescribe dilators and advise her to watch the instruction film.
B   Book examination and dilation under general anaesthetic.
C   Book her for a Fenton's procedure under general anaesthetic.
D   Arrange Botox injections to the perineal musculature.
E   Perform examination and encourage flooding.

ANSWER

E   Invasive investigations or treatments are unhelpful and can be damaging. Vaginal dilators have been shown to have little benefit in this circumstance. Psychosexual management is much more effective for this couple.

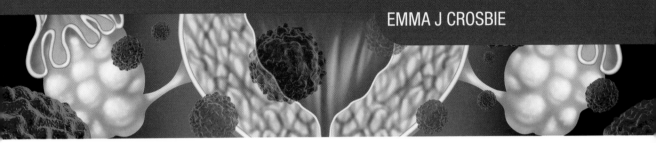

Malignant disease of the ovary

CHAPTER

14

EMMA J CROSBIE

LEARNING OBJECTIVES

- Learn how malignant disease of the ovary, Fallopian tube and peritoneum presents.
- Learn how ovarian cancer is investigated and staged.
- Learn how ovarian cancer is managed.

Introduction

Ovarian cancer is the second most common gynaecological malignancy and the major cause of death from gynaecological cancer in the UK. There are approximately 7,000 new cases and 4,000 deaths from ovarian cancer per year. When detected in its early stages, ovarian cancer has an excellent prognosis. The dismal overall survival rates from ovarian cancer reflect the advanced stage at which most women present. Screening has not been shown to be effective and there have been few advances in the development of targeted treatments for advanced disease.

Ovarian cancers

Incidence

The lifetime risk of developing ovarian cancer in the general population is 1.4% (1 in 70), and the mean age of presentation is 64 years. Ovarian cancer is more prevalent in higher income nations. There are variations in incidence with ethnicity; white women have the highest incidence at approximately 14 per 100,000, whereas Asian women have a lower incidence at 10 per 100,000. Ovarian cancer is rare in young women and only 3% of ovarian cancers occur in women under 35 years. It is now increasingly accepted that a large proportion of ovarian cancers may in fact originate in the Fallopian tube, rather than the ovarian surface epithelium as previously thought. There is a significant genetic aspect to ovarian cancer (see below). It is recognized that women with hereditary cancer present early, with a mean age at diagnosis of 54 years.

Classification of ovarian cancer

Primary ovarian cancers are epithelial (80%), sex cord stromal or germ cell. The ovary is also a common site for metastatic spread; Krukenberg tumours are

193

Table 14.1 Histological classification of malignant ovarian tumours

1 Epithelial ovarian tumours (80%)	High-grade serous Endometrioid Clear cell Mucinous Low-grade serous (Borderline)
2 Sex cord stromal tumours (10%)	Granulosa cell Sertoli–Leydig Gynandroblastoma
3 Germ cell tumours (10%)	Dysgerminoma Endodermal sinus (yolk sac) Teratoma Choriocarcinoma Mixed
4 Metastatic (including Krukenberg tumours)	

ovarian metastases associated with primary cancers of the colon, stomach and breast. *Table 14.1* shows a histological classification of ovarian tumours.

Epithelial tumours

Epithelial tumours of the ovary can be benign, malignant or borderline. Approximately 10% of epithelial tumours are classified as borderline ovarian tumours (BOTs). These tumours are well differentiated, with some features of malignancy (nuclear pleomorphism, cellular atypia) but do not invade the basement membrane. BOTs spread to other abdominopelvic structures (peritoneum, omentum) but do not often recur following initial surgery. The majority of BOTs are serous tumours. Mucinous BOTs may actually arise from appendiceal carcinomas of low malignant potential and can be associated with pseudomyxoma peritoneii.

High-grade serous carcinomas account for around 75% of all epithelial ovarian cancers; mucinous and endometrioid tumours are less common, accounting for 10%, followed by clear cell carcinomas. High-grade serous tumours are characterized histologically by concentric rings of calcification, known as 'psammoma bodies'. Mucinous carcinomas are generally large multiloculated tumours associated with pseudomyxoma peritoneii. Endometrioid carcinomas are similar in histological appearance to

endometrial cancer, are associated with endometriosis in approximately 10% of cases and also a synchronous separate endometrial cancer in 10–15%. They tend to be well differentiated and are associated with a better survival than high-grade serous carcinomas. Clear cell carcinomas can also arise from endometriosis and are characterized histologically by clear cells, much like renal cancer.

Aetiology and risk factors

Epithelial ovarian cancers include a heterogeneous group of tumours of different histological subtypes and aetiologies that affect the ovary, Fallopian tube and peritoneum.

High-grade pelvic serous carcinomas

Because most high-grade pelvic serous carcinomas present with advanced disease involving the ovary, Fallopian tube and peritoneal surfaces, it is often impossible to establish the anatomical site of origin. Assigning primary tumour site is of little clinical relevance anyway since the behaviour, prognosis and treatment of these tumours are identical. Thus the term high-grade pelvic serous carcinoma has been coined to incorporate all high-grade serous tumours arising from the ovary, Fallopian tube and/or peritoneum. Data from women with BRCA mutations who have undergone risk-reducing prophylactic bilateral salpingo-oophorectomy (BSO) suggest a Fallopian tubal precursor lesion for high-grade pelvic serous tumours. These precursors are called serous tubal intraepithelial carcinoma (STIC) lesions, and they are characterized by mutations in p53 in secretory cells of the distal Fallopian tube. As many as 30% of high-grade pelvic serous cancers have BRCA mutations, which has implications for the majority of women who present with apparently sporadic disease.

Endometrioid, mucinous, clear cell, borderline and low-grade serous ovarian carcinomas

Inclusion cysts of the ovarian surface epithelium and endometriosis give rise to neoplasms that are distinctly ovarian in origin, and can include mucinous, endometrioid, clear cell, borderline and low-grade serous carcinomas. Endometriosis-associated ovarian cancers are usually of endometrioid or clear cell histological subtype. The origin of these tumours

Table 14.2 Risk factors in ovarian cancer

Decreased risk of ovarian cancer	Increased risk of ovarian cancer
Multiparity	Nulliparity
Combined oral contraceptive pill (RR reduced by up to 50%)	Intrauterine device (RR 1.76)
Tubal ligation	Endometriosis
Salpingectomy	Cigarette smoking (mucinous tumours only)
Hysterectomy	Obesity

RR, relative risk.

involves driver mutations in *KRAS*, *PTEN*, *BRAF* and *ARID1A* rather than *TP53*. The clinical distinction between high-grade pelvic serous carcinomas and other histological subtypes is important because of differences in disease progression, response to chemotherapy and prognosis.

BRCA mutation carrier status is a risk factor for high-grade serous ovarian cancer. Most ovarian cancers, however, are sporadic and risk relates to reproductive factors that are associated with hormone treatment, contraceptive use, ovulation and pregnancy (*Table 14.2*). The 'incessant ovulation' theory holds that the repeated damage to the ovarian surface epithelium that occurs at ovulation increases the risk of mutations that drive ovarian carcinogenesis. Excess gonadotrophin secretion is also thought to drive tumorigenesis through oestrogen-stimulated epithelial proliferation and subsequent malignant transformation.

Genetic factors in ovarian cancer

It is estimated that at least 10–15% of women with epithelial ovarian cancer have a hereditary predisposition. Women with mutations in *BRCA1*, *BRCA2* and Lynch syndrome have an increased lifetime risk of epithelial ovarian cancer. The lifetime risk in the general population is one in 70 (1.4%). This rises to 1 in 20 (5%) if women have one family member affected by a defect in one of these genes and further increases to 40–50% if two first-degree relatives are affected. Hereditary cancers usually occur around 10 years before sporadic cancers and are associated with other cancers (particularly of the breast, colon and rectum).

The most common hereditary cancer is the breast ovarian cancer syndrome (BRCA), accounting for 90% of the hereditary cancers. This syndrome is due to a mutation of tumour suppressor genes *BRCA1* (80%) and *BRCA2* (15%). Lynch syndrome is hereditary non-polyposis colorectal cancer (HNPCC) and is associated with endometrial cancer and a 10% lifetime risk of ovarian cancer. Hereditary ovarian cancers tend to be adenocarcinomas, present in later stages with the exception of Lynch-associated tumours, and recent evidence supports improved survival, probably due to a better response to platinum chemotherapy.

Preventing ovarian cancer

Women who test positive for a BRCA mutation are offered risk-reducing prophylactic BSO when they have completed their families. This can usually be performed laparoscopically. Prophylactic surgery reduces the risk of ovarian cancer (by 90%) and premenopausal breast cancer (by 50%), although it does not eliminate the risk of primary peritoneal cancer. It is important to carry out risk-reducing surgery prior to the age-related surge in ovarian cancer observed in BRCA mutation carriers, which is younger in *BRCA1* (mid 30s) than *BRCA2* patients (early 40s). Another suggestion for risk reduction builds on the theory that BRCA-associated ovarian cancers actually originate in the Fallopian tube; hence performing bilateral salpingectomy with delayed oophorectomy in the 30s and early 40s may offset the morbidity associated with a surgical menopause in young women while reducing the risk of cancer. This strategy has yet to be subjected to rigorous testing and its efficacy is unknown. Recent data indicate that the opportunistic removal of the Fallopian tubes during hysterectomy for benign indications also reduces ovarian cancer risk in women at average lifetime risk of ovarian cancer. Other procedures associated with ovarian cancer risk reduction include tubal ligation (sterilization) and hysterectomy with ovarian conservation. Chemoprevention using the combined oral contraceptive pill (COCP) reduces ovarian cancer risk by up to 50% in both BRCA mutation carriers and women at average risk of ovarian cancer.

Screening

Screening using transvaginal ultrasound scan (TVUSS) and CA125 measurement has not been shown to improve survival in women with a familial predisposition to ovarian cancer. This is because the high-grade serous tumours that are associated with BRCA mutation carrier status develop rapidly and most are at an advanced stage before they can be picked up by screening. The role of screening for women of average lifetime risk of ovarian cancer remains unclear; further results from the population-based UKCTOCS randomized controlled trial are awaited, as the 2015 initial data were equivocal.

Clinical features

Most women with ovarian cancer have symptoms; however, these symptoms are non-specific and often vague. The difficulty with clinical diagnosis is the main reason that patients with ovarian cancer present with late stage disease (66% present with stage 3 disease or greater), and this has a dramatic effect on survival. The most common symptoms are:

- Increased abdominal girth/bloating.
- Persistent pelvic and abdominal pain.
- Difficulty eating and feeling full quickly.

Other symptoms such as change in bowel habit, urinary symptoms, back ache, irregular bleeding and fatigue occur frequently and any women with persistence of these symptoms should be assessed by their general practitioner (GP).

Pelvic and abdominal examination may reveal a fixed, hard mass arising from the pelvis. The differential diagnosis of a pelvic mass includes non-epithelial ovarian cancer, tubo-ovarian abscess, endometriomas or fibroids. In combination with the presence of ascites, a diagnosis of ovarian cancer is highly likely. Early-stage ovarian cancer is difficult to diagnose due to the position of the ovary, but an adnexal mass may be palpable in a slim woman. It should be noted that less than 20% of adnexal masses in premenopausal women are found to be malignant; in postmenopausal women this increases to around 50%. Chest examination is important to assess for pleural fluid and the neck and groin should be examined for enlarged nodes.

Diagnosis and investigations

If ovarian cancer is suspected, a TVUSS is the initial imaging modality of choice to check for pelvic pathology. A pelvic mass is characterized in

Table 14.3 Tumour markers used in ovarian cancer diagnosis and follow-up

Tumour Marker	Tumour type	Uses
CA 125	Epithelial ovarian cancer, (Serous) borderline ovarian tumours	Preoperative, follow-up
CA 19-9	Epithelial ovarian cancer, (Mucinous) borderline ovarian tumours	Preoperative, follow-up
Inhibin	Granulosa cell tumours	Follow-up
hCG	Dysgerminoma, Choriocarcinoma	Preoperative, follow-up
AFP	Endodermal yolk sac, Teratoma	Preoperative, follow-up

AFP, α-fetoprotein; hCG, human chorionic gonadotrophin.

terms of its size, consistency, the presence of solid elements, bilaterality, the presence of ascites and extraovarian disease, including peritoneal thickening and omental deposits. The investigation of any pelvic mass includes the measurement of tumour markers (*Table 14.3*). CA125 is a non-specific tumour marker that is elevated in over 80% of epithelial ovarian cancers. It is only raised in approximately 50% of early-stage epithelial ovarian cancers and is also commonly raised in benign conditions such as pregnancy, endometriosis and alcoholic liver disease. The Risk of Malignancy Index (RMI) is calculated from menopausal status, pelvic ultrasound features and CA125 level to triage pelvic masses into those at low, intermediate and high risk of malignancy.

Pelvic pathology at intermediate or high risk of malignancy is further imaged using computed tomography (CT) and/or magnetic resonance imaging (MRI) scans. The CT scan is particularly useful for assessment of extrapelvic disease and for staging. The MRI scan helps define tissue planes and operability. Other investigations required for preoperative work-up include chest X-ray, electrocardiography (ECG), full blood count, urea and electrolytes, and liver function tests.

If the patient presents with gross ascites or pleural effusion, paracentesis or pleural aspiration may be required for symptom relief and/or diagnosis. A sample of the fluid removed is sent for cytological assessment. If the diagnosis is uncertain or if primary chemotherapy is being considered (for advanced disease, or in patients not fit to undergo surgery), a biopsy is needed before treatment can be given. This is performed laparoscopically or radiologically (ultrasound or CT-guided biopsy). Usually the omentum is a good site for biopsy.

Staging

Ovarian cancer staging is based on clinicopathological assessment and, like other gynaecocolocial cancers, uses the FIGO staging system (*Table 14.4*). Overall, 25% of patients present with stage 1 disease, 10% stage 2, 50% stage 3 and 15% stage 4 disease. Metastatic spread is by direct spread to peritoneum and other organs and by lymphatic spread

Table 14.4 International Federation of Gynecology and Obstetrics (FIGO) staging of ovarian cancer

Stage	FIGO definition
1	Tumour confined to ovaries
1a	Limited to one ovary, no external tumour, capsule intact, no ascites
1b	Limited to both ovaries, no external tumour, capsule intact, no ascites
1c	Either 1a or 1b, but tumour on surface of ovary or with capsule ruptured or with ascites positive for tumour cells
2	Tumour confined to pelvis
2a	Extension and/or metastases to uterus or tubes
2b	Extension to other pelvic organs
2c	As 2a or 2b, but tumour on surface of ovary or with capsule ruptured or with ascites positive for tumour cells
3	Tumour confined to abdominal peritoneum or positive retroperitoneal or inguinal lymph nodes
3a	Tumour grossly limited to pelvis with negative nodes, but histologically confirmed microscopic peritoneal implants
3b	Abdominal implants <2 cm in diameter
3c	Abdominal implants >2 cm diameter or positive retroperitoneal or inguinal lymph nodes
4	Distant metastases. Must have positive cytology on pleural effusion, liver parenchyma

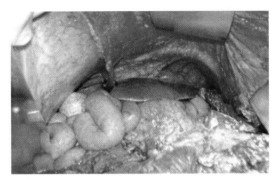

Figure 14.1 Advanced ovarian cancer illustrating diaphragmatic peritoneal disease.

to pelvic and para-aortic nodes. A high percentage of women with advanced disease have evidence of peritoneal disease on the diaphragmatic peritoneum (**Figure 14.1**). Women with early ovarian cancer (stages 1 and 2) have up to 20% metastatic spread to lymph nodes and this rises to 60% in advanced disease (stages 3 and 4).

Management

Surgery

Provided the patient is fit to undergo anaesthesia, surgery remains necessary for diagnosis, staging and treatment of epithelial ovarian cancer. If the patient is at high risk of ovarian cancer, the surgery should only be performed by a gynaecological oncologist, as this has been shown to improve outcomes. The objective of surgery is to stage accurately the disease and remove all visible tumour. This is vitally important in ovarian cancer as many studies indicate that the most important prognostic factor is no residual disease following laparotomy.

A vertical incision is required to gain access to all areas of the abdomen. Ascites or peritoneal washings are sampled and a total abdominal hysterectomy and BSO performed along with an omentectomy. Further debulking may be required, possibly including resection of bowel, peritoneal stripping or splenectomy in order to remove all tumour. Lymph node resection is important, particularly in early-stage disease where studies have found occult

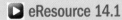 **eResource 14.1**

Surgery for epithelial ovarian cancer
http://www.routledgetextbooks.com/textbooks/tenteachers/gynaecologyv14.1.php

metastatic disease in nodes in up to 25% of patients with stage 1 tumours. Complete debulking to no visible disease varies from 40% to 80% of cases. Often in advanced epithelial ovarian cancer, there is diffuse spread of disease throughout the abdominal cavity making surgical clearance of tumour very difficult.

If a patient has been operated on outside a cancer centre and is found to have an ovarian cancer, restaging should be offered and this may be carried out laparoscopically. Occasionally, young patients who are found to have an early-stage epithelial ovarian cancer wish to have conservative, fertility-sparing surgery. In these cases, unilateral salpingo–oophorectomy, omentectomy, peritoneal biopsies and pelvic/para-aortic node dissection can be performed with endometrial sampling to exclude a synchronous tumour. Fertility-sparing surgery may also be performed in patients with borderline tumours if fertility is an issue, otherwise pelvic clearance should be performed. If a patient is unfit or unwilling to have surgery, or if preoperative assessment indicates that complete debulking is unlikely to be achievable, primary chemotherapy may be offered. If the patient responds to the chemotherapy, interval surgery can be carried out after three cycles. Recent studies indicate that this strategy may reduce postoperative morbidity but does not influence survival.

'Second-look' surgery is a planned laparotomy at the end of chemotherapy. The main function is to assess and resect any residual disease. Data on second-look surgery indicate no survival benefit and consequently it is not standard management outside clinical trials.

Following surgery, all patients with a diagnosis of epithelial ovarian cancer should be discussed at a gynaecological oncology multidisciplinary team (MDT) meeting where their history, surgical management and histology are reviewed by gynaecological oncologists, oncologists, radiologists, pathologists and nursing staff. If the cancer has been properly staged as stage 1a or b, and is histologically low grade (well or moderately differentiated), chemotherapy may be withheld. The role of chemotherapy in stage 1c disease is uncertain, but in practice most patients will be offered postoperative chemotherapy as with all other stages of epithelial ovarian cancer.

Surgical management of ovarian cancer

- Surgery combined with platinum-based chemotherapy is the mainstay of treatment for advanced ovarian cancer.
- The aim of surgery is complete or optimal cytoreduction (where <1 cm of residual macroscopic disease is left behind).
- Tumour deposits on the bowel, spleen, peritoneal surfaces and diaphragm are usually amenable to resection, while disease involving the porta hepatis and bowel mesentery are not.
- 'Supraradical ovarian cancer surgery' is appropriate in previously well, fit women with disseminated disease if complete cytoreduction is achievable; it is associated with perioperative morbidity and mortality and women must be carefully counselled.
- Three cycles of neoadjuvant chemotherapy followed by interval debulking surgery is not inferior to upfront surgery and has been shown to be associated with less morbidity.

Chemotherapy

Chemotherapy can be given as primary treatment, as an adjunct following surgery or for relapse of disease. It can be used to prolong clinical remission and survival or for palliation. First-line treatment is usually a combination of a platinum compound with paclitaxel. Most regimes are given on an outpatient basis, 3 weeks apart for six cycles.

Platinum compounds are the most effective chemotherapeutic agents in ovarian cancer. They are heavy metal agents that cause cross linkage of deoxyribonucleic acid (DNA) strands, thus arresting cell replication. Carboplatin is now the main platinum compound used as it is less renal toxic and causes less nausea than cisplatin, but is equally as effective. The dose of carboplatin is calculated according to the glomerular filtration rate (GFR) using the area under the curve (AUC).

Paclitaxol is derived from the bark of the Pacific yew and works by causing microtubular damage to the cell. This prevents replication and cell division. Pre-emptive steroids are given due to high-sensitivity reactions; side-effects of peripheral neuropathy, neutropenia and myalgia are common and dose dependent. Paclitaxol causes total loss of all body hair, irrespective of dose.

Bevacizumab, a monoclonal antibody against vascular endothelial growth factor (VEGF), inhibits angiogenesis. It has been shown to be clinically effective at improving recurrence free and overall survival when given in combination with carboplatin and paclitaxel in advanced ovarian cancer. The side-effect profile of this drug includes hypertension, delayed wound healing, gastrointestinal perforation and arterial thromboembolic events. This drug is not routinely prescribed as first-line treatment for advanced ovarian cancer on the NHS due to cost issues; however, it is available for the treatment of recurrent disease.

Following completion of chemotherapy, patients have a further CT scan to assess response to treatment. This scan can be used for comparison in the future if there is clinical or biochemical evidence of recurrence.

Follow-up of patients includes clinical examination and CA125 measurement. Studies have shown that levels of CA125 start to rise prior to onset of clinical evidence of disease recurrence; however, treating isolated rising CA125 levels does not improve survival. When disease recurs treatment is largely palliative. If the duration of remission is more than 6 months, carboplatin may be used again; otherwise taxol can be given or other chemotherapy agents, such as topotecan or liposomal doxyrubicin.

Prognosis

The survival figures depend on stage at presentation, volume of disease following surgery and the histological grade of tumour. The overall 5-year survival from ovarian cancer is 46% in the UK (2010–2011). The figures have improved due to the widespread introduction of centralized MDT care. Survival is stage dependent: overall 5-year survival for stage 1 disease is over 90% compared to 30% for stage 3 disease. Prognostic factors in ovarian cancer survival are listed in *Table 14.5*; *Table 14.6* shows the 5-year survival rates by stage at diagnosis.

Primary peritoneal carcinoma

Primary peritoneal carcinoma (PPC) is a high-grade pelvic serous carcinoma. It is histologically

Table 14.5 Prognostic factors in ovarian cancer

Stage of disease
Volume of residual disease post surgery
Histological type and grade of tumour
Age at presentation

Table 14.6 Ovarian cancer survival by stage at diagnosis

FIGO stage	5-year survival (%)
1	80–90%
2	65–70%
3	30–50%
4	15%

indistinct from tumours arising from the Fallopian tube or ovary. There are, however, morphological differences between the two groups based on clinical findings at laparotomy. Criteria for diagnosis includes:

- Normal sized or slightly bulky ovaries.
- More extraovarian disease than ovarian disease.
- Low volume peritoneal disease.

The clinical behaviour, prognosis and treatment is the same as for other high-grade pelvic serous carcinomas, although there is a trend towards using primary chemotherapy as complete surgical debulking is difficult.

Sex cord stromal tumours

These tumours account for approximately 10% per cent of ovarian tumours, but almost 90% cent of all functional (i.e. hormone-producing) tumours. Generally, they are tumours of low malignant potential with a good long-term prognosis. Some morbidity may arise from the oestrogen (granulosa, theca or Sertoli cell) or androgen production (Seroli–Leydig or steroid cell) characteristic of these tumours, resulting in precocious puberty, abnormal menstrual bleeding and an increased risk of endometrial cancer. The peak incidence is around the age of the menopause, although juvenile granulosa cell tumour usually presents in girls under 10 years of age, causing precocious puberty. Overall, granulosa cell tumours are the most common subtype, accounting for over 70% of sex cord stromal tumours.

Clinical features

A significant percentage of these tumours present with manifestations of their hormone production, typically irregular menstrual bleeding, postmenopausal bleeding or precocious puberty in young girls. Granulosa cell tumours may present as a large pelvic mass or with pain due to torsion/haemorrhage.

Sertoli–Leydig cell tumours produce androgens in over 50% of cases. Patients present with a pelvic mass and signs of virilization. Common symptoms are amenorrhoea, deep voice and hirsutism. Occasionally, this group of tumours produce oestrogen and rarely renin, causing hypertension.

Most sex cord stromal tumours present as unilateral ovarian masses, measuring up to 15 cm in diameter. Macroscopically, the tumour is often solid with areas of haemorrhage, and the cut surface may be yellow due to high levels of steroid production.

Granulosa cell tumours produce inhibin, which can be used for follow-up surveillance; levels often rise prior to clinical detection of recurrence.

Treatment

Treatment is based on the patient's age and wish to preserve fertility. If the patient is young, unilateral salpingo-oophorectomy, endometrial sampling and staging is sufficient. In the older group, full surgical staging is recommended. Granulosa cell tumours can recur many years after initial presentation and long-term follow-up is required. Recurrence is usually well defined and surgery is the mainstay of treatment as there is no effective chemotherapy regime.

Germ cell tumours

Malignant germ cell tumours occur mainly in young women and account for approximately 10% of ovarian tumours. They are derived from primordial germ cells within the ovary and because of this may contain any cell type. The emphasis of management is based mainly on fertility-preserving surgery and chemotherapy.

The most common presenting symptom is a pelvic mass; 10% present acutely with torsion or haemorrhage and due to the age incidence, some present during pregnancy. Seventy per cent of germ cell tumours are stage 1; spread is by lymphatics or blood borne.

Dysgerminomas account for 50% of all germ cell tumours. They are bilateral in 20% of cases and occasionally secrete human chorionic gonadotrophin (hCG).

Endodermal sinus yolk sac tumours are the second most common germ cell tumours, accounting for 15% of the total. They are rarely bilateral and secrete α-fetoprotein (AFP). They present with a large solid mass that often causes acute symptoms with torsion or rupture. Spread of endodermal sinus tumours is a late event and is usually to the lungs.

Immature teratomas account for 15–20% of malignant germ cell tumours and about 1% of all teratomas. They are classified as mature or immature depending on the grading of neural tissue present. About one-third of teratomas secrete AFP. Occasionally, there can be malignant transformation of a cell type within a mature teratoma. The most common cell type to transform is the epithelium, usually squamous cell carcinoma.

Non-gestational choriocarcinomas are very rare, usually presenting in young girls with irregular bleeding and very high levels of hCG.

Clinical features

Germ cell tumours should be suspected if a young woman presents with a large solid ovarian mass that is rapidly growing. Tumour markers as detailed in *Table 14.3* are measured preoperatively as this may influence the need for postoperative chemotherapy. MRI is helpful to assess morphology, particularly within teratomas. CT scaning of the abdomen allows assessment of the liver and lymph nodes. All patients should have a chest X-ray to exclude pulmonary metastases.

Treatment

Surgery is tailored to suit the patient. As most women presenting with malignant germ cell tumours are of reproductive age, fertility-sparing treatment may be preferred. An exploratory laparotomy is performed to remove the tumour and assess contralateral spread to the other ovary (20% in dysgerminoma). If there is a cyst present on the other ovary, this should be removed. Careful inspection of the abdominal cavity is required with peritoneal biopsies and sampling of any enlarged pelvic or para-aortic nodes performed. If metastatic disease is found, it should be debulked at surgery. Intraoperative frozen sections may be required to assess nodal status.

Postoperative chemotherapy depends on stage of disease. Stage 1 dysgerminomas and low-grade teratomas are treated by surgery alone and the 5-year survival is in excess of 90%. For the remainder of tumours and for patients with disease outside the ovary, chemotherapy is given. The most common regime used is a combination of bleomycin, etoposide and cisplatin (BEP), given as a course of three to four treatments, 3 weeks apart. This regime gives long-term cure rates of over 90% and also preserves fertility if required.

If the patient has recurrent disease, 90% will usually present in the first year following diagnosis; salvage chemotherapy has very good success rates.

KEY LEARNING POINTS

- Ovarian cancer tends to present late, with advanced disease because symptoms are non-specific.
- Screening has not proven effective using tumour markers or TVUSS.
- Treatment is based on removing all tumour surgically, combined with platinum-based chemotherapy.
- Prognosis is stage dependent: stage 1 disease has a 80–90% 5-year survival, whereas stage 3 disease has a 30% 5-year survival.
- Sex cord stromal tumours usually present with endocrine effects due to excess secretion of oestrogen or androgens.
- Germ cell tumours affect young women and are often cured by fertility-preserving surgery.

Further reading

Barakat RR, Bevers MW, Gershenson DM, Hoskins WJ (eds) (2002). *Handbook of Gynecologic Oncology*, 2nd edn. London: Dunitz.
Chitrathara K, Rajaram S, Maheswari A (eds) (2009). *Ovarian Cancer, Contemporary and Current Management*. Delhi: Jaypee.

Jacobs IJ, Menon U, Ryan A, *et al.* (2016). Ovarian cancer screening and mortality in the UK Collaborative Trial of Ovarian Cancer Screening (UKCTOCS): a randomised controlled trial. *Lancet* **387**(10022):945–56. Erratum *Lancet* 2016;**387**(10022):944.

Self assessment

CASE HISTORY

Mrs L is a 62-year-old woman who presents to the gynaecology clinic with non-specific abdominal pain, a change in bowel habit and bloating. Her GP arranged a pelvic ultrasound scan, which found bilateral complex solid/cystic pelvic masses, large volume ascites and omental caking.

A What is the most likely diagnosis?
B What are the key points in the examination and investigation?

Mrs L is found to have stage 3 high-grade serous ovarian cancer.

C How would you manage her?

ANSWERS

A The symptoms associated with ovarian cancer are non-specific and doctors must maintain a high index of suspicion when faced with persistent symptoms of bloating, irritable bowel and abdominal pain. The scan report shows features suggestive of advanced ovarian cancer (solid/cystic pelvic masses, ascites and extraovarian disease).

B Pelvic examination may reveal hard, fixed pelvic masses and free fluid in the abdomen (ascites) is demonstrated by shifting dullness and/or a fluid thrill. Investigations include serum CA125 levels. If the tumour secretes CA125, this can be used as a non-invasive test to monitor treatment response and subsequently screen for recurrent disease. A CT scan is needed to stage the disease and plan treatment. If there is a pleural effusion, this is generally tapped and a sample sent for cytological assessment. Sometimes there is very large volume ascites and draining this can improve symptoms in the short term as well as facilitating omental biopsy, which is more difficult when there is a lot of fluid around.

C Treatment for most women with advanced ovarian cancer is determined following discussion at the gynaecological oncology MDT meeting. If Mrs L is fit for surgery and preoperative investigations suggest that complete tumour debulking is achievable, upfront surgery followed by six cycles of adjuvant carboplatin and paclitaxel chemotherapy is generally preferred. Surgery involves a midline laparotomy, total hysterectomy (removal of uterus and cervix) and BOS (removal of both Fallopian tubes and ovaries), omentectomy, pelvic lymphadenectomy and debulking of any extraovarian tumour deposits. Sometimes surgery is avoided in the primary setting because the disease is not completely resectable, and in this scenario, three cycles of neoadjuvant chemotherapy are given and a restaging CT scan performed to decide whether surgery now is likely to remove all tumour deposits. If surgery takes place, the patient receives a further three cycles of chemotherapy afterwards.

EMQ

A High-grade pelvic serous carcinoma.
B Mucinous BOT.
C Endometrioid ovarian cancer.
D Immature teratoma.
E Dysgerminoma.
F Granulosa cell tumour.
G Choriocarcinoma of the ovary.
H Sertoli–Leydig ovarian tumour.
I Dermoid cyst.
J Krukenberg tumour.

For each description below, choose the SINGLE most appropriate answer from the above list of options. Each option may be used once, more than once or not at all.

1 Associated with STIC lesions in the Fallopian tube.
2 Commonly associated with BRCA mutation carrier status.
3 May present with amenorrhoea, deep voice, hirsutism and acne.
4 May provoke precocious puberty in young girls.
5 Associated with endometriosis.
6 Secretes inhibin.
7 Associated with appendiceal tumours and pseudomyxoma peritoneii.
8 May contain hair, teeth, bone, cartilage and sebum.
9 Metastatic ovarian tumour from colorectal or breast primary.

ANSWERS

1A The term high-grade pelvic serous carcinoma has been coined to incorporate all high-grade serous tumours arising from the ovary, Fallopian tube and/or peritoneum. There may be tubal precursors, which are called serous tubal intraepithelial carcinoma (STIC) lesions, and they are characterized by mutations in p53 in secretory cells of the distal Fallopian tube.

2A As many as 30% of high-grade pelvic serous cancers have BRCA mutations.

3H Sertoli—Leydig cell tumours produce androgens in over 50% of cases. Patients present with a pelvic mass and signs of virilization.

4F   Granulosa cell tumours frequently secrete oestrogen. Part of the work-up of girls presenting in this way would be to exclude oestrogen-secreting tumours. Granulosa cell tumours may also present as a large pelvic mass or with pain due to torsion/haemorrhage.

5C   Endometriosis-associated ovarian cancers are usually of endometrioid or clear cell histological subtype.

6F   Granulosa cell tumours produce inhibin, which can be used for follow-up surveillance; levels often rise prior to clinical detection of recurrence.

7B   Mucinous BOTs may actually arise from the appendiceal carcinomas of low malignant potential and can be associated with pseudomyxoma peritoneii.

8I   Dermoids are classically associated with tissue such as hair and teeth, and a TVUSS can be diagnostic. They are usually benign.

9J   The ovary is also a common site for metastatic spread; Krukenberg tumours are ovarian metastases associated with primary cancers of the colon, stomach and breast.

SBA QUESTIONS

1 A 34-year-old woman attends the gynaecology department because she has tested positive for a BRCA1 mutation. She wishes to lower her risk of ovarian cancer as much as possible. She is otherwise fit and well with no past medical history of note. Her cervical smears are up to date and normal.

What surgery would you recommend? Choose the single best answer.

A   Bilateral oophorectomy.

B   Bilateral salpingectomy with delayed oophorectomy.

C   BSO.

D   Subtotal hysterectomy and BSO.

E   Total hysterectomy and BSO.

ANSWER

C   Unless there are convincing reasons for hysterectomy as well, removing both Fallopian tubes and ovaries is the best way to reduce the risk of ovarian cancer (90%) and premenopausal breast cancer (50%). The downside is the surgical menopause that will ensue, but this can be effectively managed with continuous combined hormone replacement therapy (HRT). There is little evidence to suggest that this is harmful to cancer risk if there is no personal history of breast cancer (in which case, all forms of HRT are avoided).

2 A 58-year-old woman presents with a large pelviabdominal mass extending to the level of the xiphisternum. It has a heterogeneous appearance on scan with solid and cystic components. The rest of the pelvis and abdomen appears normal and there is no free fluid. The CA125 level is 430 units. She is asymptomatic.

How would you manage this patient? Choose the single best answer.

A   Laparoscopic ovarian cystectomy.

B   Laparotomy, total abdominal hysterectomy, BSO, pelvic and para-aortic lymph node sampling, omentectomy and debulking of tumour deposits.

C   Repeat scan and CA125 in 3 months to check for interval change.

D   Six cycles of neoadjuvant carboplatin and paclitaxel-based chemotherapy followed by restaging CT scan at 3 months.

E   Ultrasound-guided transcutaneous aspiration of ovarian cyst fluid and cytological assessment.

ANSWER

B   This patient has a high risk of malignancy index (RMI) and therefore should undergo a full staging laparotomy and complete debulking. If the ovarian mass is the only abnormal finding at laparotomy, intraoperative frozen sections can be used to direct further surgical effort, since pelvic and para-aortic lymphadenectomy is not required if the cyst is benign. Aspiration of the cyst is avoided when malignancy is suspected, to prevent 'seeding' malignant cells in the peritoneal cavity.

EMMA J CROSBIE

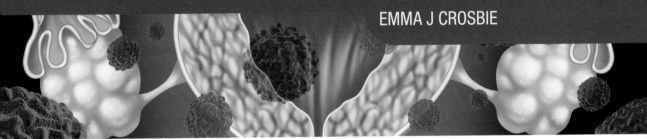

LEARNING OBJECTIVES

- Describe the classification of uterine malignancy.
- Learn how malignant disease of the uterus presents.
- Describe which investigations are needed for women with suspected endometrial cancer.

- Know the International Federation of Gynecology and Obstetrics (FIGO) staging of endometrial cancer.
- Understand how endometrial cancer is managed.

Introduction

Uterine cancer refers to tumours that arise from the uterine corpus (body of the uterus). By far the most common are endometrial tumours that originate from the lining of the uterine cavity (endometrium). Tumours arising from the myometrium (sarcomas) are rare.

Endometrial cancer

Incidence

Endometrial cancer is the most common gynaecological malignancy affecting UK women with an age-related incidence of 95 per 100,000 women. The life-time risk of developing endometrial cancer is approximately 1 in 46. The mean age of diagnosis is 62 years, although cancers can be diagnosed in women throughout their reproductive life.

Approximately 25% of endometrial cancers occur before the menopause.

The incidence of endometrial cancer has risen steadily over the past 20 years as a consequence of the ageing population, the trend away from hysterectomy for benign gynaecological disease and the obesity epidemic.

Classification

Endometrial cancer usually arises from the glandular component of the endometrium and stromal tumours are exceedingly rare. Endometrial cancers are classified as type 1 or type 2, depending on their histological subtype (**Figure 15.1**) and are graded 1–3, with 3 being high grade (mostly abnormal cells). Type 1 tumours are endometrioid adenocarcinomas that are oestrogen driven and arise from a background of endometrial hyperplasia. Type 2 tumours include high-grade serous and clear cell histological subtypes and arise from an atrophic endometrium.

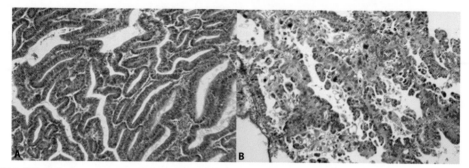

Figure 15.1 Histological comparison of endometrial adenocarcinoma (**A**) with endometrial serous carcinoma (**B**).

Aetiology

The risk factors for type 1 endometrial cancer are well established (*Table 15.1*). Most of these reflect an increased life-time exposure to oestrogen. Oestrogen causes endometrial cells to proliferate when it is unopposed by progesterone. Therefore, hyperoestrogenic states increase endometrial cancer risk, while cyclical or continuous progestin-containing hormone treatments reduce risk. Obese women are at risk of endometrial cancer because they are more likely to have anovulatory menstrual cycles and less likely to get pregnant. Furthermore, the aromatization of androgens to oestrogen by adipose tissue provides a continuous postmenopausal supply of oestrogen. Besides oestrogen, insulin and insulin-like growth factor stimulate endometrial proliferation, which is why endometrial cancer is more common in diabetic women. Other risk factors include treatment with tamoxifen, a selective oestrogen receptor modulator (SERM) used to prevent recurrent breast cancer, which is antioestrogenic in the breast but stimulatory in the endometrium. New generation SERMs, such as raloxifene, have a lesser effect on the endometrium. Hereditary predisposition to endometrial cancer is increasingly appreciated as genetic services and tests are being developed. The most common association is with Lynch syndrome, an autosomal dominant condition caused by mutations in one of the mismatch repair genes *MLH1*, *MSH2*, *MSH6* or, less commonly, *PMS2*. The life-time risk of endometrial cancer in women with Lynch syndrome is 40–60%. Other tumour associations include colorectal, ovarian and urothelial tumours, depending on the mutation responsible. The risk factors for type 2 endometrial cancer are less well understood.

Table 15.1 Risk and protective factors for type 1 endometrial cancer

Factors that increase endometrial cancer risk	Factors that protect against endometrial cancer
Obesity	Hysterectomy
Diabetes	Combined oral contraceptive pill
Nulliparity	Progestin-based contraceptives, including injectables
Late menopause >52 years	Intrauterine device, including Cu-IUD and LNG-IUS
Unopposed oestrogen therapy	Pregnancy
Tamoxifen therapy	Smoking
Family history of colorectal and endometrial cancer	

Prevention

Hormonal contraceptives and intrauterine devices reduce the risk of endometrial cancer (*Table 15.1*). Women with Lynch syndrome are offered prophylactic hysterectomy following completion of childbearing.

Screening

There is currently no evidence to support screening for endometrial cancer in high-risk groups or the general population.

Clinical features

Endometrial cancer usually presents at an early stage following the onset of postmenopausal bleeding (PMB) (see also Chapter 4, Disorders of menstrual bleeding). Approximately 5–10% of women with PMB have an underlying gynaecological malignancy and this 'red flag' symptom should always be investigated. Abnormal bleeding is the most common presenting complaint in premenopausal women too, who variously complain of heavy, irregular or intermenstrual bleeding (IMB). Women at more advanced stages of disease present with abdominal pain, urinary dysfunction, bowel disturbances or respiratory symptoms.

Sometimes endometrial cancer is picked up incidentally on a cervical smear, which shows 'abnormal glandular cytology'. Signs of endometrial cancer include bleeding from the cervical os on speculum examination and a bulky uterus on bimanual pelvic examination. In most women with endometrial cancer, however, pelvic examination is completely normal.

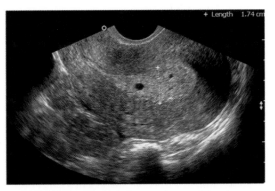

Figure 15.2 Transvaginal ultrasound scan of the uterus showing thickened endometrium.

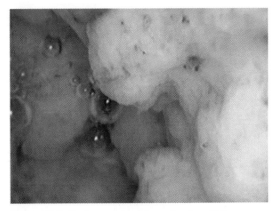

Figure 15.3 Hysteroscopic picture of endometrial carcinoma.

Postmenopausal bleeding

- PMB is a 'red flag' symptom for gynaecological cancer and should always be taken seriously.
- Careful inspection of the external genitalia followed by speculum examination will exclude vulval, vaginal and cervical cancer as the underlying cause.
- Physical examination may be normal in women with endometrial cancer, which can only be excluded by transvaginal ultrasound scan (TVUSS), hysteroscopy and/or endometrial biopsy.
- Benign causes of PMB include unscheduled bleeding on hormone replacement therapy (HRT) and vaginal atrophy.

Diagnosis and investigation of PMB

Many hospitals have a one-stop clinic dedicated to the urgent investigation of women with PMB. The mainstays of diagnosis are TVUSS, hysteroscopy and endometrial biopsy.

TVUSS allows a quick and accurate assessment of endometrial thickness (**Figure 15.2**). If the endometrium measures less than 4 mm, cancer is very unlikely and further investigation is not needed.

Any measurement greater than this requires further evaluation by hysteroscopy and/or biopsy.

Hysteroscopy is performed in the outpatient setting under local anaesthetic where possible. A general anaesthetic is required in patients with cervical stenosis or where hysteroscopy is poorly tolerated. A thin camera is passed into the uterine cavity, allowing visualization of the endometrium and directed biopsy of any abnormal areas (**Figure 15.3**). In addition, an endometrial sampler is used for histological assessment of the endometrium as described in Chapter 2, Gynaecological history, examination and investigations.

The histology report describes the type (endometrioid or other histological subtype) and grade of tumour. Complex hyperplasia with atypia is a premalignant condition that frequently coexists with low-grade endometrioid tumours of the endometrium. The risk of progression to endometrial cancer is 25–50%.

Staging

The extent of disease (stage) is determined by magnetic resonance imaging (MRI) scan (**Figure 15.4**) and FIGO staging uses this information (*Table 15.2*). Patients with high-grade tumours undergo a computed tomography (CT) scan of the chest, abdomen and pelvis to exclude distant metastases. In the UK, women with early stage (stage IA or IB) endometrioid tumours are offered surgery at their local hospital. Women with high-grade or high-stage (stage II or above) tumours undergo surgery in a cancer centre, as this has been shown to improve outcomes.

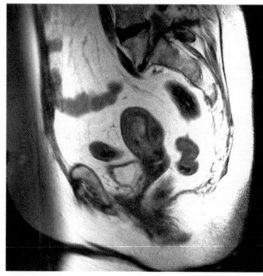

Figure 15.4 Magnetic resonance imaging of stage 1B endometrial carcinoma.

Table 15.2 International Federation of Gynecology and Obstetrics (FIGO) staging of carcinoma of the uterus

I	Confined to uterine body
IA	Less than 50% invasion
IB	More than 50% invasion
II	Tumour invading cervix
III	Local and or regional spread of tumour
IIIA	Invades serosa of uterus
IIIB	Invades vagina and/or parametrium
IIIC	Metastases to pelvic and/or para-aortic nodes
IV	Tumour invades bladder ± bowel ± distant metastases

Pathological terminology in endometrial cancer

Type

- Endometrial tumours are classified histologically as type 1 endometrioid adenocarcinomas (comprising 75–80% of all tumours) or type 2, including high-grade serous and clear cell tumours.
- Type 2 are more aggressive and carry a worse prognosis.

Grade

- Histological analysis differentiates between low-grade and high-grade (grade 3) tumours, of which the higher grade is more aggressive.

Stage

- FIGO staging describes the size and spread of the tumour and is used with the above to give prognostic information to patients.

Management

Surgery

Surgery is the mainstay of treatment for endometrial cancer. The extent of surgery depends on several factors including grade and stage of disease, and the patient's comorbidities.

Standard surgery is total hysterectomy and removal of both Fallopian tubes and ovaries (bilateral salpingo-oophorectomy, BSO). This can be performed abdominally or laparoscopically (total, vaginally assisted or robotically). If the MRI suggests cervical involvement, a modified radical hysterectomy is performed, which also removes a cuff of vagina, paracervical and parametrial tissue to ensure adequate excision margins (**Figure 15.5**). If the tumour is high grade (grade 3) or of type 2 histology, many centres perform pelvic and para-aortic node dissection because nodal disease (to either pelvis or para-aortic lymph node chains) is seen in one-third of patients. The role of nodal dissection remains contentious; a large scale UK study (ASTEC) failed to show a survival benefit in endometrial cancer patients who

 eResource 15.1

Surgical treatment of endometrial cancer
http://www.routledgetextbooks.com/textbooks/tenteachers/gynaecologyv15.1.php

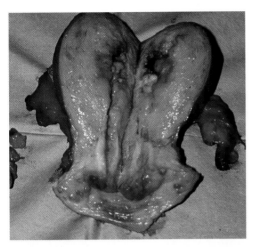

Figure 15.5 Radical hysterectomy showing cervical invasion of endometrial cancer.

had pelvic node dissection. Critics of the study argue that it was underpowered to show survival benefit in those at highest risk of nodal disease.

Adjuvant treatment

Postoperative radiotherapy reduces local recurrence rate but does not improve survival. Different units treat following surgery or only treat if the cancer recurs. Strategies include local radiotherapy to the vaginal vault over a short period of time (brachytherapy) for local disease, or brachytherapy combined with external beam radiotherapy for locally advanced disease (stage III). Chemotherapy is given for advanced or metastatic disease, although there is currently little evidence to support its use.

Hormone treatment

Some women are not fit for surgery and others wish to avoid it for fertility-sparing reasons. Treatment with high-dose oral or intrauterine progestins is successful for some women with complex atypical hyperplasia and low-grade stage IA endometrial tumours, but relapse rates are high.

Endometrial cancer and fertility

- Primary infertility due to polycystic ovary syndrome (PCOS) is a risk factor for premenopausal endometrial cancer.
- Women diagnosed with endometrial cancer during investigation for primary infertility face two devastating diagnoses at once.

- Alternatives to hysterectomy for premenopausal women are only possible for precancer or early-stage low-grade endometrial cancers.
- Hormone therapy (oral progestagens or LNG-IUS) is associated with moderate response and high relapse rates.
- Women faced with losing their fertility should be referred to a specialist to discuss ovarian conservation and/or stimulation for egg retrieval and surrogacy.

Prognosis

The overall 5-year survival rate for endometrial cancer is 80%, although this varies depending on tumour type, stage and grade of tumour (*Table 15.3*). In stage I disease, overall 5-year survival ranges from 93% for patients with low-grade IA disease to 66% in patients with high-grade IB disease.

Adverse prognostic features include advanced age, grade 3 tumours, type 2 histology, deep myometrial invasion, lymphovascular space invasion, nodal involvement and distant metastases.

Table 15.3 Five-year survival for women with endometrial cancer

Stage	5-year survival (%)
I	88
II	75
III	55
IV	16

Sarcomas of the uterus

These are rare tumours accounting for approximately 5% of all uterine cancers. They are classified into pure sarcomas, mixed epithelial sarcomas and heterologous sarcomas. The most common types are leiomyosarcomas and carcinosarcomas.

Pure sarcomas

This group includes endometrial stromal sarcomas and leiomyosarcoma. Endometrial stromal sarcomas occur in perimenopausal women presenting with irregular bleeding and a soft, enlarged uterus. The majority are low grade and surgery is the main treatment.

Leiomyosarcomas are rare tumours of the myometrium. Rarely (0.75%), they are associated with malignant transformation of benign fibroids and present with a rapidly growing pelvic mass and pain. Preoperative diagnosis is difficult, but may be aided by MRI, which can delineate areas of necrosis within the fibroid, suggestive of malignant change. The uterus is enlarged and soft on palpation. Surgery is the main treatment and adjuvant treatment may be considered if the mitotic count is high (above 10 mitoses per high powered field). Metastatic spread is usually vascular to distant sites, such as lung and brain.

Mixed epithelial sarcomas (carcinosarcoma)

This group of tumours, formerly known as malignant mixed Müllerian tumours, contain both carcinomatous and sarcomatous elements. The carcinomatous component is usually glandular and the sarcomatous component is homologous (endometrial, stromal and/or smooth muscle) or heterologous (tissues not normally found in the uterus, including bone, cartilage and skeletal muscle). The majority present after the menopause and sometimes there is a history of previous pelvic irradiation. There is usually a history of PMB and a fleshy mass is often seen protruding from the cervix along with an enlarged soft uterus. Treatment is surgery followed by postoperative radiotherapy. The 5-year survival is 73% if confined to the uterus, but only 25% if the tumour has spread outside the uterus.

Heterologous sarcomas

This rare group of tumours consists of sarcomatous tissue not usually found in the uterus, such as striated muscle, bone or cartilage. The most common is rhabdomyosarcoma, which may present in children as a grape-like mass protruding from the cervix with a watery discharge. Histology reveals primitive rhabdomyoblasts. Recurrence rates are high with distant metastases.

KEY LEARNING POINTS

- Endometrial cancer is the most common gynaecological malignancy.
- The majority of cancers present with stage I disease and the overall 5-year survival is 80%.
- Type 2 and high-grade tumours have the worst prognosis.
- Obesity and other hyperoestrogenic states play a major aetiological role.
- The majority of patients present with PMB; however, 25% of cases occur in premenopausal women.
- 5–10% of women with PMB will have an underlying gynaecological malignancy.
- Endometrial biopsy ± hysteroscopy is the gold standard for diagnosis, while MRI defines the extent of disease.
- Total hysterectomy and BSO is the treatment of choice for most patients.

Further reading

MacKintosh ML, Crosbie EJ (2013). Obesity-driven endometrial cancer: is weight loss the answer? *BJOG* **120**:791–4.

Morice P, Leary A, Creutzberg C, Abu-Rustum N, Darai E (2015). Endometrial cancer. *Lancet* **387**:1094–108.

Self assessment

CASE HISTORY

Mrs P is a 65-year-old woman who presents to the gynaecology clinic with PMB. She is obese and suffers from type 2 diabetes. She has no children, has never taken HRT and does not smoke. Her cervical smears have always been normal.

A What is the most likely diagnosis?

B What are the key points in the examination and investigation?

Mrs P is found to have a grade 1 stage 1A endometrioid adenocarcinoma.

C How would you manage her?

ANSWERS

A   PMB is a red flag symptom for gynaecological cancer. Cancers of the endometrium, cervix, vagina and vulva all present with abnormal bleeding. Mrs P's medical history and risk factor profile make endometrial cancer the most likely diagnosis.

B   Mrs P has several risk factors for endometrial cancer, including obesity, type 2 diabetes and nulliparity. A normal, up-to-date cervical smear history makes cancer of the cervix extremely unlikely. Cancers of the vulva, vagina and cervix should be excluded by careful inspection. Blood coming from the cervical os indicates uterine bleeding. Bimanual pelvic examination may find a bulky uterus or pelvic mass, although a normal examination does not exclude endometrial cancer.

C   Treatment for most women with endometrial cancer involves total hysterectomy (removal of uterus and cervix) and BSO (removal of both Fallopian tubes and ovaries). It is important to assess fitness for anaesthetic as many women with endometrial cancer have comorbidities, including obesity, type 2 diabetes, hypertension, cardiovascular disease, sleep apnoea and poor mobility, that limit their ability to tolerate general anaesthesia. Laparoscopic surgery is now standard of care for women with endometrial cancer but this may be difficult to achieve in women with morbid obesity who cannot tolerate the prolonged head-down tilt required or where previous abdominal surgery has resulted in adhesions and scarring. All women with endometrial cancer should be discussed at the central gynaecological oncology multidisciplinary team (MDT) meeting. Women with low-grade early-stage disease may undergo surgery in their local hospital while high-risk cases are referred centrally for care. All women are offered support from gynaecological oncology clinical nurse specialists or Macmillan nurses, who provide a single point of contact for continuity of care as well as written information, contact phone numbers and emotional support.

EMQ

A   Simple hyperplasia of the endometrium.
B   Complex hyperplasia of the endometrium with atypia.
C   Endometrioid adenocarcinoma of the endometrium.
D   Serous uterine carcinoma.
E   Clear cell carcinoma of the uterus.
F   Carcinosarcoma of the uterus.
G   Leiomyosarcoma of the uterus.
H   Endometrial stromal sarcoma.
I   Rhabdomyosarcoma.

For each description below, choose the SINGLE most appropriate answer from the above list of options. Each option may be used once, more than once or not at all.

1   Most common uterine malignancy.
2   Rare tumour of myometrium.
3   Rare uterine tumour derived from skeletal muscle.
4   Precursor lesion of endometrioid adenocarcinoma of the endometrium.

ANSWERS

1C 75–80% of endometrial tumours are type 1, which are endometrioid adenocarcinomas. The rest are type 2, including high-grade serous and clear cell histological subtype.

2G Leiomyosarcomas are rare tumours of the myometrium. Carcinosarcomas contain both carcinomatous and sarcomatous elements.

3I This rare tumour may be diagnosed in children; it is a heterologous sarcoma as it contains sarcomatous tissue not usually located in the uterus.

4B The type 1 endometroid adenocarcinomas are hormone dependent and develop from hyperplasia of the endometrium. In contrast, type 2 tumours may develop from an atrophic endometrium.

SBA QUESTIONS

1 A 54-year-old woman attends the gynaecology department with PMB. A TVUSS measures her endometrial thickness as 8 mm. An endometrial biopsy shows moderately differentiated adenocarcinoma cells.

What is the most appropriate staging investigation? Choose the single best answer.

A   Chest X-ray.

B   CT scan of her thorax, abdomen and pelvis.

C   Hysteroscopy.

D   MRI scan of her pelvis.

E   Transabdominal ultrasound scan.

ANSWER

D   MRI is used to determine the extent of the tumour for staging. It is possible to tell how far through the myometrium the tumour has spread, so surgery can then be planned. No other imaging modality will give this information accurately. An ultrasound scan is too subjective and a CT scan does not have ideal enhancement of tissue types.

2 A fit 72-year-old woman has an MRI after an endometrial biopsy shows endometrioid adenocarcinoma of the endometrium. Staging from the MRI is stage II. What management is indicated? Choose the single best answer.

A   Carboplatin-based chemotherapy.

B   Total abdominal hysterectomy with bilateral salpingo-oophrectomy.

C   External beam radiation therapy to the pelvis.

D   Modified radical hysterectomy.

E   Brachytherapy.

ANSWER

D   If the MRI suggests cervical involvement, a modified radical hysterectomy is performed, which also removes a cuff of vagina, paracervical and parametrial tissue to ensure adequate excision margins. Simple hysterectomy would have a high relapse rate. Chemotherapy or brachytherapy is not indicated. However, in very elderly unfit for surgery women, these options could be explored. External beam radiotherapy would also not be a first-line treatment and there is no evidence that it would prevent progression of the tumour.

Premalignant and malignant disease of the lower genital tract

EMMA J CROSBIE

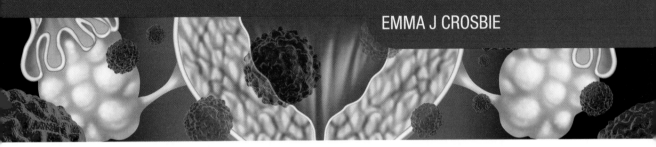

LEARNING OBJECTIVES

- Understand the pathogenesis of lower genital tract malignancy.
- Understand primary prevention of cervical cancer through human papillomavirus (HPV) vaccination and cervical screening.
- Understand the diagnosis, International Federation of Gynecology and Obstetrics (FIGO) staging and management of premalignant and malignant disease of the lower genital tract, including cervix, vagina and vulva.

Introduction

Cancer of the cervix in higher income countries is relatively uncommon due to screening. Cancers of the vagina and vulva are far less common than cervical cancer in both higher and lower income countries. This chapter covers premalignant and malignant disease of the lower genital tract.

Premalignant disease of the cervix

Introduction

Cervical screening has been shown to reduce both the incidence and the number of deaths from cervical cancer in higher income countries. It has been estimated that cervical screening prevents around 5,000 deaths every year in the UK alone.

Epidemiology and aetiology

Cervical cancer is caused by persistent high-risk HPV infection. HPV is a small, double-stranded deoxyribonucleic acid (DNA) virus of which there are more than 100 different types. These are classified as low-risk or high-risk types, depending on their ability to cause cancer. Low-risk types HPV 6 and 11 cause benign warts, while high-risk types HPV 16, 18, 31, 33 and 45 cause cervical cancer. HPV infection is spread during sexual intercourse. Infection is very common following the onset of sexual activity and up to 80% of adults show serological evidence of previous infection. Infection is usually transient and of no clinical consequence, but a minority of individuals develop a persistent genital infection that predisposes them to premalignant and malignant change (see below under Natural history of CIN). Smoking reduces the efficiency with which the virus is cleared by the immune system and increases the risk of persistent infection. Women who are immunocompromised, for example those with human immunodeficiency virus (HIV) and transplant recipients on long-term immunosuppressive therapy, are particularly at risk of premalignant and malignant disease of the cervix.

Pathophysiology

The tubular cervix is composed of stromal tissue covered by by squamous epithelium in the vagina (ectocervix) and columnar epithelium within the cervical canal (endocervix). The endocervix contains many deep folds, called crypts, that are lined by columnar epithelium. The meeting of the two types of epithelium is called the squamocolumnar junction (SCJ) and this is usually on the ectocervix (**Figure 16.1**). The position of the SCJ varies throughout life. In children it lies at the external cervical os, at puberty it extends outwards onto the ectocervix as the cervix enlarges, and in adult life it returns to the external cervical os through the process of metaplasia, which is the physiological transformation of columnar epithelium to squamous epithelium. The so-called 'transformation zone' (TZ) is defined as the area between the original SCJ and the current SCJ where the epithelium changes from columnar to squamous epithelium over time. Sometimes the columnar epithelium is covered by squamous epithelium, leading to retention of mucus – this is called a nabothian follicle (**Figure 16.2**). The TZ is the site where premalignancy and malignancy develop.

When HPV infection persists in certain individuals, it triggers an oncogenic process in the region of the TZ where metaplasia occurs. Integration of HPV DNA into the basal epithelial cells leads to immortalization and rapid cellular turnover. This disordered immaturity within the epithelium is called 'cervical intraepithelial neoplasia' (CIN) and is truly an intraepithelial condition (cancer is diagnosed when this process breaks the basement membrane). Immature cells are hyperchromatic with large nuclei, minimal cytoplasm and abnormal mitotic figures. CIN is classified as either low-grade (CIN 1) or high-grade disease (CIN 2 and 3), depending on whether the abnormal cells are seen in the bottom third or top two-thirds of the cervical epithelium, respectively.

Natural history of CIN

Regression and progression of CIN may occur. Spontaneous regression of low-grade disease is not uncommon and is likely to occur through the patient's own cell-mediated immunity. This is the argument for observational follow-up in patients with low-grade abnormality. High-grade disease is less likely to regress spontaneously and requires treatment, as there is a risk of progression to cancer. If left untreated, around 20% of patients with high-grade abnormalities develop cancer of the cervix. Reasons for this remain unclear but may include high-risk HPV types, reduced host immunity and smoking. There is a convincing link between CIN and cancer of the cervix, as

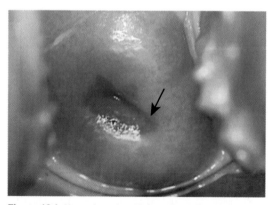

Figure 16.1 Normal cervix with transformation zone.

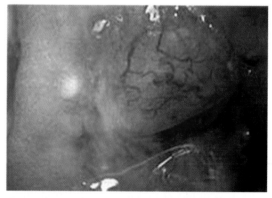

Figure 16.2 Normal cervix with nabothian follicle.

nearly all microscopic cancers of the cervix coexist with CIN.

Diagnosis and investigations

Cervical cytology

Cells exfoliated from the cervix can be examined under the microscope and this acts as a good screening test. Originally the 'Pap smear' was introduced by Papanicolou, where cells were removed from the cervix using a wooden spatula and placed on a glass slide and fixed. The Pap smear has now been superseded by liquid-based cytology (LBC), whereby a small brush is used to sample cells from the TZ and the brush head placed in fixative. This is then spun down and the cellular aspect of the specimen examined under the microscope. For more than 95% of women, cervical cytology is normal and normal squamous cells are seen (**Figure 16.3**). Abnormal cervical cytology shows squamous cells at different stages of maturity (dyskaryosis). Like CIN, cervical cytology is classified as low grade (minor cytological abnormalities showing mild dyskaryosis or borderline change) or high grade (moderate and severe dyskaryosis) (**Figure 16.4**). There is some correlation between the grade of cytological abnormality and the extent of CIN found on the cervix, but this is not totally reliable. Cervical cytology triages patients to the colposcopy clinic for further assessment (see below under Colposcopy). The sensitivity of a single cervical smear for high-grade CIN detection is between 40% and 70%; however, as there is slow progression for most women with CIN to cancer, if a lesion is missed then this should be picked up on a subsequent test. Women who attend regularly for cervical cytology have a very low risk of developing cervical cancer.

The role of HPV testing in cervical screening

High-risk HPV testing improves the sensitivity of cervical screening. Its value lies in its extremely high negative predictive power, which means that if a woman tests high-risk HPV negative, her risk of developing cervical cancer over the next 5–10 years is exceptionally low. The majority of women (around 95%) have normal cervical cytology and are placed on routine recall. Women with high-grade cytology (2%) are referred urgently for colposcopic assessment. Women with minor cytological abnormalities undergo reflex testing with high-risk HPV. HPV-negative women are returned to routine recall, while high-risk HPV-positive women are referred for colposcopy. Many countries, including the UK, are now moving towards primary HPV screening; that is, testing all cervical cytology specimens for high-risk HPV first, and carrying out reflex cytological assessment on those that test positive. This will reduce the costs of the screening programme, since HPV testing is automated and achieves a high throughput, while cytological assessment is manual and requires a skilled workforce.

The National Cervical Screening Programme

Since 1988, the UK has offered population-based cervical screening. Women aged 25–64 are invited every 3–5 years to take part in the screening programme. Invitations for cervical screening and the handling of results are coordinated by the National Health Service Cervical Screening Programme (NHSCCP). The coverage in the UK is around

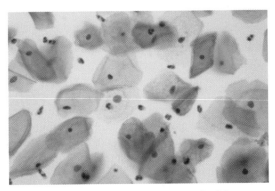

Figure 16.3 Liquid-based cytology – normal cytology.

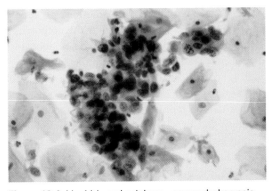

Figure 16.4 Liquid-based cytology – severe dyskaryosis.

70–85% of the population. There has been a recent trend for a fall in uptake of cervical screening in the 25–34 age group, which is worrying. Reasons for this remain unclear, but may include ignorance and a lack of education about the importance of screening.

Global view

The main burden of cervical cancer is in low income countries, where it is a common killer of women during their reproductive years. This 'hidden' cancer can take away young mothers who are head of their family unit, causing considerable emotional and economic upset. In higher income countries, cervical cancer is an uncommon malignancy due to screening, education and access to good medical care.

Colposcopy

Colposcopy is the examination of the magnified cervix using a light source (**Figure 16.5**). It is used for both diagnosis and treatment. The woman undresses and places her legs in the semi-lithotomy position. A speculum is placed in the vagina and the cervix examined with a light source, under magnification (5–20-fold). The application of acetic acid and iodine solutions highlights abnormal areas of the cervix that can be biopsied. Acetic acid causes nucleoproteins within cells to coagulate temporarily; therefore, areas of increased cell turnover, including CIN, appear white (**Figure 16.6**). Areas of CIN lack intracytoplasmic glycogen and fail to stain brown when iodine is applied. CIN is a preneoplastic process and the process of angiogenesis (new blood vessel formation) is apparent in CIN when viewed through the colposcope (**Figure 16.7**). If CIN is present, the colposcopist determines whether the appearances are low or high grade. The latter can be treated in the clinic on the same visit (known as 'see and treat'); the former can be monitored with a subsequent colposcopy and cytology 6 months later. A biopsy usually helps make the decision if unsure ('select and treat'). All doctors and nurses carrying out colposcopy are required to undergo a period of

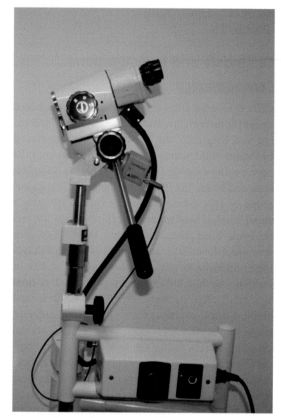

Figure 16.5 Colposcope.

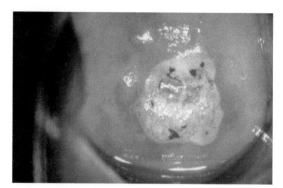

Figure 16.6 Cervix with acetic acid.

training and examination to ensure high quality and standards of care are met. In addition, each colposcopy service undergoes a rigorous external quality assurance assessment every 5 years to ensure high standards.

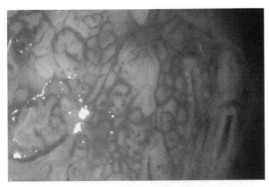

Figure 16.7 Cervix with cervical intraepithelial neoplasia and new vessels.

Treatment of premalignant disease of the cervix

The aims of treatment are to effectively eradicate CIN, ensuring that post-treatment cytology is negative, while minimizing harm to the patient from the treatment. High-grade CIN requires treatment, usually with excision or ablation. Low-grade CIN regresses spontaneously in up to 60% of cases; therefore, close follow-up with colposcopy and cytology 6 months after initial diagnosis is favoured as this avoids overtreating lesions that might have regressed. In the UK, the favoured method of treatment for higher-grade CIN is loop diathermy (large loop excision of transformation zone, LLETZ). Under local anaesthetic, a diathermy wire loop is used to remove a portion of the cervix that includes the TZ with the area of CIN (**Figure 16.8**). CIN can develop within the crypts of the epithelium and therefore excisional techniques need to be at least 7 mm deep. The procedure takes 15 minutes under local anaesthetic. The advantages of this excisional technique are that it is clinically effective (95% of patients have negative cytology at 6 months), cost-efficient (patients can be treated at the first hospital visit) and it provides a specimen for pathological assessment (1% of loop biopsies have an unsuspected microscopic cancer). The disadvantage relates to its potential impact on obstetric outcome. Small excisional treatments are unlikely to have obstetric consequences; however, if a large excision or repeat excisions remove a substantial proportion of the cervix, there is an increased risk of midtrimester miscarriage and preterm delivery in subsequent pregnancies. This concern relates to young women who have not completed their family.

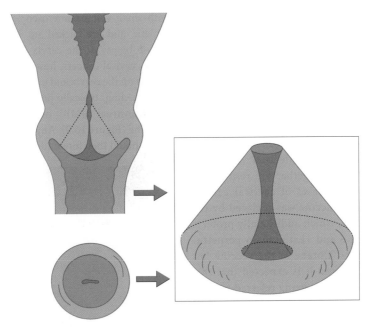

Figure 16.8 Large loop excision of transformation zone.

Recognizing the potential for overtreatment has been the main reason why women under 25 are not screened, as many lesions in this group of women are associated with HPV infection and simply regress with observational follow-up.

Other options have been suggested for the treatment of CIN including cold coagulation and cone biopsy. The term 'cold coagulation' is a misnomer as the treatment involves placing a hot probe on the cervix in outpatients under local anaesthetic. It is a destructive treatment, is effective for both high- and low-grade CIN but does not provide a specimen. Cone biopsy involves cutting away a portion of the cervix under general anaesthetic and produces a specimen, like a LLETZ. Its disadvantage relates to the need for a general anaesthetic and 5% of patients may develop cervical stenosis or incompetence, which has obstetric implications. It has been largely superseded by loop diathermy.

Patients who have received treatment for CIN undergo a 'test of cure' 6 months later. This includes a high-risk HPV test and cytological assessment. If negative, the woman is returned to routine recall; that is, cervical screening in 3 years time. If positive, repeat colposcopy is indicated to identify any residual, untreated CIN. A woman with a history of CIN has an increased life-time risk of recurrent CIN and cervical cancer.

HPV vaccination

HPV vaccines have been shown to be safe and effective at preventing persistent high-risk HPV infection CIN. School-based immunization in the UK is aimed at 12–13-year-old girls so it will take many years to know if HPV vaccination can reduce deaths from cervical cancer. The bivalent vaccine prevents persistent infection with HPV types 16 and 18, which together are responsible for more than 70% of cases of cervical cancer. In 2011, the bivalent vaccine was replaced by the quadrivalent vaccine, which additionally protects against HPV types 6 and 11, the main perpetrators of genital warts. Uptake of the vaccine has been good (75–85%) and it is expected that this will result in fewer women being referred for colposcopy when they reach screening age. Current vaccination strategies are unlikely to result in the eradication of cervical cancer because other high-risk HPV types are not included and uptake is not universal. Future strategies will increase efficacy by vaccinating adolescent boys and the development of new polyvalent vaccines that provide protection against more high-risk HPV types.

KEY LEARNING POINTS

- Cervical cancer is now considered a preventable disease in countries where resources permit.
- Prophylactic HPV vaccination can prevent infection with high-risk HPV types that cause cancers of the cervix and other lower genital tract sites.
- Regular screening by cervical cytology allows premalignant disease to be detected and treated before it undergoes malignant transformation.
- Women who are treated for high-grade CIN are at increased risk of cervical cancer in their lifetime compared to other women, but regular cervical screening will pick up residual or recurrent disease that can be treated.

Malignant disease of the cervix

Clinical presentation

The clinical presentation is variable. Many patients with small volume microscopic disease are asymptomatic and are picked up incidentally following a loop biopsy of the cervix for preinvasive disease. Most cervical cancers, however, are friable, vascular masses on the cervix and patients present with abnormal bleeding, typically postcoital (PCB), prolonged, intermenstrual (IMB) or postmenopausal (PMB) bleeding (**Figure 16.9**). Any woman with these symptoms should therefore undergo a pelvic examination,

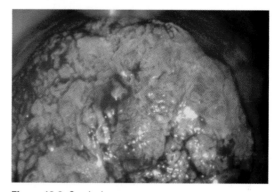

Figure 16.9 Cervical cancer.

including visualization of the cervix. In advanced disease (stages III–IV), patients may experience a number of distressing symptoms including pain (malignant infiltration of the spinal cord), incontinence (due to vesicovaginal fistulae), anaemia (from chronic vaginal bleeding) and renal failure (from ureteric blockage).

A pelvic and speculum examination usually clinches the diagnosis as there is often a cervical mass that bleeds on contact and if advanced disease, a hardness and fixity of the tissues. A biopsy should be taken in the outpatient setting. Very occasionally, the diagnosis can be missed as some tumours are endophytic rather than exophytic and therefore less clinically revealing. The clinician therefore needs to retain a level of clinical suspicion in the presence of unexplained symptoms and investigate patients with persistent problems.

Pathophysiology

The majority (70%) of cervical cancers are squamous cell carcinomas, with adenocarcinomas making up most of the remainder. In higher income countries with screening programmes, there has been a relative fall in the numbers of squamous tumours and a relative rise in the incidence of adenocarcinomas. In the UK, 30% of tumours are adenocarcinomas and are less likely to be picked up on cervical screening. Precursors of adenocarcinoma, known as cervical glandular intraepithelial neoplasia (CGIN), can also be detected at colposcopy, although lesions reside within the endocervical canal and may be difficult to visualize. Often CGIN is found incidentally in loop excision biopsies carried out for high-grade CIN; it is not uncommon for the two precursors to coexist. Cervical tumours are locally infiltrative in the pelvic area, but also spread via lymphatics and, in the late stages, via blood vessels. The tumour can grow through the cervix to reach the parametria (anatomical area lateral to the cervix), bladder, vagina and rectum. Metastases can occur, therefore, in pelvic (iliac and obturator) and para-aortic nodes and, in the later stages, liver and lungs.

Investigation and the importance of staging

Assessing the stage of the disease is crucial for planning treatment. The stage of disease also correlates with prognosis. Staging for cervical cancer is given in *Table 16.1*. Patients are staged according to the FIGO system. A biopsy is crucial to confirm malignancy and assess the tumour type. Magnetic resonance imaging (MRI) of the abdomen and pelvis will assess the local spread of the disease in the cervix and will detect enlarged lymph nodes in the pelvic area. A chest X-ray is vital to exclude lung metastases. An examination under anaesthetic may be helpful when, despite the above tests, the clinician is still unclear whether the tumour is operable. Doing a rectovaginal examination under anaesthetic can give crucial information on the tumour including size of disease, fixity and vaginal involvement, and a cystoscopy can help eliminate bladder involvement. Small mobile tumours favour a surgical approach, whereas larger fixed tumours favour the use of radiotherapy. The FIGO staging includes an intravenous urogram to ensure the integrity of the ureters; however, this is not standard practice in higher income countries, where MRI has superseded such tests. The staging of the disease is based on clinical findings, unlike other gynaecological tumours where there is a reliance on surgery and pathology to give the ultimate stage. The reasons for this are that radiotherapy is used in advanced disease and it still remains possible to stage patients in low income countries where most of the disease occurs.

Treatment

Treatment for cervical cancer depends on the stage of the disease, the requirement for future fertility and the patient's performance status. Ideally, all cancer patients should be discussed within the context of a multidisciplinary team (MDT) of doctors (surgeons, radiotherapists, radiologists and pathologists) and nurses, so that the most appropriate treatment can be offered to the patient. The fitness of the patient is crucial before embarking on treatment as radical surgery may not be appropriate in an unfit patient.

Preclinical lesions: stage IA

These microscopic tumours have a low volume of cancer and are usually picked up as incidental findings after loop excision for precancerous disease. Small lesions must be removed with a clear margin of excision, and the preinvasive disease (CIN) that invariably coexists should also be completely excised

Table 16.1 Staging and prognosis of cervical cancer

Stage	Extent of disease	5-year survival rate (%)
I	Tumour confined to the cervix	83
	IA: Microscopic disease. Maximum horizontal dimension is 7 mm and depth of invasion is 5 mm	
	IA1: Maximum horizontal dimension is 7 mm and depth of invasion is 3 mm	
	IA2: Maximum horizontal dimension is 7 mm and depth of invasion between 3 and 5 mm	
	IB: Clinical lesions confined to the cervix or preclinical lesions greater than 1A	
	IB1: Clinical lesions no greater than 4 cm in size	
	IB2: Clinical lesions greater than 4 cm in size	
II	Tumour extends beyond the cervix and involves the vagina (but not the lower third) and/or the parametrium (but not reaching the pelvic side wall)	65
	IIA: Tumour involves the vagina	
	IIB: Tumour infiltrates the parametrium	
III	Tumour involves the lower third of the vagina and/or extends to the pelvic side wall	36
	IIIA: Tumour involves the lower third of the vagina	
	IIIB: Tumour extends to the pelvic wall and/or hydronephrosis or non-functioning kidney due to ureteric obstruction caused by tumour	
IV	IVA: Tumour involves the mucosa of the bladder or rectum and/or extends beyond the true pelvis	10
	IVB: Spread to distant organs	

(According to the International Federation of Gynecology and Obstetrics [FIGO] staging system.)

as the cancer is often multifocal. If the preinvasive disease is not completely excised then a repeat loop biopsy or knife cone biopsy must be carried out. For microscopic lesions (stage IA1), local excision with good clear margins is all that is required. This allows fertility to be preserved and a hysterectomy is not necessary.

Clinical invasive cervical carcinoma: stages IB–IV

The tumour volumes are much greater in patients with stage 1B disease and therefore fertility-preserving treatment for this group of patients is more challenging. When small volume disease is confined to the cervix (stage IB1), radical hysterectomy and bilateral pelvic node dissection (Wertheim's hysterectomy) is standard of care. For young women who have not completed their families, radical trachelectomy (surgical removal of the cervix and upper part of the

vagina) and bilateral pelvic node dissection is an alternative (see Chapter 17, Gynaecological surgery and therapeutics).

It is important to remember that in early stage IB disease, pelvic radiotherapy has similar success rates to surgery and therefore this treatment is considered in women who are too overweight for radical surgery or who are anaesthetically unfit.

When the disease is beyond the cervix (stages II–IV disease), radiotherapy (with or without chemotherapy) becomes the optimal treatment. Surgery in isolation is problematic as complications can occur (severe haemorrhage) and also achieving clearance of the tumour is unlikely. Incomplete excision of cancer by surgery requires adjuvant postoperative radiotherapy and the combined treatments can lead to high complication rates. As an oncological rule it is not wise to cut through cancer.

Surgery

The standard surgical operation for stage IB tumours is a radical hysterectomy and pelvic lymph node dissection. This involves removal of the cervix, upper third of the vagina, uterus and the paracervical tissue. Pelvic lymph node removal includes the obturator, internal and external iliac nodes. The ovaries in premenopausal women can be spared. There is higher morbidity with this procedure over the standard total abdominal hysterectomy. Bladder dysfunction (atony), sexual dysfunction (due to vaginal shortening) and lymphoedema (due to removal of the pelvic lymph nodes) are not uncommon. An atonic bladder is frequent in the immediate postoperative period due to neuronal damage from the surgery, and intermittent self-catheterization may be required until the bladder tone returns.

Lymphoedema is variable and is described by patients as a wooden, heavy feeling to the legs with swelling and reduced mobility. Management includes leg elevation, good skin care (e.g. avoid shaving), massage and occasionally compression stockings. Despite these potential problems, surgery is the preferred treatment as the cure rate is high, ovarian tissue can be preserved and the patient avoids the complications of radiotherapy (see below).

KEY LEARNING POINTS

- Cervical cancer affects young women who may not have completed their families.
- Many cervical tumours are picked up when they are microscopic or very small volume, making fertility-sparing treatment a possibility.
- Cone biopsy or radical trachelectomy with bilateral pelvic lymphadenectomy allows preservation of the ovaries and uterus, permitting pregnancy in the future.
- The long-term cure rate of radical trachelectomy is less well established than radical (Wertheim's) hysterectomy.

Radiotherapy

The aim of radiotherapy is to deliver a lethal dose of radiation to the tumour and minimize damage to the surrounding tissues. Treatment is overseen by a radiotherapist and team. Treatment is delivered in two ways: external beam radiotherapy (as teletherapy) and internal radiotherapy (brachytherapy).

In external beam radiotherapy, the source of the radiation is from a machine called a linear accelerator, and radiation is delivered to the pelvis a distance from the patient (**Figure 16.10**). The dose of radiotherapy is carefully calculated according to the patient and the tumour, and is usually administered as 45 Gy in total. This is given in several treatments or 'fractions' as an outpatient over 4 weeks. Although this treatment is given daily, the time of each fraction is no more than 10 minutes. Brachytherapy is a radiotherapy technique where the radiation is delivered internally to the patient. The source of the radiation is usually selenium and patients generally have to undergo an examination under anaesthetic to insert the rods into the uterus. These rods are then attached to the radiotherapy source; the patient receives this internal treatment in isolation to protect the staff. Brachytherapy delivers a high dose of radiation to the tumour source and its harmful effects on the bladder and bowel are minimized as its effects are targeted only 5 mm from the rod.

Patients frequently suffer lethargy with treatment and may experience both bowel and bladder urgency, which is due to the initial inflammatory effects of the radiation. Skin erythema-like sunburn is not uncommon after external beam radiotherapy. Symptomatic treatment is usually required, such as anti-inflammatory creams for skin. Around 5% of patients experience a serious side-effect that might interrupt treatment, for example bowel perforation. There are many long-term complications of radiotherapy that affect only a minority of patients but do have a significant impact on patients' quality of life.

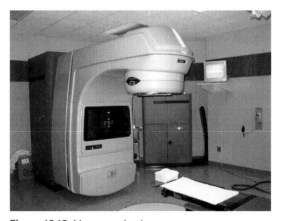

Figure 16.10 Linear accelerator.

The initial inflammatory process is replaced by fibrosis in the long term. Vaginal stenosis can cause sexual pain, bladder damage can lead to cystitis-like symptoms, haematuria and bowel damage lead to malabsorption and mucous diarrhoea. None of these complications can be managed easily. Patients who are premenopausal will undergo a radiotherapy-induced menopause as the ovaries are very sensitive to small doses of irradiation.

Chemotherapy (cisplatin) is ideally given in conjunction with the radiotherapy, as this combination increases cure rates more than when radiotherapy is used in isolation. It probably works by enhancing the effects of radiotherapy and might also address micrometastases that are outside the radiotherapy field.

Palliative treatment

When it is not possible to offer curative treatment, palliation of symptoms becomes important and early involvement of the palliative care team is essential for symptom control. The disease can be hidden from family and friends even in the late stages of the disease; patients may be experiencing a number of symptoms from local infiltration of the pelvis by the cancer. Malignant pain, recto and/or vesicovaginal fistulae and bleeding may occur. Distant spread is often a very late stage of the disease. Radiotherapy may be considered with a palliative intent; for example, a one-off treatment may be used for symptomatic bone metastases.

Malignant disease of the vagina

Epidemiology and aetiology

Vaginal cancer is rare, accounting for just 1–2% of gynaecological malignancies. The majority of vaginal tumours arise from metastatic spread from the endometrium and cervix. Primary cancers of the vagina are usually squamous cell carcinomas, although clear cell adenocarcinomas and malignant melanomas occur occasionally. The peak age of incidence is 60–70 years of age. Sarcoma botryoides is a rare vaginal tumour affecting young girls, with a peak incidence at 8 years of age.

More than 60% of primary vaginal tumours are HPV associated and risk factors for the disease include previous malignant and premalignant disease of the cervix, and vaginal intraepithelial neoplasia (VaIN), a premalignant disease with a 10% risk of progression to invasive disease. Vaginal cancer is also sometimes seen in women with a previous history of pelvic radiotherapy.

Clinical presentation and diagnosis

Abnormal bleeding or blood-stained vaginal discharge is the most common presenting complaint. Speculum examination reveals a mass or an ulcer, usually at the top of the vagina. Advanced disease presents with haematuria, constipation, pelvic pain or tenesmus, a feeling of incomplete emptying of the rectum. Diagnosis is confirmed by biopsy. Staging of vaginal cancer uses the FIGO system (*Table 16.2*). An examination under anaesthetic, cystoscopy and sigmoidoscopy defines local spread. An MRI scan of the pelvis confirms clinical findings and a computed tomography (CT) scan of the thorax and abdomen establishes whether distant metastases are present.

Treatment

Most vaginal cancer is treated by primary radiotherapy, although early-stage tumours may be managed surgically. Prognosis depends on stage.

Table 16.2 Staging and prognosis of vaginal cancer

Stage	Extent of disease	5 year survival rate
I	Tumour confined to vagina	75%
II	Tumour invades the subvaginal tissue	40%
III	Tumour invades the pelvic side wall	30%
IV	Tumour involves bladder or bowel mucosa or extends beyond the true pelvis	0–20%

(According to the International Federation of Gynecology and Obstetrics [FIGO] staging system.)

Malignant disease of the vulva

Epidemiology and aetiology

Vulval cancer is uncommon, with just 1,000 new diagnoses every year in the UK. It was previously a disease that exclusively affected older women, but recent years have witnessed rising incidence rates among young women in their 4th, 5th and 6th decades of life.

Almost 90% of vulval cancers are squamous cell carcinomas, with malignant melanoma, basal cell carcinoma and adenocarcinoma of the Bartholin gland making up the remainder. It is generally accepted that squamous cell carcinoma of the vulva is a disease of two separate aetiologies: high-risk HPV-associated cancers, which arise on a background of multifocal high-grade vulval intraepithelial neoplasia (VIN 3), often in younger women; and non-HPV-associated tumours, affecting older women and associated with the premalignant vulval condition lichen sclerosus (*Table 16.3*).

Clinical presentation

Vulval cancer presents as a lump or ulcer associated with bleeding or discharge that may be painful or painless. Women may present late due to embarrassment and reluctance to be examined. Clinical assessment should include an evaluation of the patient's performance status and general fitness for anaesthetic.

On examination, a well-demarcated raised or ulcerated lesion that is hard and craggy and bleeds on touch is highly suspicious for vulval cancer (**Figure 16.11**). There is often associated premalignant change, specifically VIN in younger women, and lichen sclerosus in older women. Examination includes an assessment of the size of the lesion, its position on the vulva and its proximity to important midline structures, particularly the urethra and anus. Vulval tumours spread locally and metastasize first via the inguinofemoral lymph nodes, before involving pelvic lymph nodes. Haematogenous spread to liver and lungs is a late event. It is therefore important to examine the groins for lymph node metastases, which are palpable as hard, craggy and fixed subcutaneous lymph node swellings.

Investigation

Patients with vulval cancer are managed by specialist gynaecological oncology MDTs in cancer centres, where there is sufficient experience and expertise

Table 16.3 Premalignant conditions of the vulva

	Aetiology	Characteristics	Symptoms	Treatment	Risk of malignancy
VIN	High-risk HPV	Multifocal leukoplakic, erythematous or pigmented lesions	Itch, irritation, asymptomatic	Surgical excision, laser treatment, imiquimod cream	10% – may be higher in immunocompromised women (e.g. HIV, renal transplant recipients on immunosuppressive treatments)
Lichen sclerosus	Unknown	Leukoplakia of the vulval skin in a 'figure of eight' distribution, with loss of vulval architecture	Itch, irritation, asymptomatic	Superpotent steroid cream if symptomatic	10%
Extramammary Paget's disease of the vulva	Unknown	Well-demarcated erythematous lesion affecting the vulva with 'cake icing' effect	Itch, irritation, asymptomatic	Surgical excision aiming for wide margin of healthy skin to reduce risk of recurrence	10% risk of invasive vulval disease at presentation, 30% risk of associated internal malignancy (of urethra, bladder, uterus, vagina or bowel)

HIV, human immunodeficiency virus; HPV, human papillomavirus; VIN, vulval intraepithelial neoplasia.

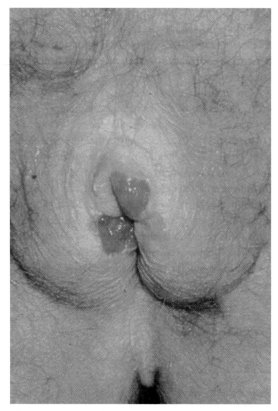

Figure 16.11 Vulval cancer.

in the management of this relatively rare condition. The team includes gynaecological cancer surgeons, clinical oncologists, specialist radiologists, histopathologists and clinical nurse specialists who guide the investigation and treatment of the patient according to nationally agreed guidelines.

A biopsy is needed to confirm the diagnosis. For large tumours, this should incorporate the edge of the lesion with the transition to normal epithelium, as this aids histological assessment. For smaller tumours, where biopsy would effectively excise the lesion, it is important to take a clinical photograph first. The vulva heals well and it can be difficult to locate the scar if further excision is necessary. Alternatively, the patient may be referred prior to biopsy if there is a small but clinically suspicious lesion. An examination under anaesthetic is sometimes useful to assess the suitability of the tumour to resection, particularly if the tumour is very large and involving midline structures.

Most patients do not require preoperative imaging, apart from a chest X-ray to confirm suitability

for surgery. Imaging of the groins is unreliable in the detection of groin node metastases, although the high negative predictive power of an MRI scan of the groins can sometimes spare very unfit, elderly women from the morbidity associated with full groin lymphadenectomy. A staging CT scan of the thorax, abdomen and pelvis is necessary for large vulval tumours or those with obvious groin node disease, to exclude distant metastases. Staging is according to FIGO (*Table 16.4*).

Treatment

Vulval excision

Radical surgical excision aiming for a clear surgical margin of at least 10 mm is standard of care. Margins less than 5 mm are associated with unacceptably high recurrence rates and necessitate further excision or radiotherapy. Where lesions impinge on the urethra or anus, achieving good surgical clearance is more challenging. Sometimes it is appropriate to shrink very large or midline tumours with neoadjuvant radiotherapy, often given in combination with chemotherapy, prior to surgery. This allows better preservation of urinary or bowel function than upfront radical surgical excision. For small lesions, primary closure is straightforward but larger lesions necessitate vulval reconstruction using 'flaps' of skin, subcutaneous tissue and blood vessels, usually from the buttock crease or inner thigh.

Sentinel lymph node biopsy and groin lymphadenectomy

Untreated groin lymph node metastases are invariably fatal but it is not possible to predict whether groin nodes are involved using current radiological techniques. The standard approach until recently has been to carry out full inguinofemoral lymphadenectomy; that is, to remove all the lymph nodes in the groin for all patients where the tumour depth of invasion exceeds 1 mm. Tumours with less than 1 mm depth of invasion are extremely unlikely to have groin node metastases (less than 5%). Lymph drainage for lateral vulval tumours is to the ipsilateral groin nodes, but lesions within 10 mm of the midline drain to nodes on either side of the groin, necessitating bilateral groin lymphadenectomy. Groin lymphadenectomy is a highly morbid

Table 16.4 Staging and prognosis of vulval cancer

Stage	Extent of disease	5-year survival rate
Stage I	Tumour confined to vulva	90%
IA	≤2 cm in size, stromal invasion ≤1 mm, no nodes	
IB	>2 cm in size or stromal invasion >1 mm, no nodes	
Stage II	Tumour extending to lower 1/3 urethra or vagina, or anus	50%
Stage III	Positive inguinofemoral lymph nodes	30%
IIIA1	1 lymph node metastasis ≥5 mm	
IIIA2	1–2 lymph node metastases <5 mm	
IIIB1	≥2 lymph node metastases ≥5 mm	
IIIB2	≥3 lymph node metastases <5 mm	
IIIC	Extracapsular spread	
Stage IV	Tumour invading regional or distant sites	15%
IVA1	Upper urethra/vaginal mucosa, bladder or rectal mucosa, fixed to pelvic bone	
IVA2	Fixed or ulcerated inguinofemoral lymph nodes	
IVB	Distant metastases including pelvic lymph nodes	

(According to the International Federation of Gynecology and Obstetrics [FIGO] staging system.)

procedure, associated with significant postoperative and long-term complications, including wound healing problems, infection, venous thromboembolism, prolonged hospital stay, lymphocyst and chronic lymphoedema. Since groin node metastases affect just 15% of patients undergoing surgery for vulval cancer, many women are being exposed to the unnecessary risks and long-term sequelae of groin lymphadenectomy without receiving any direct benefit from it.

Sentinel lymph node biopsy is an attempt to address this issue. The sentinel node is the first node in the lymph node basin to receive lymphatic drainage from a tumour. The theory states that if the sentinel lymph node is negative then the rest of the lymph node basin must be negative for metastatic disease too. Therefore, if the sentinel lymph node can be identified and carefully checked for metastatic disease, full groin lymphadenectomy can be reserved for those patients who really need it. Removing the sentinel lymph node is a far less morbid procedure than full groin lymphadenectomy. The sentinel lymph node principle has been established in tumours originating from other anatomical sites, including breast cancer and malignant melanoma. The data in vulval cancer look extremely promising and sentinel lymph node biopsy is likely to replace full groin lymphadenectomy as standard of care for carefully selected patients in the near future.

Small vulval tumours (<4 cm) with greater than 1 mm depth of invasion are injected with radioactive nucleotide on the day before surgery. Intraoperative identification of the sentinel node is by gamma probe detection. This is facilitated by injection of blue dye into the tumour immediately preoperatively. The sentinel node is the 'hot', blue node or nodes. It is important to identify bilateral sentinel lymph nodes where tumours impinge on the midline. Careful assessment of the sentinel node(s) identifies the presence or absence of metastatic disease; if the sentinel node is positive for metastatic disease, full groin lymphadenectomy is indicated as a secondary procedure. False-positive nodes are unlikely but false-negative nodes have been described in the literature and threaten the safety of the procedure; it is essential that high standards are achieved through strict adherence to sentinel node protocols to reduce this risk.

Radiotherapy

Adjuvant radiotherapy, given after surgery with curative intent, is indicated when vulval excision margins are close or involved or in the presence of two or more groin node metastases. Adjuvant radiotherapy is given to reduce the risk of recurrence. Neoadjuvant radiotherapy, given before surgery to shrink the tumour and render it operable, is used for very large vulval tumours, particularly those that involve the urethra or anus and where adequate surgical effort would have functional urinary or bowel implications. Occasionally, radical radiotherapy is given instead of surgery in women who are not fit for an anaesthetic due to severe medical comorbidities (see previous section). Chemoradiotherapy is associated with improved cure rates compared to radiotherapy alone. Treatment of recurrent disease and palliative treatment follows the same principles as for cervical malignancy discussed in the previous section

schools is likely to reduce rates further, but this will take many years to show benefit.

- All patients with abnormal bleeding should undergo speculum and pelvic examinations to exclude malignant disease.
- Early-stage malignant disease of the lower genital tract is treated by surgical excision. The principle of surgery in this context is to remove all the tumour with adequate surgical margins.
- Fertility-sparing treatment is possible in early-stage cervical tumours in young women who have not completed their families.
- Most lower genital tract tumours are radiosensitive, but surgery is preferred as first-line treatment due to a lower toxicity profile.
- Chemotherapy is used alongside radiotherapy to improve response rates and in the setting of metastatic disease.

KEY LEARNING POINTS

- Cervical cancer is a disease commonly affecting women in low income countries. Most women never see a health professional in their life and die from their disease in their community.
- Population-based cervical screening of adult women has prevented 70% of cases of cervical cancer developing in the UK. HPV vaccination of children in

Further reading

Crosbie EJ, Brabin L (2010). Cervical cancer: problem solved? Vaccinating girls against human papillomavirus. *BJOG* **117**:137–42.
Crosbie EJ, Einstein MH, Franceschi S, Kitchener HC (2013). Human papillomavirus and cervical cancer. *Lancet* **382**:889–99.
Kitchener HC, Denton K, Soldan K, Crosbie EJ (2013). Developing role of HPV in cervical cancer prevention. *BMJ* **347**:f4781.

Self assessment

CASE HISTORY

Mrs S is an 88-year-old woman who presents to the gynaecology clinic with a vulval lump. It has been bleeding intermittently. It is very sore and she is finding it difficult to sit down. She is frail and lives in sheltered accommodation.

A What is the most likely diagnosis?
B What are the key points in the examination and investigation?

Mrs S is found to have a 6 cm vulval tumour involving the clitoris, right labium majorum and the introital margin. It extends to a few millimetres away from the external urethral meatus. Her staging CT scan excludes distant metastases.

C How would you manage her?

ANSWERS

A   A new vulval lump in an elderly woman is vulval cancer until proven otherwise. It is not unusual for elderly women to put off consulting their GP because of embarrassment and reluctance to be examined.

B   It is important to inspect the vulva, noting the size of the lesion, its position on the vulva and its proximity to the urethra and anus. A biopsy in the outpatient setting will expedite diagnosis but may be difficult if the lesion is exquisitely tender, as the history suggests. An examination under anaesthetic including biopsy may be necessary. Assessment of the groins is important since enlarged, hard, fixed nodal masses may not be resectable. If distant metastases are suspected, a CT scan of the thorax, abdomen and pelvis is important for treatment planning.

C   It is important to establish up front what treatment the patient wants and whether she is fit for general anaesthetic and the morbidity of radical vulval cancer surgery. From an oncological point of view, the best treatment is radical vulval excision with flap reconstruction of the vulva and bilateral groin lymphadenectomy. This may be followed by adjuvant radiotherapy if surgical margins are close or two or more groin nodes are positive. If proximity of the tumour to the urethra prohibits good surgical clearance without rendering Mrs S incontinent, it may be appropriate to consider neoadjuvant (chemo)radiotherapy to shrink the tumour prior to surgery. Radical vulval surgery and placement of a permanent suprapubic catheter is another option. If Mrs S is not fit or does not wish to have surgery, radical radiotherapy with/without chemotherapy is the treatment of choice. All decisions are made following full consultation with the patient and her family and after discussion with the specialist gynaecological oncology MDT.

EMQ

A   Cryotherapy.
B   Directed punch biopsy.
C   High-risk HPV test.
D   LLETZ.
E   Referral for colposcopy.

F   Repeat cervical cytology in 3 months.
G   Repeat cervical cytology in 6 months.
H   Repeat cervical cytology in 3 years.
I   Test of cure.

For each description below, choose the SINGLE most appropriate answer from the above list of options. Each option may be used once, more than once or not at all. What is the appropriate follow-up for:

1   Inadequate cervical cytology.
2   Mild dyskaryosis.

3   CIN 2 on directed punch biopsy.
4   Negative test of cure.

ANSWERS

1F   The sensitivity of a single cervical smear for high-grade CIN detection is between 40 and 70%; however, as there is slow progression for most women with CIN to cancer, if a lesion is missed then this should be picked up on a subsequent test. Women who attend regularly for cervical cytology have a very low risk of developing cervical cancer.

2C   Women with minor cytological abnormalities undergo reflex testing with high-risk HPV. HPV-negative women are returned to routine recall, while high-risk HPV-positive women are referred for colposcopy. Women with high-grade abnormalities are referred direct to colposcopy.

3D   LLETZ is intended to be curative to remove the area of abnormality with margins.

4H   Patients who have received treatment for CIN undergo a 'test of cure' 6 months later. This includes a high-risk HPV test and cytological assessment. If negative, the woman is returned to routine recall; that is, cervical screening in 3 years time. If positive, repeat colposcopy is indicated to identify any residual, untreated CIN. A woman with a history of CIN has an increased life time risk of recurrent CIN and cervical cancer.

SBA QUESTIONS

1 A 48-year-old woman attends the gynaecology department with prolonged vaginal bleeding. Her last cervical smear was 8 years previously. A speculum examination reveals a suspicious-looking cervix that bleeds on contact.

What is the most appropriate initial investigation? Choose the single best answer.

A   Cervical biopsy.
B   LLETZ.
C   Hysteroscopy.
D   MRI scan of her pelvis.
E   Transabdominal ultrasound scan.

ANSWER

A   Cervical biopsy is required to make a histological diagnosis first, before imaging to stage or surgical treatment.

2 A 32-year-old woman is diagnosed with a 3 cm stage IB1 squamous cell carcinoma of the cervix. She is devastated because she and her partner would like to start a family.

What fertility-sparing treatment would you recommend? Choose the single best answer.

A   Cold knife cone biopsy.
B   LLETZ.
C   Radical hysterectomy with bilateral pelvic lymphadenectomy.
D   Radical radiotherapy with cisplatin chemotherapy.
E   Radical trachelectomy with bilateral pelvic lymphadenectomy.

ANSWER

E   IB1 lesions are greater than 4 cm in size but confined to the cervix. Radical hysterectomy and bilateral pelvic node dissection (Wertheim's hysterectomy) is the standard of care. However, radical trachelectomy with bilateral pelvic lymphadenectomy allows preservation of the ovaries and uterus, permitting pregnancy in the future.

Gynaecological surgery and therapeutics

DOUGLAS TINCELLO

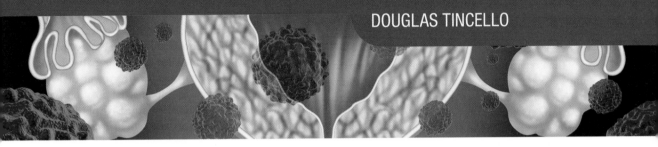

LEARNING OBJECTIVES

- Revise the key points of surgical anatomy applied to gynaecology.
- Understand the relative risks and benefits of abdominal and vaginal hysterectomy as well as laparoscopic hysterectomy.
- Understand the advantages and principles of minimal access surgery.
- Understand the advantages and disadvantages of common incisions.
- Understand the purpose of careful preassessment and postoperative care.

- Be aware of how to minimize surgical risk during and immediately after surgery.
- Recognize the importance of fully informed consent.
- Be aware of the common gynaecological procedures and their risks.
- Describe the common hormonal and non-hormonal drugs used in gynaecology, and understand the principles of safe prescribing.

Gynaecological surgery

Introduction

In this chapter, the principles of good surgical practice as they relate to gynaecology will be discussed. Various procedures that have been discussed in other chapters are examined in more detail here, as are therapeutics. For more detailed descriptions see Further reading.

Gynaecology is a surgical specialty; before obstetrics and gynaecology was recognized as a speciality in its own right, most gynaecological procedures were performed by surgeons.

Key surgical anatomy

Anatomy has been discussed in Chapter 1, The Development and anatomy of the female sexual organs and pelvis. A thorough knowledge of pelvic anatomy is essential for safe surgical practice. The major vessels supplying the uterus and adnexae are the ovarian vessels (arising in the abdomen from the aorta and renal artery), which enter the pelvis over the sacroiliac joints in the infundibulopelvic ligament (a fold of peritoneum), and the uterine vessels. The uterine arteries are branches from the posterior trunk of the internal iliac artery and run medially in the base of the broad ligament to turn upwards and course along the lateral border of the uterus on each side. At the base of the broad ligament, the uterine artery runs 1 cm above and 1 cm lateral to the ureter, where it is at risk of injury if care is not taken. This is much more likely if there is scarring in the pelvis from endometriosis, or if the anatomy is distorted by any gynaecological cancers or ovarian cysts.

The ureter runs from the kidney over the psoas muscle in line with the lateral processes of the lumbar vertebrae and enters the pelvis over the sacroiliac joint. It runs in the posterior leaf of the broad ligament to the level of the ischial spine, where it turns inwards and forwards to enter the bladder. In order to safely dissect the uterine arteries away from the ureter, the bladder is reflected downwards at an abdominal hysterectomy or upwards at a vaginal hysterectomy. The bladder is emptied before open and laparoscopic surgery to protect it from injury. The bladder is intimately associated with the anterior vaginal wall and the front of the uterine cervix and isthmus. The vesicouterine fold of peritoneum must be opened to allow the bladder to be reflected before clamping the uterine arteries during hysterectomy. It is for these reasons that bladder and ureteric injuries may occur during gynaecological surgery. If there is any doubt as to the position of the ureter, the broad ligament can be opened by dividing the round ligament, and the ureter can always been seen on the reflected peritoneum.

The sigmoid colon runs along the left side wall of the abdomen and pelvis and becomes retroperitoneal midway along its passage through the pelvis. In a healthy pelvis the rectum falls away when the uterus is lifted, to allow clear identification of the rectum and posterior vagina in the pouch of Douglas. Scarring (particularly from endometriosis) can obliterate the pouch of Douglas and increase the risk of rectal injury considerably. Also, after hysterectomy, the anatomical planes between vagina and rectum are less easily seen and so rectal injury can occur at the time of sacrocolpopexy.

For a discussion of the anatomy of the ligaments and fascial supports relevant to prolapse see Chapters 1, The Development and anatomy of the female sexual organs and pelvis, and

Chapter 10, Urogynaecology and pelvic floor problems.

Hysterectomy

Hysterectomy is one of the commonest surgical procedures in gynaecology and therefore given special mention here. Other routine gynaecological operations are described more briefly later. Hysterectomy is commonly performed for heavy or painful or irregular periods, when medical treatment or less invasive surgery such as endometrial ablation has failed. When the uterus is enlarged by fibroids or significant adhesions are expected, or it is planned to remove the ovaries, hysterectomy is usually performed abdominally. Although a complete description of abdominal hysterectomy is outside the scope of this chapter, the procedure involves taking three pedicles:

- The infundibulopelvic ligament, which contains the ovarian vessels.
- The uterine artery.
- The angles of the vault of the vagina, which contain vessels ascending from the vagina; the ligaments to support the uterus can be taken with this pedicle or separately.

In vaginal hysterectomy, the same steps are taken but in the reverse order. If the uterus is of normal size, hysterectomy can be performed vaginally, even in the absence of significant prolapse. In prolapse surgery, hysterectomy is commonly performed vaginally as part of the correction of anatomical prolapse, although there is an increasing awareness that the uterus is an innocent 'passenger' in the prolapse process and prolapse surgery can be done without removing the uterus.

The choice of abdominal or vaginal route for hysterectomy has to balance the benefits and risks of each approach (*Table 17.1*). Published data have failed to demonstrate a lower morbidity after vaginal surgery, but many studies have included women undergoing prolapse who are older with more comorbidities. It is now generally agreed that vaginal surgery requires a shorter time in hospital and less recovery time before full mobility and activity is resumed. Increasingly, laparoscopy is used to aid vaginal surgery, termed laparoscopic-aided vaginal hysterectomy (LAVH)

Table 17.1 Hysterectomy routes

Procedure	Key points	Advantages	Disadvantages
Abdominal hysterectomy	Abdominal incision Uterus, cervix removed Tubes and ovaries can be removed together at the same procedure Can be performed laparoscopically	Allows full inspection of pelvis Oophorectomy is straightforward Can remove large fibroid uterus	Abdominal incision More pain Longer recovery period *TLH/LAVH will offset these disadvantages*
Vaginal hysterectomy	Vaginal incision Cervix and uterus removed Ovaries and Fallopian tube not removed Can be combined with vaginal wall surgery Can be assisted laparoscopically	No abdominal incision Rapid recovery Suitable for spinal anaesthesia Appropriate for frail/eldery	Ovaries not removed Surgical access can be limited Not suitable for large fibroid uterus

LAVH, laparoscopic-aided vaginal hysterectomy; TLH, total laparoscopic hysterectomy.

in which the first two steps are completed laparoscopically and the third vaginally. The entire operation can be performed laparoscopically, with the uterus removed through the vagina and the open vault closed with laparoscopic sutures, termed total laparoscopic hysterectomy (TLH). Although at the moment the procedure time and hence anaesthetic may be longer, postoperative pain and recovery time will be less. As the specialty of minimal access surgery (MAS) evolves, newer and more effective laparoscopic tools and energy modalities are being developed, which will further reduce the operative time.

Hysterectomy by any route carries some specific complications. Some risks can be minimized by careful surgical planning and preoperative preparation. It should be remembered that removal of the ovaries is not essential if hysterectomy is being performed for benign indications, and the decision about whether to do so should be made in discussion with the patient. For postmenopausal women undergoing surgery, oophorectomy may be a sensible option because it removes the low risk of later ovarian cancer. For a woman who is still menstruating regularly, then it would be usual to leave the ovaries *in situ*, to preserve endogenous ovarian function and prevent early onset of menopausal symptoms and osteoporosis. For women in the perimenopausal years who may have some early menopausal symptoms and a degree of menstrual irregularity, the decision about removing the ovaries should be individualized in relation to personal preferences

regarding hormone replacement therapy (HRT) use and any risk factors for later cancer of the ovary. In general, there is a move towards conservation of the ovaries.

Complications of hysterectomy

- Haemorrhage (intra- or immediate postoperative).
- Deep vein thrombosis (pelvic surgery).
- New bladder symptoms (both overactive bladder and stress incontinence).
- Higher incidence of vaginal prolapse after hysterectomy for any cause.
- Bladder injury (uncommon).
- Ureteric injury (rare).
- Rectal injury (rare).
- Vesicovaginal or rectovaginal fistula (consequence of injury) (very rare).
- Early onset of menopausal symptoms (if ovaries left *in situ*).
- Immediate onset of menopausal symptoms (if ovaries removed in a premenopausal woman).
- Thromboembolism.

A word of caution when considering oophorectomy for a patient with significant menstrual cycle pain: in the absence of proven endometriosis it is wise to be careful, since some non-gynaecological conditions can cause pain in a cyclical manner (e.g. irritable bowel syndrome). In these cases a 3-month trial of gonadotrophin releasing hormone (GnRH) analogues to suppress ovarian function prior to surgery can be useful to be confident that oophorectomy will alleviate the pain if it is relieved by the medication. On the other hand, if one is sure the pain is related to the ovaries, then performing hysterectomy without oophorectomy can leave a patient with ongoing pain, and later oophorectomy can be technically difficult, with adhesions and with the ovary adherent to the pelvic side wall and ureter.

Exceptions to the principle of ovarian conservation in young patients would be a woman with significant and debilitating premenstrual syndrome where oophorectomy would alleviate this, or a woman with severe endometriosis, where oophorectomy is necessary to achieve a cure. Oophorectomy in young women will usually require immediate recourse to systemic HRT, which is not always without complications (see Chapter 8, The Menopause and postreproductive health).

KEY LEARNING POINTS

- The bladder and ureters are closely related to the uterus, cervix and uterine vessels and are at risk of injury during hysterectomy.
- Abdominal hysterectomy has a longer recovery time than vaginal hysterectomy but makes removal of large fibroids and ovaries easier.
- Hysterectomy by any route increases the risk of new urinary and prolapse symptoms.
- Oophorectomy is not mandatory at the time of hysterectomy.
- The decision whether to remove the ovaries should consider the patient's age, presence of menopausal symptoms, pain and the individual risk of later ovarian cancer.

Preassessment

In modern medical practice, patients are admitted for as short a time as is practical and safe for the patient. As a result, the presurgical preparation of patients in now often performed in a preassessment clinic (PAC) up to 2 weeks before the date of surgery. At preassessment a clinical review is undertaken, usually by a junior doctor or specialist nurse, to confirm the patient's medical condition is still present and to identify any new or existing medical comorbidities that may affect the risks of anaesthesia or increase the risk of intra- and postoperative complications. All patients will have a full blood count (FBC) and blood group and serum save (or a full cross-match in advance if significant bleeding is anticipated), and patients over the age of 50 or thereabouts, plus those with known cardiac, renal or respiratory problems, will also have serum biochemistry measured (urea, electrolytes, renal function, hepatic function), a chest X-ray and electrocardiography (ECG) performed. These results will be available for the surgeon and anaesthetist in advance of the surgery.

The PAC is a valuable opportunity to arrange additional investigations and make specific surgical plans for high-risk patients. For instance, patients with significant cardiac failure or severe respiratory disease may require echocardiography or lung function test. Patients with known coagulation disorders, or those taking long-term anticoagulants such as warfarin, can be reviewed by the haematologist and a detailed bridging plan prepared. Many hospitals support their PACs with consultant anaesthetists who provide expert review of high-risk patients even before the decision for surgery has been made, and who can make detailed plans for the care of the very high-risk patient, including the provision of a high dependency or intensive care bed in the immediate postoperative period.

The risk of thromboembolism is best assessed at the PAC so that plans can be made for postoperative thromboprophylaxis. The combined oral contraceptive pill (COCP) should be stopped 4 weeks prior to surgery and alternative contraception used. HRT should also be stopped, although there is some disagreement about this. Covering women with low-molecular weight heparin (LMWH) even for minor surgery would be an option if HRT is continued. All women must be mobilized early after surgery, and giving women the expectation that this will be the case is useful. All women are given thromboembolic stockings (TEDS) and kept hydrated. LMWH is given according to standard risk assessment.

Thromboprophylaxis in surgery

- Low risk: surgery less than 30 min without risk factors.
- Moderate risk:
  - use TEDS and LMWH;
  - surgery more than 30 min, high body mass index (BMI), varicose veins, sepsis, immobility, comorbidity.
- High risk:
  - use TEDS and LMWH for 5 days or until mobile;
  - cancer, prolonged surgery, previous thromboembolic event, thrombophilia or >3 of moderate risk factors.

PACs are also an opportunity for the patient to discuss any remaining concerns or questions she may have about her impending surgery, and it is considered good practice to use preassessment appointments as an opportunity to obtain written consent from the patient at a time slightly distant from the anxieties of the day of surgery (see below).

Surgical practice and decision making

Safe surgical practice and careful decision making begins in the outpatient clinic. With the exception of cancer, most gynaecology conditions we treat affect quality of life and are not life-threatening. It is important, therefore, to work with the patient to ensure that all available conservative and non-medical interventions have been tried or at least discussed before considering surgery. Although in the modern world anaesthesia and surgery are safe, any surgical procedure does carry risks and complications, some of which can rarely be life-threatening or cause significant physical morbidity. It is one of the duties of a professional to ensure that his or her patients are made aware of all the issues. Many patients seem to consider surgery to be the only intervention that will make a lasting difference and can be overoptimistic about the likely outcome. The best way to avoid surgical complications and mishaps is not to operate!

Having made the decision to perform an operation, one must be careful to consider the alternatives, to arrive at the best operation for that patient with that condition. Abdominal surgery requires longer recovery than vaginal surgery, and involves longer incisions usually, while laparoscopic surgery requires a patient to endure a longer anaesthetic (often) while in a steep Trendelenburg position (head down). So, for instance, one might decide to avoid an abdominal approach on a very frail elderly patient with comorbidities in favour of a laparoscopic or vaginal approach. One might decide to avoid complex laparoscopic surgery in a morbidly obese woman, or one might decide against bilateral oophorectomy in a patient known to have had several previous laparotomies, extensive endometriosis and intra-abdominal adhesions. In complex cases, it is often prudent to seek the views of colleagues, either in an informal discussion or more recently in the format of multidisciplinary team (MDT) meetings as best practice. At the MDT meeting the patient can be discussed and the views and expertise of surgeon, anaesthetist, specialist nurse (e.g. oncology or urogynaecology) and other specialists (e.g. medical oncologist, pathologist, urologist, colorectal surgeon) can be shared to decide on the safest and most likely to be effective procedure. MDTs are extremely valuable in gynaecological oncology, urogynaecology and severe endometriosis.

During surgery, careful tissue handling throughout is a prerequisite. Careful dissection of tissues and gentle handling of other organs and the abdominal wall will both minimize the risk of surgical trauma but will also reduce the release of acute phase proteins and inflammatory mediators. This is very likely to make the patient feel better and less fatigued in the immediate postoperative period. Careful and methodical surgery is the key to successful outcomes, particularly when faced with difficult surgery and distorted anatomy. The key principles are to restore the anatomy to as close to normal as possible by dividing adhesions and mobilizing adjacent organs before doing one's standard procedure. In the modern era, there is no place for cavalier 'have a go' attitudes in surgery, and if one encounters difficulty and complexity, it is sound practice to call an experienced colleague to assist you before things become too challenging.

Common incisions

For vaginal surgery, there are really only two incisions to consider. For vaginal prolapse the surgical incision is usually a midline one in whichever wall is affected. This allows the skin to be reflected and to gain access to the fascia and underlying tissues. For vaginal hysterectomy the vaginal mucosa around the cervix is excised to gain access to the uterosacral ligaments and vesicouterine space and pouch of Douglas. The morbidity associated with vaginal incisions is very low; many patients experience almost no pain after vaginal surgery. Occasionally, adhesion bands can form between the anterior and posterior vagina, which can be troublesome and interfere with intercourse. These can often be broken down with the fingers but sometimes an examination under anaesthesia is required.

For abdominal gynaecological surgery the choice of incision is usually between a transverse lower abdominal incision (Pfannenstiel incision) and a subumbilical midline incision (**Figure 17.1**). Pfannenstiel incisions are ideal for uncomplicated gynaecological procedures. The incision is quick to make and open, since there is no posterior rectus sheath at the level of the incision, it being below the arcuate line. It is a strong incision, which is not prone to herniation and is cosmetically attractive. The major drawback with the Pfannenstiel is that it cannot be easily extended, so in situations where the anatomy is unexpectedly distorted, or some unanticipated pathology is encountered, the surgeon is forced to make an inverted T incision to improve access, which is neither strong in repair, nor attractive.

Pfannenstiel incision

- Transversely, two finger breadths above the pubic symphysis.
- Strong when repaired with low risk of herniation or dehiscence.
- Not very painful (limited to one or two dermatomes).
- Cosmetically attractive (lower than the 'underwear line').
- Cannot be easily extended or made larger.
- Surgical access limited to pelvic organs.

Midline incision

- Vertically from pubic symphysis up to umbilicus.
- Less strong; prone to herniation or dehiscence.
- More painful (involves several dermatomes).
- Cosmetically unattractive.
- Can easily be extend around umbilicus up to the xiphisternum.
- Gives excellent surgical access.

A midline (or paramedian) incision is often favoured by oncologists, and also when significant surgical difficulty is anticipated (e.g. from adhesions, large fibroids or ovarian cysts). Although less strong than a Pfannenstiel incision, the major advantage of the midline incision is that is can easily be extended to provide excellent surgical access. A large incision will of course cause more postoperative pain, which can increase the risk of respiratory infection by limiting breathing and coughing efforts. The author recommends a vertical incision in emergency cases when the exact underlying diagnosis is not entirely clear (e.g. a pelvic mass in a pyrexial patient) to allow flexibility of access should the findings be unexpected.

Laparoscopic surgery holds several advantages over open abdominal surgery. Laparoscopic entry wounds are usually less than 1 cm in length and thus cause much less postoperative pain than an

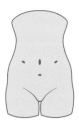
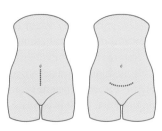

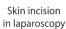
Skin incision in laparoscopy   Traditional skin incisions

Figure 17.1 Incisions used in gynaecological surgery.

open wound. The risk of herniation is very low. The lack of pain and extensive external wounds mean that patients become mobile after surgery very quickly and most laparoscopic procedures (even hysterectomy) allow for hospital discharge within 24–48 hours. The laparoscopic approach allows for enhanced visibility for some pelvic procedures, especially those deep in the pelvis, such as excision of infiltrating endometriosis or performing the mesh attachment at a laparoscopic sacrocolpopexy. Although the operating time may be longer than with open surgery, the more rapid discharge from hospital makes laparoscopic surgery more cost-effective in general, although there are limited data suggesting it also leads to better surgical outcomes.

> ### 🔑 KEY LEARNING POINTS
>
> - Surgical preassessment is an important part of patient care and allows personalized plans of care to be made for those with comorbidities.
> - Multidisciplinary review of planned cases can be helpful in deciding on the safest approach to complex or medically unfit patients.
> - Surgical incisions should be made after consideration of the requirements for surgical access and potential difficulties, but also the strength and recovery time for each type of incision.
> - Many gynaecological procedure are performed by minimal access techniques, thereby minimizing incisional pain and recovery.

Sutures

Surgical suture materials are essential elements for surgical practice, necessary for tying off vascular pedicles, closing the vaginal vault at hysterectomy and repairing abdominal and vaginal incisions. The ideal suture material is one that allows secure knot tying without slippage, provokes little tissue reaction, does not increase the risk of infection, retains enough tensile strength until the healing process has laid down enough collagen and connective tissue to restore integrity of the tissues and can be wholly reabsorbed by the body. Such a material does not exist! The choice of suture for any particular purpose will depend on which of the above characteristics are considered most important. Broadly, sutures can

Table 17.2 Examples of sutures used in gynaecology

	Absorbable (>50% strength retention)	Non-absorbable
Multifilament	Polyglactin (Vicryl®) (21 days)	Silk Braided Nylon Braided polyester/dacron (Ethibond®)
Monofilament	Catgut (rarely used) (7–10 days) Polyglactin (Vicryl®) (14–21 days) Poliglecaprone (Monocryl®) (7 days) Polydioxanone (PDS®) (28 days)	Nylon Polyester/dacron Polypropylene (Prolene®) Stainless steel (rarely used in gynaecology)

be characterized by two properties: monofilament versus multifilament, and absorbable versus non-absorbable (*Table 17.2*).

Multifilament sutures are generally more secure in knot tying than monofilament sutures, due to greater friction from the braided filaments, and so will require fewer throws to secure the knot and thus reduce the amount of suture material used. Suture volume is relevant to the risk of surgical site infection, as more foreign material increases this risk. Conversely, multifilament sutures carry a greater risk of infection than monofilament sutures, because the spaces between the filaments retain bacteria. Monofilament sutures will generally cause less tissue reaction.

For most indications in gynaecology, absorbable sutures will be preferred to non-absorbable sutures. Most modern sutures are polymers of synthetic material that can be broken down by tissue enzymes and macrophages over time. The time taken to degrade is material dependent but is also influenced by inflammation, infection and the general health of the patient. The choice of which material is used depends on the length of time for which tensile strength is required. Non-absorbable 'permanent' sutures are not absorbed so retain their strength indefinitely, but carry a risk of erosion through the skin or vaginal epithelium in the long term.

Non-absorbable sutures are reserved for specific situations where long-term strength is required. In gynaecology, this is most often for the closure of midline abdominal incisions, incisions in cases of malignancy or in a patient with major chronic illness compromising healing (e.g. chronic kidney disease, diabetes), or in a patient where the same incision has been opened more than once before. Other situations where non-absorbable sutures may be used are for colposuspension for incontinence or for attachment of the mesh during sacrocolpopexy.

Consent and surgical risk

Obtaining valid consent for surgery is an integral step of the care of the patient. Patients must be provided with all the relevant information about the planned procedure including the likely success rate or outcome, as well as the usual recovery time and any particular measures to be observed during that recovery. Additionally, patients need to be made aware of the potential complications of surgery, and how such events may affect the patient's recovery and eventual outcome. Complications that can be deemed common (usually an incidence of 1% or more) should always be discussed with the patient, and any serious complications (i.e. those with risk of long-term adverse effects, including death, long-term morbidity or disability) should also be mentioned, even if rare.

From a legal perspective, consent is considered to be a continuous process rather than a single event. Written consent is usually obtained, but it should be remembered that the process is much more than completing the form. The physician has a duty to ensure that the patient has been provided with all the relevant information in a way that she can understand, and should be able to demonstrate understanding of this information. It is good practice to ask the patient to repeat back her understanding of what she has been told. Doctors are often anxious to avoid creating unnecessary anxiety by discussing rare complications, but as long as one explains the context and relatively rarity of such events, it is important to be as comprehensive as possible and to ensure the discussion has been carefully and completely documented. The discussion and, where possible, local- or surgeon-specific success rates and complication rates, should be written in the patient's case notes in addition to the completion of the consent form. It is also good practice to record that the patient has been able to repeat the information to demonstrate understanding. The person obtaining consent should ideally be someone competent to undertake the procedure, who understands what is involved and the risks, rather than delegating the task to the most junior member of the surgical team.

Thus, it can be seen that obtaining and recording consent can be a time-consuming process and so ideally should be concluded and documented before the time of admission; for example, during an outpatient consultation. It is very easy to fall into the habit of obtaining written consent on the day of surgery, but this is not ideal, although is acceptable as long as the procedure, outcome and risks have been discussed previously. Careful counselling and accurate, detailed record keeping is essential.

The issue of mental capacity to consent is occasionally encountered. Mental capacity is the ability of a person to make decisions for themselves about things that influence their lives, from simple one, to complex decisions, including the decision to undergo medical or surgical treatment. In a legal context it refers to decisions that may have legal consequences for the individual or for others. In terms of surgical practice, capacity is usually obvious from contact with the patient, but in cases of long-term mental illness or dementia, the issue of whether the patient has capacity is important and requires to be formally evaluated.

From a legal perspective, a person lacks capacity when at the time of decision making he or she is unable to make or communicate that decision due to an 'impairment of, or a disturbance in the function of the mind or brain'. Assessing capacity has two stages: firstly, is there an impairment or disturbance to the mind or brain; and secondly, is this sufficient to render the person unable to make this decision. It should be remembered that capacity is task and time specific. Thus, a person with dementia, for example, may have capacity for simple decisions (e.g. to have a cup of tea), but not for a complex decision, or that capacity might vary from day to day.

The key issue for health professionals is to ensure that capacity has been assessed. Legally, having capacity is distinct from the nature of the decision made, and individuals with capacity may well make decisions that others regard as rash, foolish or dangerous. However, if capacity can be demonstrated, the individual can make whatever decision they wish! Where capacity is in doubt, the responsibility to ascertain capacity lies with the health care professional, and sometimes it may be necessary to seek the opinion of more than one practitioner. Many hospitals have a formal process where a panel will make the decision. Where capacity is absent or unclear, clinical decisions have to be made on the basis of what is in the patient's best interests. This can be difficult to establish and will often require discussion with family members or friends who can advise on what the patient would usually wish or any previous expressions or views made when the patient had capacity. An individual will be protected by law when making a clinical decision where they have 'reasonable belief' that the person lacks consent and that the course of action is in the person's best interest. This is limited by certain things, including any advance decision by the individual (e.g. a 'living will'), or by a legal judgement. In many cases, the issue of capacity is easy to determine, but sometimes it can be difficult, and identifying the patient's 'best interests' can also be difficult. If in doubt, clinicians should seek advice from their employer's legal team. Occasionally, decisions on care need to be made by court ruling.

On the day of surgery, the surgical MDT must work together to ensure that the anaesthetic, surgical procedure and recovery occurs efficiently and without complications or adverse events. Communication within the team is of paramount importance and will often begin before the day of surgery with discussion between the surgeon and anaesthetist regarding issues identified at preassessment.

The World Health Organization (WHO) has developed a safe surgery checklist that is recommended for use for all surgical activities. It is a written checklist developed to minimize surgical adverse events. Worldwide the crude mortality rate after surgery is between 0.5% and 5% and postoperative complications occur in up to 25% of cases. In higher income countries, nearly half of adverse events in hospital relate to surgical care, one-half of which are considered to have been avoidable. The checklist is a validated and tested tool to reduce these risks, which includes specific tasks before,

during and after surgery to ensure the whole team is aware of issues relating to the specific case about to be performed (**Figure 17.2**). It includes elements to ensure anaesthesia safety, identification of the correct surgical site and confirmation of the procedure planned, discussion of any specific or non-standard elements to the procedure and attention to careful postoperative care in the immediate recovery period.

KEY LEARNING POINTS

- Consent for surgery is a continuous process, and should be fully documented.
- Where possible, local figures for cure and complications should be given to the patient and included in the written notes recorded.
- Mental capacity is required to give consent.
- Assessing mental capacity where doubt exists is a formal process and must be carefully documented. Formal legal advice may be necessary.
- Where capacity is lacking, treatment decisions can only be made if they can be shown to be in the patient's best interests.

Postoperative care and recovery

The first 48–72 hours after surgery are when the patient is most at risk of immediate surgical complications. Nursing and medical care is focussed on identifying early signs of sepsis, and the source of any infection, haemorrhage or thromboembolic disease. The patient will have regular (usually 4 hourly) observations of temperature, pulse and blood pressure in the first 24 hours to identify the clinical signs of infection or hypovolaemic collapse. Most patients will be given intravenous fluids for the first 12–24 hours after surgery until they can resume eating and drinking, but the timing of resumption of oral intake will vary depending on the length of surgery, whether the abdominal cavity was opened and whether there were any intraoperative complications that might require delayed oral feeding.

The postoperative ward round is a daily (or twice daily) opportunity to review the patient's progress. The patient should be asked about the presence and site of any pain, particularly pain that is more than one would expect from a recent surgical wound or which is in a different site. The pulse, temperature and blood pressure should be checked, and signs of conjunctival

Before induction of anaesthesia

(With at least nurse and anaesthetist)

Has the patient confirmed his/her identity, site, procedure, and consent?
- ☐ Yes

Is the site marked?
- ☐ Yes
- ☐ Not applicable

Is the anaesthesia machine and medication check complete?
- ☐ Yes

Is the pulse oximeter on the patient and functioning?
- ☐ Yes

Does the patient have a:

Known allergy?
- ☐ No
- ☐ Yes

Difficult airway or aspiration risk?
- ☐ No
- ☐ Yes, and equipment/assistance available

Risk of >500 ml blood loss (7 ml/kg in children)?
- ☐ No
- ☐ Yes, and two IVs/central access and fluids planned

Before skin incision

(With nurse, anaesthetist and surgeon)

- ☐ **Confirm all team members have introduced themselves by name and role.**

- ☐ **Confirm the patient's name, procedure, and where the incision will be made.**

Has antibiotic prophylaxis been given within the last 60 minutes?
- ☐ Yes
- ☐ Not applicable

Anticipated critical events

To surgeon:
- ☐ What are the critical or non-routine steps?
- ☐ How long will the case take?
- ☐ What is the anticipated blood loss?

To anaesthetist:
- ☐ Are there any patient-specific concerns?

To nursing team:
- ☐ Has sterility (including indicator results) been confirmed?
- ☐ Are there equipment issues or any concerns?

Is essential imaging displayed?
- ☐ Yes
- ☐ Not applicable

Before patient leaves operating room

(With nurse, anaesthetist and surgeon)

Nurse verbally confirms:
- ☐ The name of the procedure
- ☐ Completion of instrument, sponge and needle counts
- ☐ Specimen labelling (read specimen labels aloud, including patient's name)
- ☐ Whether there are any equipment problems to be addressed

To surgeon, anaesthetist and nurse:
- ☐ What are the key concerns for recovery and management of this patient?

Note: This checklist is not intended to be comprehensive. Additions and modifications to fit local practice are encouraged.

Figure 17.2 WHO surgical safety check list. (Adapted from WHO, 2009.)

pallor or a thready pulse should be sought, as young patients may often compensate for blood loss with minimal changes in pulse rate or blood pressure at first. For all cases of either abdominal or vaginal surgery, the abdomen should be palpated for localized tenderness (suggesting a haematoma or focus of infection), peritonism or distension, and bowel sounds should be checked (for return of peristalsis and exclude obstruction or ileus). The abdominal wound should be checked for inflammation, bruising or discharge. If drains are present, these should be checked. If there are any concerns about bleeding or infection after vaginal surgery, a gentle pelvic examination is appropriate to exclude a haematoma or collection. Routine blood sampling for haemoglobin concentration can be done on the second postoperative day, and urea and electrolytes will need to be checked for those patients who remain on intravenous fluids.

Generally patients should be encouraged to mobilize as soon as possible and oral intake resumed at the earliest opportunity. Single-dose antibiotic prophylaxis is usually give intraoperatively for all gynaecological surgery, but one should be mindful of avoiding empirical prescription of antibiotics in the postoperative period. It is common to see a low-grade pyrexia in the first 12–24 hours as a manifestation of the release of acute phase proteins, particularly interleukin-1, and this will usually settle without intervention. Persistent pyrexia, or pyrexia above 39°C, should be treated. After clinical examination to exclude obvious wound infection or chest infection, a screen should be undertaken by means of urine culture, vaginal swabs and blood cultures before commencing antibiotics in all patients, to ensure that appropriate antibiotic sensitivities can be checked. Where the focus of infection is identified or suspected, liaison with microbiology will ensure appropriate choice of antibiotic based on local resistance patterns, and this is even more important when no source of infection has been identified. Remember that intravenous cannulae or central lines can often be the source of infection.

Wound dressings should be removed by 48–72 hours after surgery and abdominal wound sutures are usually removed on day 5 for Pfannenstiel incisions or day 7–10 for midline incisions. Thromboprophylaxis commences on the day of surgery until discharge, in the form of TEDs and LMWH. In patients with gynaecological malignancy, this will often be continued for longer. There is growing evidence that the risk window for thromboembolic disease can last for up to 6 weeks, so many clinicians recommend their patients continue to wear antiembolic stockings for that length of time. The postoperative review is lastly a good opportunity to debrief the patient about her surgery and to address any remaining concerns about wound care and recovery after discharge, resumption of normal activity and intercourse, and the need or not for HRT. Usually 6 weeks is recommended before resumption of full activity and intercourse after major surgery, based on the time required for scar tissue to regain full strength, but there is little evidence supporting this recommendation. For less major surgery a gradual resumption of activity from about 4 weeks is acceptable.

Common gynaecological procedures

Full details of each procedure are beyond the scope of this book, but a brief summary of the most common procedures, indications and complications are presented in *Table 17.3*.

Hysteroscopy (Figures 17.3, 17.4)

Hysteroscopy involves passing a small-diameter telescope, either flexible or rigid, through the cervix to directly inspect the uterine cavity. Excellent images can be obtained. A flexible hysteroscope may be used in the outpatient setting. Rigid instruments employ circulating fluids and therefore can be used to visualize the uterine cavity even if the woman is bleeding.

Indications

Any abnormal bleeding from the uterus can be investigated by hysteroscopy, including:

- Postmenopausal bleeding.
- Irregular menstruation, intermenstrual bleeding and postcoital bleeding.
- Persistent heavy menstrual bleeding.

Table 17.3 Common gynaecological surgeries

	Procedure	Key points	Short description	Complications
For prolapse	Anterior vaginal repair (colporrhaphy)	For anterior vaginal prolapse NOT a procedure of stress incontinence	Sutures to reinforce fascia between vaginal and bladder	Risk of bladder injury Relatively high recurrence
	Posterior vaginal repair (colporrhaphy)	For posterior vaginal prolapse Can improve obstructed defaecation Risk of recurrence is low	Sutures to reinforce fascia between vaginal and rectum	Risk of rectal injury Associated with postoperative dyspareunia
	Vaginal repair with polypropylene mesh	Usually reserved for recurrent prolapse Surgical repair reinforced with a sheet of mesh Very low recurrence rates Excellent anatomical result	Mesh can be an inlay (not fixed) or fixed to the pelvic ligaments to mimic the native uterosacral ligaments and fascial attachments	Mesh erosion through vagina (5%) Mesh erosion to bladder/rectum (<5%) Dyspareunia Chronic pelvic pain Excision of mesh is difficult
For incontienence	TVT or TOT	For stress incontinence	Tape inserted running either through both obturator fossa under bladder neck, or through retropubic space	Mesh erosion Bladder damage Voiding problems
	Colposuspension	For stress incontinence	Open procedure to elevate bladder neck and replace intrabdominally	Haemorrhage Infection Bladder damage Voiding difficulty
For asssessment of uterine cavity	Hysteroscopy	Uterus distended with saline or glycine to view cavity Performed as day case or outpatient	Cervix is dilated to enable introduction of hysteroscope. Cavity and ostia are viewed Can be used for surgical removal of polyps, septum, submucous fibroids Can be used for directed endometrial biopsy	Bleeding Perforation Infection

(Continued)

Table 17.3 (Continued) Common gynaecological surgeries

	Procedure	Key points	Short description	Complications
For miscarriage	Evacuation of retained products of conception	Now termed surgical completion of miscarriage To remove pregnancy tissue retained after miscarriage Procedure for STOP is identical	Cervix is dilated Suction curette used to evacuate uterus	Bleeding Perforation Infection Need for further procedure
For cervical abnormality	LLETZ and cone biopsy	To remove transformation zone of cervix when CIN present	Transformation zone removed under local anaesthetic (LLETZ) using diathermy Or cut away under general anaesthetic with benefit of histological confirmation of excision	Haemorrhage and secondary haemorrhage from infection Preterm delivery
For assessment of pelvis	Laparoscopy	Minimal access surgery through umbilical port to view and treat pelvic organs Can be route of surgery for oophorectomy, division of adhesions, ligation or clipping or removal of tubes, removal of ovarian cysts, treatment of endometriosis Route of preference for salpingectomy or salpingostomy for ectopic pregnancy Also used for laparoscopic hysterectomy or myomectomy	CO_2 is insufflated through a Veress needle to expand the abdominal cavity and instruments are then introduced	Haemorrhage Infection Damage to pelvic organs Perforation of uterus
For fibroids	Myomectomy	Abdominal operation to remove uterine fibroids Can also be performed laparoscopically	Individual fibroids are 'shelled' out of the myometrium of the exposed uterus, which is sutured closed	Haemorrhage and haematomas requiring transfusion Adhesion formation

CIN, cervical intraepithelial neoplasia; LLETZ, large loop excision of transformation zone; STOP, surgical termination of pregnancy; TOT, transobturator tape; TVT, transvaginal tape.

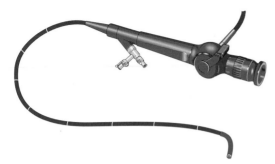

Figure 17.3 Flexible fibreoptic hysteroscope.

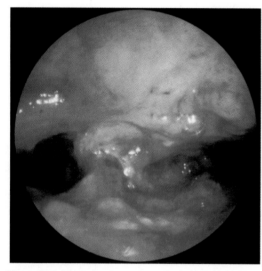

Figure 17.4 View of endometrial cavity demonstrating Asherman's adhesions.

- Persistent discharge.
- Suspected uterine malformations.
- Suspected Asherman's syndrome.
- Essure hysteroscopic sterilization.

Complications

- Perforation of the uterus.
- Cervical damage – if cervical dilatation is necessary.
- If there is infection present, hysteroscopy can cause ascending infection.

An operating hysteroscope can also be used to resect endometrial pathology such as fibroids and polyps and uterine septums.

Laparoscopy (Figures 17.5–17.7)

Laparoscopy allows visualization of the peritoneal cavity. This involves insertion of a needle called a Veress needle into a suitable puncture point in the umbilicus. This allows insufflation of the peritoneal cavity with carbon dioxide so that a larger instrument can be inserted. The majority of instruments used for diagnostic laparoscopy are 5 mm in diameter, and 10 mm instruments are used for operative laparoscopy. More recently, a 2 mm laparoscope has become available.

Indications

- Suspected ectopic pregnancy.
- Ovarian cyst accident and acute pelvic pain.
- Undiagnosed pelvic pain.
- Tubal patency testing.
- Sterilization.

Operative laparoscopy can be used to perform ovarian cystectomy or oophorectomy and to treat endometriosis with cautery or laser. As discussed above, more extensive laparoscopic work is now performed for hysterectomy, lymph node biopsy, omentectomy and myomectomy.

Complications

Complications are uncommon, but include damage to any of the intra-abdominal structures, such as bowel and major blood vessels. The bladder is always emptied prior to the procedure to avoid bladder injury. Incisional hernia has been reported.

 eResource 17.1

Laparoscopy
http://www.routledgetextbooks.com/textbooks/
tenteachers/gynaecologyv17.1.php

Cystoscopy (Figures 17.8, 17.9)

Cystoscopy involves passing a small-diameter telescope, either flexible or rigid, through the urethra into the bladder. Excellent images of both these structures can be obtained. A cystoscope with an operative channel can be used to biopsy any abnormality, perform bladder neck injection, retrieve stones and resect bladder tumours.

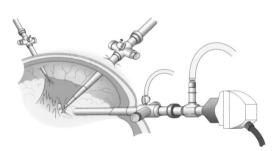

Figure 17.5 Schematic diagram showing laparoscope.

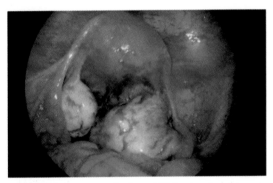

Figure 17.6 Laparoscopic view of bilateral endometriomas.

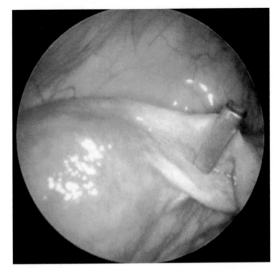

Figure 17.7 Laproscopic view showing Filshie clip on the right Fallopian tube.

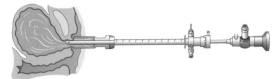

Figure 17.8 Diagram showing the cystoscopic procedure.

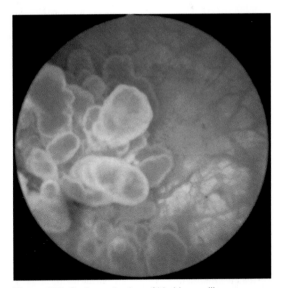

Figure 17.9 Cystoscopic view of bladder papilloma.

Indications

- Haematuria.
- Recurrent urinary tract infection.
- Sterile pyuria.
- Short history of irritative symptoms.
- Suspected bladder abnormality (e.g. diverticulum, stones, fistula).
- Assessment of bladder neck.

Complications

- Urinary tract infection.
- Rarely, bladder perforation.

Therapeutics

The drugs used for particular conditions have been described in the relevant chapters. For reference these are summarized here in *Table 17.4*. Readers are advised to refer to the British National Formulary (BNF) for further information and contraindications.

Table 17.4 Common gynaecological therapeutic agents

Agent	Action	Use
Antifibrinolytics (tranexamic acid)	Reduce blood loss through antifibrinolysis in small capillaries of endometrium	HMB, reducing blood loss by 50%
NSAIDs (e.g. mefenamic acid)	Inhibit prostaglandin synthesis	Reduce blood loss by 30% and aid dysmenorrhoea
GnRH (e.g. Zoladex®)	After an initial flare block receptors in pituitary and cause ovarian suppression via hypogonadotrophism	Suppression of menstrual cycle in endometriosis or fibroids prior to surgery
Osterogens: Ethinyl oestradiol is synthetic and used in most OCPs. Natural oestrogens oestradiol and oestrogen are used in HRT and have less metabolic effect	Simulate oestrogenic activity on end-organs of bone, endometrium and many others, such as skin, mucosa, neutrons, etc	For HRT or contraception. Delivered in various ways: orally, transdermally, vaginally
Progestogens: There are three generations of progestogens with varying androgenic activity. Levonorgestrel is delivered by the LNG-IUS at 20 µg per day	Suppression of endometrium and ovulation in some cases	For HMB, contraception, HRT
Tibolone A synthetic steroid converted *in vivo* to have activity of all three steroid groups	Conserves bone mass and improves libido	For use with long-term GnRH suppression to preserve bone strength
Clomiphene citrate	Ovulation induction	Antioestrogen at level of hypothalamus and pituitary, leading to increased release of FSH and LH, hence initiating folliculogenesis

FSH, follicle-stimulating hormone; GnRH, gonadotrophin-releasing hormone; HMB, heavy menstrual bleeding; HRT, hormone replacement therapy; LH, luteinizing hormone; LNG-IUS, levonorgestrel intrauterine system; NSAID, non-steroidal anti-inflammatory drug; OCP, oral contraceptive pill.

Further reading

Jayson GC, Kohn EC, Kitchener HC, Ledermann JA (2014). Ovarian cancer. *Lancet* **384**(9951):1376–88.
Mental capacity advice from the British Medical Association: http://bma.org.uk/practical-support-at-work/ethics/mental-capacity.
British National Formulary http://www.bnf.org.
The UK Mental Capacity Act: http://www.mentalhealth.org.uk/help-information/mental-health-a-z/M/mental-capacity-act-2005/.
RCOG Guide to Consent https://www.rcog.org.uk/guidelines.
WHO Safe Surgery Checklist website: http://www.who.int/patientsafety/safesurgery/en/.

Self assessment

CASE HISTORY

A 34-year-old woman has been seen in clinic with severe dysmenorrhoea and pelvic pain and a possible diagnosis of endometriosis. She would also like to become pregnant. An ultrasound has shown a normal uterus and 'kissing ovaries', with a 6-cm endometrioma on the right ovary. She would like to undergo a laparoscopy for diagnosis and treatment.

A What additional points in the history should be sought?

B What preoperative checks and tests should be made for this woman?

C What consent process should take place?

ANSWERS

A The gynaecological history should cover length of symptoms, severity, interference with normal function and her expectations of surgery. In particular, symptoms of dyschexia are important to assess likelihood of recto-vaginal nodes.

The length of time trying for a pregnancy, treatments tried and partner's fertility assessment are vital here, as they may affect a decision to treat tubal or ovarian disease. The balance of fertility issues and symptomatology are crucial in surgery for endometriosis (for example, if she is about to undergo in-vitro fertilization, then minimal intervention is advised beyond draining large endometriomas if they will affect egg collection).

As in all surgery past medical history is important, as is previous surgery on the abdomen, which may make laparoscopic surgery more hazardous.

The woman reveals that she has not yet tried for a pregnancy but has just come off the pill and is awaiting a period. She has been tricycling this for 2 years since endometriosis was suspected from symptoms. Initially she felt better but her pain is returning. She has developed new abdominal swelling over the last year, and attributes this to the endometrioma. She does not have dyspareunia or dyschexia. At the moment her symptoms are of greatest importance.

She reveals that she has asthma, although she rarely takes an inhaler. However, she was once hospitalized after contracting the 'flu, requiring nebulizers.

B She requires referral for anaesthetic assessment for her asthma. She requires a FBC and group and save for surgery. A pregnancy test is very important, and she must use contraception in the cycle in which her surgery will fall.

C Initial informed consent will cover the procedure and the risks of surgery. Written information should be given. Common complications are written down (or printed) on the consent form including perforation of uterus, damage to bladder, bowel or viscera, procedures to repair damage and laparotomy.

It is good practice to record details of the consultation that are covered, which should include insertion of a levonorgestrel intrauterine system (LNG-IUS) (but not appropriate if she wishes to conceive), complications that are more likely with endometriosis and the extent of procedure planned. For example, it is useful to record that a discussion has taken place that if the pelvis is frozen and inoperable, the procedure will end without full treatment of the endometriosis. In this situation a referral to the nearest endometriosis centre should be made, where elective surgery with a general surgeon might be planned.

On the day of procedure confirmation of consent will be completed, and further questions answered.

EMQ

A   Internal iliac artery.
B   Uterus.
C   Fallopian tube.
D   Uterine artery.
E   Ovaries.

F   Pudendal artery.
G   Aorta.
H   Ovarian artery.
I   Cervix.

For each description below, choose the SINGLE most appropriate answer from the above list of options. Each option may be used once, more than once or not at all.

1   Contained in the infundibulopelvic ligament.
2   The origin of the uterine artery.

3   Should always be removed at hysterectomy to cure endometriosis.
4   The ureter is at surgical risk where it runs close to this structure.

ANSWERS

1H   The ovarian vessels arise from the aorta just below the renal artery. At the level of the pelvic brim the ovarian vessels cross in front of the ureter and pass into the infundibular-pelvic fold of the broad ligament.

2A   The uterine artery originates from the anterior branch of the internal iliac, as do the other vessels supplying the pelvis.

3E   When hysterectomy and pelvic clearance is performed to provide relief from endometriosis, it is advisable to remove the ovaries. Not doing so may allow continued hormonal cycling and recurrence of pelvic endometriosis. Further surgery to remove the ovaries later would be high risk, due to the presence of adhesions around the ovaries that tend to seal to the pelvic side wall.

4D   The ureter is closely related to the uterine artery at the level of the cervix. During a hysterectomy the bladder is carefully dissected away from the uterus and pushed down, so that the ureters are also moved out of the way. The ureter is visualized or palpated to ensure it is out of the way before clamping is applied to the uterine artery pedicle.

SBA QUESTIONS

1   A 38-year-old woman underwent total abdominal hysterectomy for heavy menstrual bleeding yesterday, with ovarian conservation. On your morning ward round you find that she is pale, with a blood pressure of 110/68 mmHg and a pulse of 88. Her temperature is 36.8°C. Her abdomen is soft, but there is considerable tenderness in the left lower quadrant. Her urine output since surgery has been 350 ml. The nurse caring for the patient reports that the patient was very dizzy and light headed, and vomited when she was taken out of bed that morning.

Which of the following statements describes the most appropriate management? Choose the single best answer.

A   Ensure the patient has adequate analgesia and prescribe extra intravenous fluids and an antiemetic.

B   Take a urine sample and commence intravenous antibiotics.

C   Arrange an urgent FBC and ask for review by your consultant.

D   Explain that the patient does not require hormone replacement therapy and review her that afternoon.

ANSWER

C The signs of paleness, tachycardia and dizziness suggest blood loss. Blood pressure is often maintained in healthy women. The site of a possible intra-abdominal bleed is the left side. Always keep your consultant informed. FBC will confirm if there is blood loss as expected, then further imaging will identify the size of the collection. Subsequently, her clinical status and serial blood picture will identify further management. The FBC will identify whether blood transfusion is needed, but meanwhile intravenous crystalloid should be given to maintain blood pressure and urine output. The site of the bleeding is often the vaginal angle.

2 A 56-year-old woman with endometrial cancer diagnosed on outpatient biopsy attends her preassessment appointment for her planned laparoscopic hysterectomy and bilateral salpingo-oophorectomy. She has hypertension, hyperlipidaemia, ischaemic heart disease and a BMI of 39. She smokes 25 cigarettes day.

Which of the following statements is not correct? Choose the single best answer.

A She will require a high-dependency anaesthetic bed to be available after surgery.

B Early mobilization and antiembolic stockings will be sufficient thromboprophylaxis.

C You will arrange a chest X-ray, ECG, urea and electrolytes.

D She should be counselled about the possible need for laparotomy as part of her surgical consent process.

ANSWER

B She is at high risk for thromboembolic events and will require low-molecular weight heparin for a minimum of her inpatient stay and possibly for 6 weeks.

Index

Note: Page numbers in *italic* refer to tables or boxes; those in **bold** refer to figures